A Clinical Guide to Osteoarthritis

A Clinical Guide to Osteoarthritis

Editor: Shawn McLean

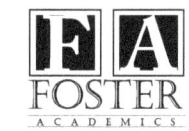

FOSTER
ACADEMICS

www.fosteracademics.com

www.fosteracademics.com

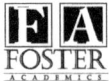

Cataloging-in-Publication Data

A clinical guide to osteoarthritis / edited by Shawn McLean.
    p. cm.
Includes bibliographical references and index.
ISBN 978-1-64646-143-1
1. Osteoarthritis. 2. Osteoarthritis--Guidebooks. 3. Osteoarthritis--Treatment--Guidebooks. I. McLean, Shawn.
RC931.O67 C55 2022
616.722 3--dc23

Foster Academics,
118-35 Queens Blvd., Suite 400,
Forest Hills, NY 11375, USA

ISBN 978-1-64646-143-1 (Hardback)

Contents

Preface

The disease that affects the joints in the body is referred to as osteoarthritis. It is the most common chronic condition of the joints. It is characterized by the breakdown of the cartilage, thus causing pain, swelling and limited mobility. The joints on one side of the body are usually more affected. Osteoarthritis can be classified into spondylosis, trapeziometacarpal osteoarthritis, knee osteoarthritis, hip osteoarthritis and wrist osteoarthritis. It may be caused due to a combination of mechanical stress on the joint and inflammatory processes. Its diagnosis is based on the presentation of signs and symptoms alone, and in some cases it is guided by X-ray results. The treatment of osteoarthritis includes pain medications, weight loss, exercise and resting. In extreme instances of pain which deters normal activities, joint replacement surgery is considered a viable treatment. This book is compiled in such a manner, that it will provide an in-depth case-based approach to the study of osteoarthritis. It strives to provide a fair idea about the diagnosis and management of osteoarthritis. With state-of-the-art inputs by acclaimed experts of orthopedics, this book targets students and professionals.

After months of intensive research and writing, this book is the end result of all who devoted their time and efforts in the initiation and progress of this book. It will surely be a source of reference in enhancing the required knowledge of the new developments in the area. During the course of developing this book, certain measures such as accuracy, authenticity and research focused analytical studies were given preference in order to produce a comprehensive book in the area of study.

This book would not have been possible without the efforts of the authors and the publisher. I extend my sincere thanks to them. Secondly, I express my gratitude to my family and well-wishers. And most importantly, I thank my students for constantly expressing their willingness and curiosity in enhancing their knowledge in the field, which encourages me to take up further research projects for the advancement of the area.

Editor

Increased synovial lipodystrophy induced by high fat diet aggravates synovitis in experimental osteoarthritis

Ane Larrañaga-Vera[1], Ana Lamuedra[1], Sandra Pérez-Baos[1], Ivan Prieto-Potin[1], Leticia Peña[2], Gabriel Herrero-Beaumont[1*] and Raquel Largo[1]

Abstract

Background: Metabolic syndrome (MetS) may be associated with knee osteoarthritis (OA), but the association between the individual components and OA are not well-understood. We aimed to study the effect of hypercholesterolemia on synovial inflammation in knee OA.

Methods: OA was surgically induced in rabbits fed with standard diet (OA group, $n = 10$) or in rabbits fed with high fat diet (OA-HFD, $n = 10$). Healthy rabbits receiving standard diet (Control, $n = 10$) or fed with HFD (HFD, $n = 6$) were also monitored. Twelve weeks after OA induction, synovial membranes were isolated and processed for studies.

Results: Animals fed HFD showed higher levels of total serum cholesterol, triglycerides and C-reactive protein than control rabbits. Twelve weeks after OA induction, synovial membrane inflammation and macrophage infiltration were increased in rabbits with OA, particularly in the OA-HFD group. Extensive decrease of synovial adipose tissue area, adipocyte size and perilipin-1A synthesis were observed in the OA-HFD group in comparison to the OA and control groups. The HFD further increased the proinflammatory mediators IL-1β, IL-6 and TNF in the OA synovium. However, the synovial gene expression of adipokines, such as leptin and adiponectin, were markedly decreased in the rabbits with OA, especially in the OA-HFD group, in correlation with adipose tissue loss. However, circulating leptin was upregulated in the HFD and OA-HFD groups.

Conclusion: Our results indicate that a HFD is an aggravating factor worsening synovial membrane inflammation during OA, guided by increased infiltration of macrophages and removal of the adipose tissue, together with a remarkable presence of proinflammatory factors. Synovial adipocytes and dyslipemia could probably play pivotal roles in OA joint deterioration in patients with MetS, supporting that the link between obesity and OA transcends mechanical loading.

Keywords: Osteoarthritis, Hypercholesterolemia, Synovial inflammation, Metabolic syndrome, Macrophages, Synovial adipose tissue, Adipokines

Background

Osteoarthritis (OA) is the most common joint disorder worldwide, characterized by joint pain, impaired mobility and structural changes in the joints. Although cartilage destruction is the main feature of the disease, every joint structure such as the synovium, bone, meniscus or muscle is affected, leading to the recognition of OA as a whole-organ disease [1]. Synovial inflammation is present in a substantial population of patients with OA and has been associated with different signs and symptoms of the disease, including increased pain and joint effusion, which could promote more rapid cartilage degeneration [2, 3]. Elevated thickness of the lining layer and greater presence and activation of synovial macrophages have been identified in cartilage degradation and osteophyte formation in both human and experimental OA [4–6].

OA is not merely a local disease, but there are different systemic processes that determine its progression. The concept of metabolic OA, coined in recent years, identifies a syndrome whereby the contribution of metabolic

* Correspondence: gherrero@fjd.es
[1]Bone and Joint Research Unit, IIS-Fundación Jiménez Díaz UAM, Avda. Reyes Católicos, 2, Madrid 28040, Spain
Full list of author information is available at the end of the article

dysregulation and low-grade systemic inflammation to the progression of the disease has been firmly pointed out [7, 8]. The metabolic syndrome (MetS) comprises a cluster of conditions, including glucose intolerance, high blood pressure, hypercholesterolemia and hypertriglyceridemia, and obesity [9, 10]. The accumulation of the different components of MetS has been related to both the occurrence and progression of knee OA [11, 12]. However, little is known about the specific contribution of each of these metabolic alterations in OA progression, and specifically in the synovial damage associated with OA.

The contribution of obesity to OA progression is probably the most extensively studied association [7, 13]. In fact, obesity has been pointed out as the main contributing factor for the association between OA and MetS, in studies showing a markedly attenuated association after adjustment for body mass index [14]. However, OA is also common in non-weight bearing joints of obese persons, suggesting a systemic mechanism rather than a simply mechanic phenomenon [7].

The possible role of hyperlipidemia in mediating obesity-related effects on OA has been explored in different studies. Contradictory results have been published on the relationship between serum lipids and OA incidence in humans, probably due to the presence of obesity and being overweight as confounding factors [15]. In turn, different experimental studies have suggested that hypercholesterolemia could be mainly associated with osteophyte generation rather than to aggravation of cartilage lesions [16, 17]. Macrophages, endothelial cells and fibroblasts are dominant cells within the synovium, together with abundant adipose tissue that constitute the synovial stroma, and every component is sensitive to changes in lipid levels [17, 18].

Adipokines have been considered at least partially responsible for the link between systemic metabolic alterations and OA [19–21]. Adipokines are essentially released by adipocytes and exhibit pleiotropic functions both in central and peripheral systems, including blood pressure control, hemostasis, food intake, energy expenditure, cell metabolism and inflammation, among others [19–21]. They are also synthesized by joint cells during OA, mainly by the synovium, cartilage and intra-articular fat tissue, and have been demonstrated to play proinflammatory and catabolic or anabolic roles in OA pathophysiology. It has been hypothesized that the altered circulating patterns of adipokines induced by obesity could be responsible for the deleterious effect of this disease on OA. However, it is not known whether expression and release of adipokines in the joint could be modulated by metabolic factors during OA, thus contributing to disease progression.

Therefore, this work aimed to study the effect of hypercholesterolemia, without any other component of the MetS, on synovial inflammation in an experimental model of knee OA. We have also determined the synovial expression and systemic concentration of adiponectin and leptin, two adipokines involved in joint deterioration associated with metabolic OA.

Methods
Animal model

Thirty-six New Zealand male white rabbits, 13–15 weeks of age, weighing 2.5–3.0 kg (Granja San Bernardo, Navarra, Spain) were housed individually in cages with transparent walls (0.5 m cage height and 0.6 m^2 floor space) exposed to a 12-hour light/dark cycle.

After 2 weeks of adaptation to our facilities, 16 rabbits started receiving a high fat diet (HFD) (0.5% cholesterol + 4% peanut oil; S9504-S010; 22% kJ from fat, 20% kJ from proteins and 58% kJ from carbohydrates; Ssniff, Soest, Germany) administered *ad libitum* (Fig. 1a, time point 0). At this time point, there were no significant differences between the group on HFD and the one that remained at standard diet (112; 10% kJ from fat, 17% kJ from proteins; 73% kJ from carbohydrates; Safe-Diets, Augy, France) regarding body weight or age, as can be observed in Fig. 1b. Six weeks later, bilateral osteoarthritis (OA) was surgically induced in 10 of these 16 animals (OA-HFD group, $n = 10$) by anterior cruciate ligament transection and partial medial meniscectomy [22] (week 6, Fig. 1a). At this time point, OA was also induced in 10 rabbits fed with standard diet (OA group, $n = 10$). The surgery was always performed in the morning after overnight fasting, under general anesthesia (intramuscular administration 20 mg/ml xylazine (Rompun, Bayer, Kiel, Germany) and 50 mg/ml ketamine (Ketolar, Pfizer, Hameln, Germany) in a 3:1 ratio), under aseptic conditions in an operating room. Besides, 10 rabbits fed with standard diet (control group, $n = 10$), and six rabbits fed with the HFD (HFD group, n=6) underwent no experimental intervention.

Two animals in the OA-HFD group died during the time of the study due to OA surgery complications. Weight gain was monitored every week. Systolic blood pressure (SBP) was measured before OA surgery and 1 week before euthanasia, using a High Definition Oscillometry unit (DVM Solutions Houston TX, USA) adapted to the hind paw of the rabbits. This non-invasive method for SBP measurement has been validated in cats, an animal physiologically and anatomically similar to rabbits [23].

Twelve weeks after OA induction (Fig. 1), overnight-fasted rabbits were bled from their marginal ear vein in the morning and killed by an intracardiac injection of pentobarbital (50 mg/kg, Tiobarbital, Braun medical S.A. Barcelona, Spain). The articular cavity of each rabbit was

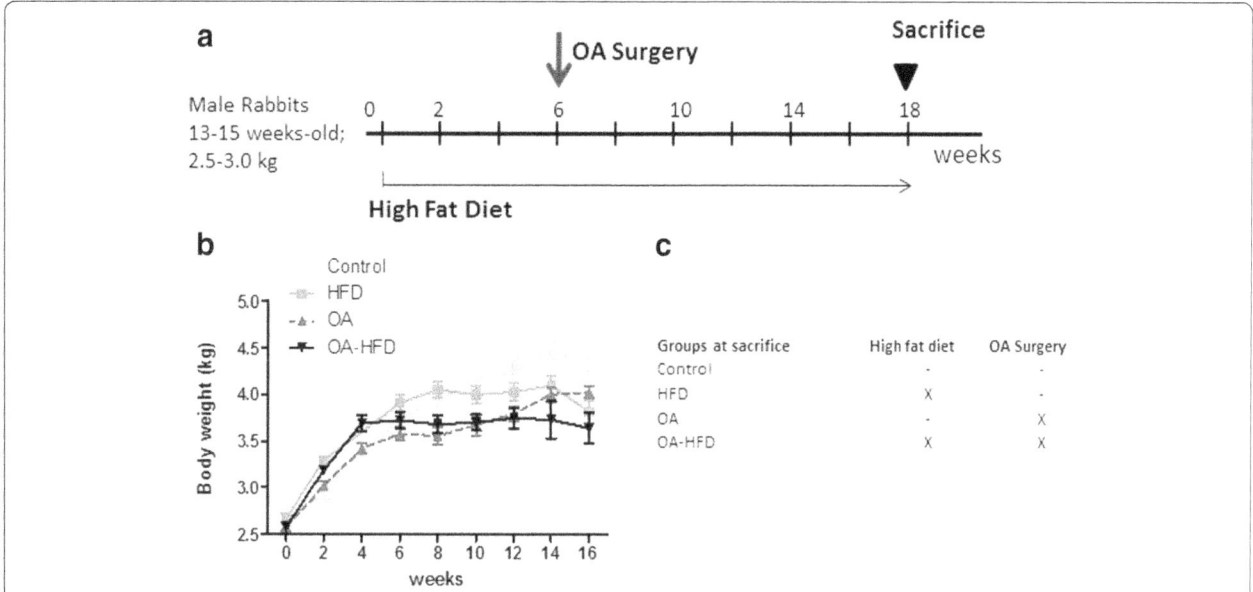

Fig. 1 Animal model. **a** Schematic representation of the experimental model. *Arrow* indicates the time of osteoarthritis (OA) induction by surgical partial medial meniscectomy plus anterior cruciate ligament transection. *Arrowhead* indicates the end of the study, when all animals were killed and samples extracted. **b** Change in body weight during follow up. **c** Scheme of the interventions in each group studied. HFD, high-fat diet

accessed by sectioning the patellar tendon and taking out the patella, thus the entire infrapatellar synovial membrane (SM) was collected by the same operator (AL-V), always taking the same specimen from each animal (Additional file 1: Figure S1). The SM was not separated from the adipose tissue [24, 25]. Half of the SM containing both stroma and lining was then fixed in 4% paraformaldehyde for 24 h and then was embedded in paraffin for histological studies; the other portion was immediately frozen and used for molecular biology studies. Femoral condyles were also removed and fixed in 4% buffered paraformaldehyde, decalcified for 4 weeks in a solution of 10% formic acid plus 5% paraformaldehyde, and embedded in paraffin [26]. The left and right SM and condyles were analyzed as independent samples.

Serum and synovial measurements
Glucose, total cholesterol, HDL cholesterol and triglyceride levels were assayed by automatic techniques as previously described [27, 28]. Adiponectin, leptin and plasma C-reactive protein (CRP) were measured by ELISA using commercial specific kits (SEA605Rb and SEA084Rb, respectively, USCN, Houston TX, USA and ab157726, Abcam, Cambridge, UK). Both adiponectin and leptin were measured in synovial tissue homogenates. For this purpose, total protein from the SM was extracted as described elsewhere [28, 29], and equal amounts of proteins diluted in the same volume for each knee were tested by specific ELISA for each adipokine.

Histological synovitis grading
The SM from both knees of each rabbit were sectioned 5-μm thick and stained with hematoxylin and eosin, and Masson's Trichrome. Synovitis was evaluated according to the Krenn score [30] as previously described [28], assessing lining hyperplasia, activation of synovial stroma related to fibrosis, and tissue infiltration. Each item was evaluated by a blinded observer using a subscale of 0– 3 points, where 0 indicated absence, 1 mild, 2 intermediate and 3 strong evidence of synovitis. The total score was obtained from the sum of partial grades with a maximum total score of 9.

Histological cartilage grading
The decalcified femurs were cleaved in a sagittal plane along the central portion of the articular surface of each medial femoral condyle corresponding to the weight-bearing area, and subsequently embedded in paraffin wax. Cartilage was sectioned 5-μm thick and stained with hematoxylin/eosin and alcian blue to evaluate cartilage abnormalities. These samples were evaluated using a modified version of Mankin's grading score system, which analyses four different parameters with a total score up to 21: structure (0–8), proteoglycan staining (0–6), loss of chondrocytes (0–4), and clone formation (0–3) [25, 31].

Immunohistochemical analysis
SM infiltrating macrophages were visualized using mouse anti-rabbit macrophage monoclonal antibodies

(mAb) (RAM11; Dako, Glostrup, Denmark) as previously described [27], whereas adipocytes were identified with anti-perilipin A1 (PLIN, Abcam, ab61682, 1/100 dilution) antibody. To evaluate RAM11-positive immunoreactivity, five photographs were obtained using a Leica DMD108 digital micro-imaging instrument (Leica, Microsystems, Inc. Buffalo Grove, IL, USA) at × 10 magnification ensuring constant light exposure. Each image was analyzed with ImageJ software (NIH, Bethesda, MD, USA), and the percentage of positive area was calculated with the Color Deconvolution plugin [32] in relation to the total tissue area. For each SM, the percentage of positive staining was calculated as the mean of these five images corresponding to the same SM [28].

Adipose tissue area (%ATA) and adipocyte size were analyzed in PLIN-stained slides using the Coreo Iscan Au Scanner (Ventana Medical Systems, USA) and ImageJ software. Five representative images at × 20 magnification were used to identify stained adipocyte boundaries. Every white area showing no immunoreactivity to PLIN was manually removed. Finally, the area of each adipocyte was measured and the average size was calculated for each SM sample.

Western blot
Briefly, total protein was extracted from the SM as described elsewhere [28, 29]. Protein extracts were separated by SDS-PAGE and transferred to a polyvinylidene fluoride membrane. The following primary antibodies were applied overnight at 4 °C: anti-human collagen type I (Col I, Merck Millipore, Billerica, MA, USA); anti-human PLIN (Abcam), anti-rabbit IL-1, anti-rabbit IL-6, anti-rabbit TNF (Cloud-Clone Corp, Houston TX, USA), and anti-human cyclooxygenase-2 (COX-2) (Santa Cruz Biotechnology, Dallas TX, USA). Loading control was performed employing EZBlue gel staining reagent (Sigma-Aldrich). Results were normalized relative to total protein presence and expressed as arbitrary densitometric units [28] (AU).

Gene expression
Total RNA was extracted from SM using TriPure Isolation Reagent (Roche Diagnostics, Indianapolis, IN, USA), according to the manufacturer's instructions. RNA was reverse-transcribed and RNA expression was quantified using the StepOnePlus™ detection system and StepOne™ software v2.2 (Applied Biosystems) as previously described [27, 33]. TaqMan® primers and probes were used to measure adiponectin (Oc03823307_s1), leptin (Oc03395809_s1) and Glyceraldehyde-3-phosphate dehydrogenase (GAPDH Oc03823402_g1) as endogenous control. Target genes were normalized relative to the expression of the endogenous control.

Statistical analysis
Histological analyses were carried out by two observers (AL-V and RL) in a blinded fashion. Scoring and quantitative analyses were averaged for the images and sections from the same SM to calculate the value per sample for statistical analyses. Each limb was analyzed as an independent sample for the studies of synovial tissue. All statistical analyses were performed using GraphPad Prism version 5.0 for Windows (GraphPad Software, San Diego, CA, USA). We employed the non-parametric Kruskal-Wallis test with a post-hoc correction for (Dunn's procedure) for comparisons between multiple groups, and the Mann-Whitney U test for comparisons between two groups. P values less than 0.05 were considered significant. Data are expressed as the mean ± 95% confidence interval (CI).

Results
Metabolic profile
We first studied the effect of the HFD in rabbits over an 18-week period in order to ensure the different characteristics that have been associated with MetS, such as being overweight, hypertension, basal glucose and dyslipidemia. There were no significant differences between the different groups in weight gain at week 6, the time point of surgery to induce OA (Fig. 1b). At the end of the study after 18 weeks of HFD feeding, rabbits fed a HFD gained less weight than controls (Table 1). Animals in the OA and OA-HFD groups also gained less weight than controls, probably due to discomfort associated with knee surgery. Rabbits in the HFD, OA and O-HFDA groups maintained similar SBP to control animals during the whole study period (Table 1). After 18 weeks of HFD, rabbits did not have any alteration in basal

Table 1 Characterization of the rabbit model

Group	Weight gain (kg)	SBP (mmHg)	Basal glucose (mg/dl)	Cholesterol (mg/dl)	Triglycerides (mg/dl)	HDL (mg/dl)	CRP (µg/ml)
Control (n = 10)	1.9 (1.7–2.0)	100 (93–107)	109 (101–116)	32.2 (8.9–55.5)	48 (32–64)	11.1 (8.6–13.6)	15.95 (8.2–23.7)
HFD (n = 6)	1.5* (1.1–1.7)	103 (87–119)	105 (98–112)	1876* (1139–2613)	253* (4–502)	12.5 (6.9–18.1)	39.14 (1–77.3)
OA (n = 9)	1.5* (1.2–1.8)	108 (96–119)	105 (94–115)	28.3 (18.2–38.4)	67.3 (40–95)	13.8 (10.2 17.3)	6.9 (3.8–10.0)
OA-HFD (n = 8)	0.7* (-0.12–1.6)	106 (96–117)	104 (98–111)	2050* (1587–2514)	290* (99–480)	15.6 (11.0–20.3)	18.1 (5.5–30.7)

Measures were obtained from serum or plasma samples taken just before animals were killed. Values represent mean with 95% confidence interval
HFD high-fat diet, OA osteoarthritis, SBP systolic blood pressure, HDL high-density lipoprotein, CRP C-reactive protein
*P < 0.05 vs. Control

glucose levels or in oral glucose tolerance (data not shown) in comparison to control animals (Table 1). However, there was increased total serum cholesterol and triglycerides in the rabbits fed HFD in comparison to controls. Although no significant differences were observed in circulating CRP levels between either the HFD or OA-HFD groups and controls (Table 1), there was a significant increase in CRP in animals fed with HFD vs. those fed with the standard diet, as a result of grouping rabbits into HFD plus OA-HFD and control plus OA (27.1 ± 7.3 vs 10.5 ± 1.9, $p = 0.026$).

Histological synovial inflammation and cartilage damage

Rabbits fed HFD had mild lining hyperplasia, discrete presence of infiltrating cells and a slight increment in stromal fibrosis, and thus the synovitis score was significantly higher than that observed in healthy controls (Fig. 2b, 2i). The OA group had a higher synovitis score than the control and HFD groups, with similar lesions to those described in synovitis in humans with advanced OA: mild to moderate lining hyperplasia, discrete presence of inflammatory cells, and stromal activation. The OA-HFD group had mild lining thickening, a clear increment in stromal cellularity, presence of infiltrating cells and inflammatory foci. All samples had enlarged stroma with an intense cell density (Fig. 2d). The synovitis score in the OA-HFD group was significantly higher than in the other groups (Fig.2i).

The HFD administration did not modify the histological appearances of cartilage damage, with the HFD group having a similar score to control animals (HFD 2.8 ± 1.5 vs. control 2.9 ± 1.0; p not significant (NS)). In addition, HFD did not significantly modify the histopathological damage in the cartilage in the OA-HDF group in comparison to the damage observed in the OA group (OA 15.2 ± 2.1 vs. OA-HFD 14.0 ± 2.7; p NS).

Macrophage infiltration and presence of foam cells

There was moderate presence of macrophages in the SM of rabbits fed HFD, which were especially localized in the lining layer (Fig. 2f, j). Lipid droplets were identified in their cytoplasm and their morphological shape resembled to pro-atherosclerotic foam cells, as previously described [5, 28] (Fig. 2f). RAM11 staining was scarce in the SM in the OA group, whereas there was extensive infiltration of RAM11-positive cells in the OA-HFD group to a much greater extent than in the HFD and OA groups (Fig. 2g, h, j). They were both consistently localized in the lining and sub-lining layers in every sample, and had the characteristic phenotype of foam cells [5, 28] (Fig. 2h).

Characterization of synovial stroma

Whereas healthy SM was mainly composed of adipocytes with little surrounding matrix, we observed patchy distribution of some fibrotic areas in the HFD group (Fig. 3a, b). OA membranes had a highly vascularized fibrotic stroma with some lax and dense stents, green-colored on Masson's Trichrome staining (Fig. 3). OA-HFD samples also had highly vascularized fibrotic membranes. The quantification of col I protein revealed a clear increase in the fibrotic content of the SM in the OA and OA-HFD groups (Fig. 3e-f) in comparison to control and HFD groups.

Adipose tissue area and adipocyte size in the SM

We quantified the adipose tissue fraction using PLIN staining, a distinguishing marker of adipocytes [34, 35]. A clear diminution in the percentage of adipose tissue area (%ATA) in the SM in the OA and OA-HFD samples in comparison to control and OA groups was observed, which was even lower in the OA-HFD than in the OA group (Fig 4a-e). Furthermore, SM adipocytes were significantly smaller in both the OA and OA-HFD groups than in the controls (Fig. 4f). The shape of these cells in control tissues was regular (Fig. 4a), whereas we observed high heterogeneity in the appearance of these cells in the SM in the OA and OA-HFD groups (Fig. 4c, d). Adipocyte size further decreased in the SM in the OA-HFD group in comparison to the OA group (Fig. 4f). PLIN content in the SM was also evaluated by western blot. In correlation with the %ATA, there was diminution in the SM PLIN in the OA and OA-HFD groups in comparison to the controls (Fig. 4g, h). Of note, the synthesis of PLIN was also significantly diminished in the OA-HFD group in comparison to the OA group.

Adipokine gene expression and concentration in SM and serum

Rabbits in both the HFD and OA groups had a clear decrease in leptin and adiponectin gene expression in the SM in comparison to controls (Fig. 5a, b). We observed an additive effect of these interventions in the OA-HFD group, where the gene expression of both leptin and adiponectin was significantly lower to that observed in the HFD and OA groups (Fig. 5). Interestingly, there was significant correlation between adipokine gene expression and the %ATA ($R = 0.746$; $p = 0.001$ for leptin expression; $R = 0.732$; $p = 0.002$ for adiponectin expression). Leptin levels in the SM measured by ELISA were decreased in the HFD group in comparison to controls, and it was also significantly reduced in the SM in the OA-HFD group in comparison to controls, the HDF and the OA groups (Fig. 5c). Adiponectin concentration only significantly diminished in the HFD group in comparison to controls (Fig. 5d). There was no correlation between the presence of these proteins and the %ATA in the SM.

However, HFD increased the circulating concentration of both adipokines, and there were no significant

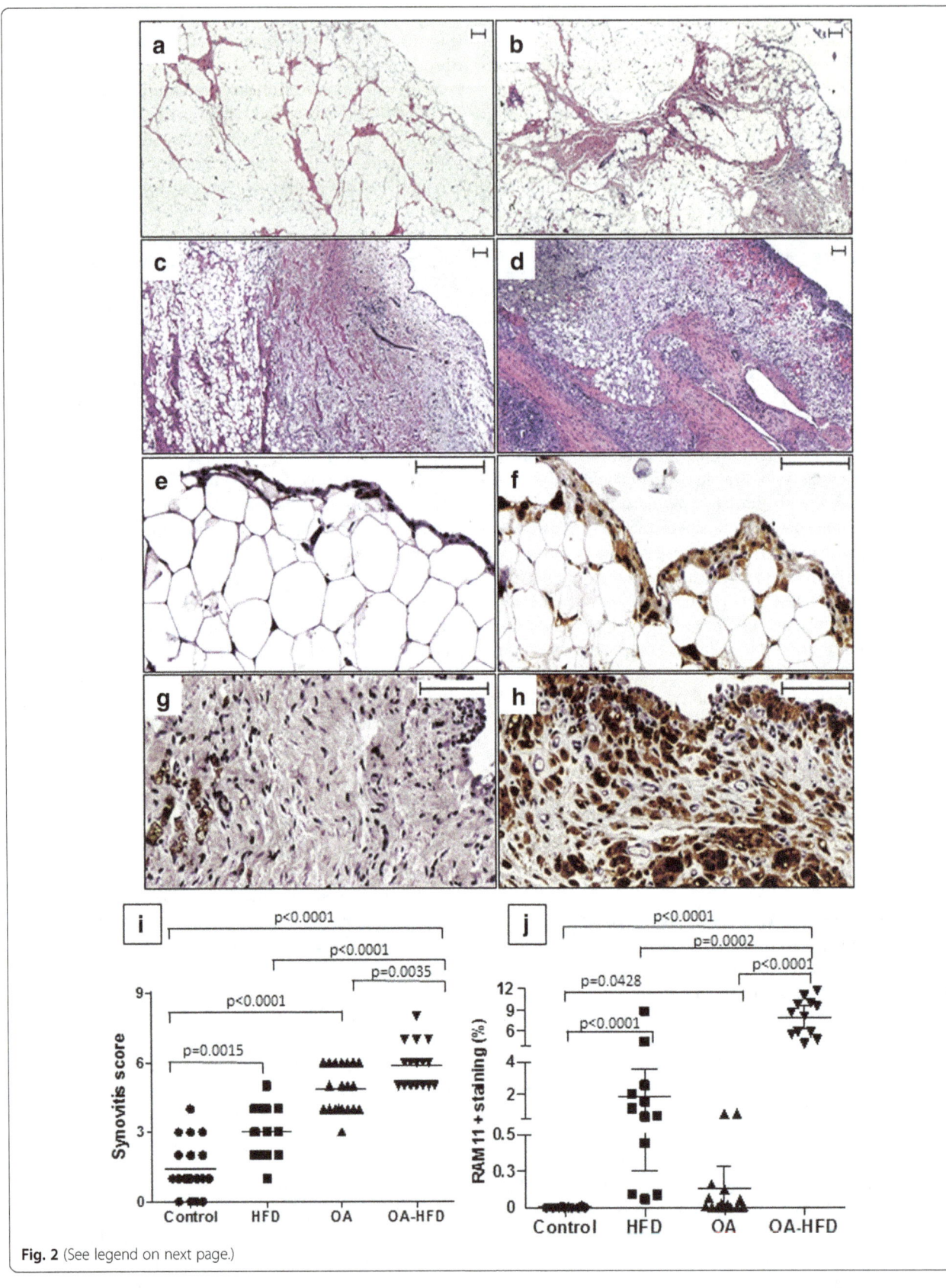

Fig. 2 (See legend on next page.)

(See figure on previous page.)
Fig. 2 Histopathological and macrophage analysis in the synovial membrane (SM). **a-d** Representative sections of SM stained with hematoxylin-eosin or **e-h** stained with a monoclonal anti-rabbit macrophage antibody (RAM11) from Control rabbit (**a** and **e**); rabbit fed with a high-fat diet (HFD) (**b** and **f**); osteoarthritic (OA) rabbit (**c** and **g**); and OA rabbit fed with a HFD (OA-HFD) (**d** and **h**). **a-d** Scale bar = 100 μm. **e-f** Scale bar = 100 μm. **i** Synovitis score quantified as described in "Methods. **j** Quantification of RAM11-positive area represented as percentage of total area. Data from individual measurements and mean for each group are shown. $n = 12–20$ SM per group for histopathological analysis; $n = 10–16$ SM per group for RAM11 analysis

differences between the HFD and OA-HFD group in the serum concentration of these mediators (Fig. 5e, f).

Synovial proinflammatory mediators

We then explored whether the HFD was able to modify the presence of different proinflammatory cytokines, such as IL-1β, IL-6, TNF and COX-2 in the SM of rabbits in the OA group. As expected, western blot studies that OA induced a marked increase in the presence of all the studied proinflammatory mediators in comparison to control animals. The presence of hyperlipidemia further increased the presence of IL-1 β, IL-6 and TNF in the SM in the OA-HFD group in comparison to the OA group (Fig. 6).

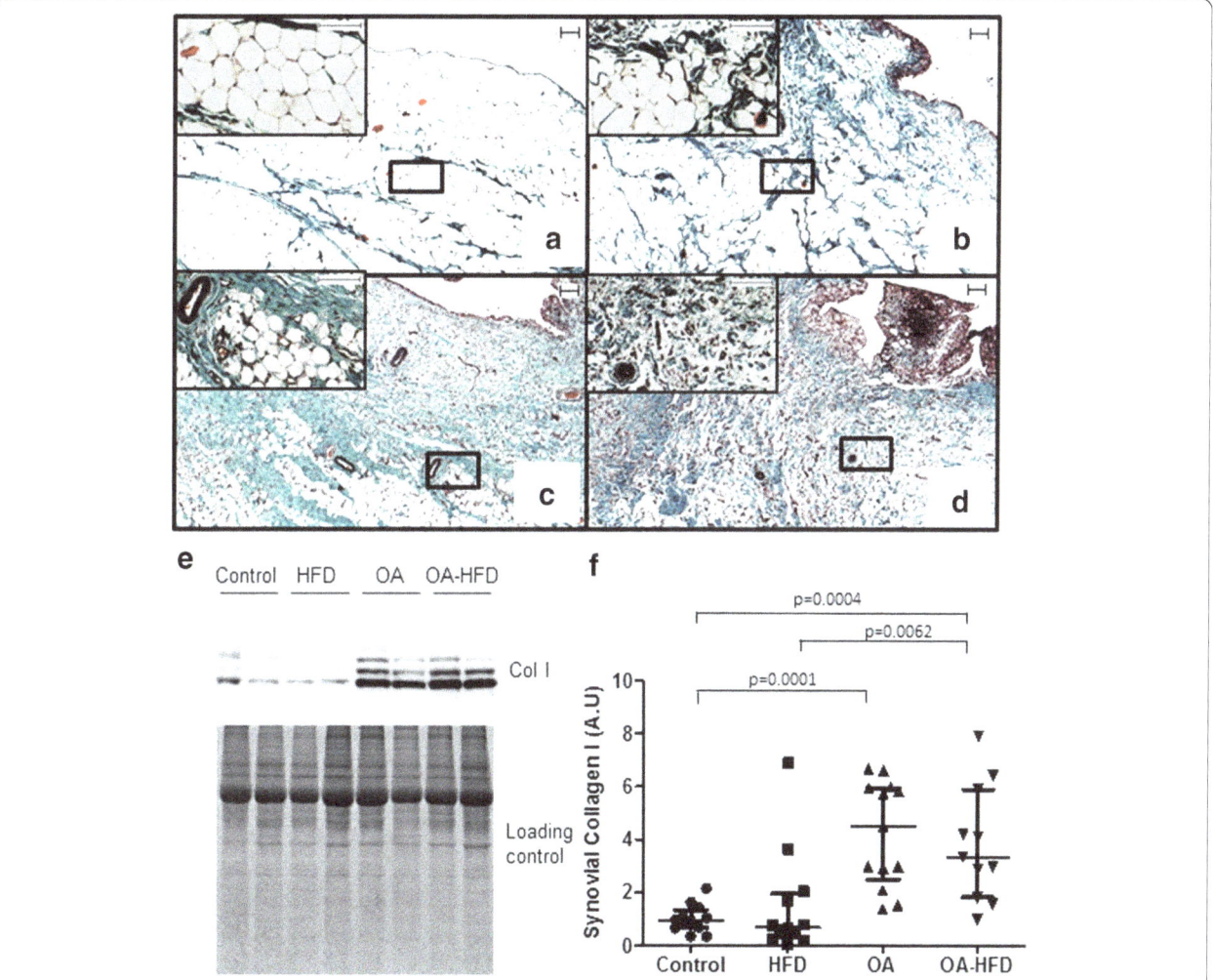

Fig. 3 Characterization of synovial stroma. Representative sections of synovial membranes stained with Masson's Trichrome. Magnification of the selected area is also shown. **a** Control healthy rabbit; **b**, rabbit on a high-fat diet (HFD); **c** osteoarthritic (OA) rabbit; **d** OA rabbit fed with HFD (OA-HFD); scale bar = 100 μm. **e** Representative western blot of collagen I (Col I) in the synovial membrane (SM) of the rabbits. EZ blue staining was used as protein loading control. **f** Densitometric analysis of Col I measured by western blot. Results are expressed as fold induction. Data from individual measurements and mean and 95% CI are shown ($n = 10–14$ SM per group)

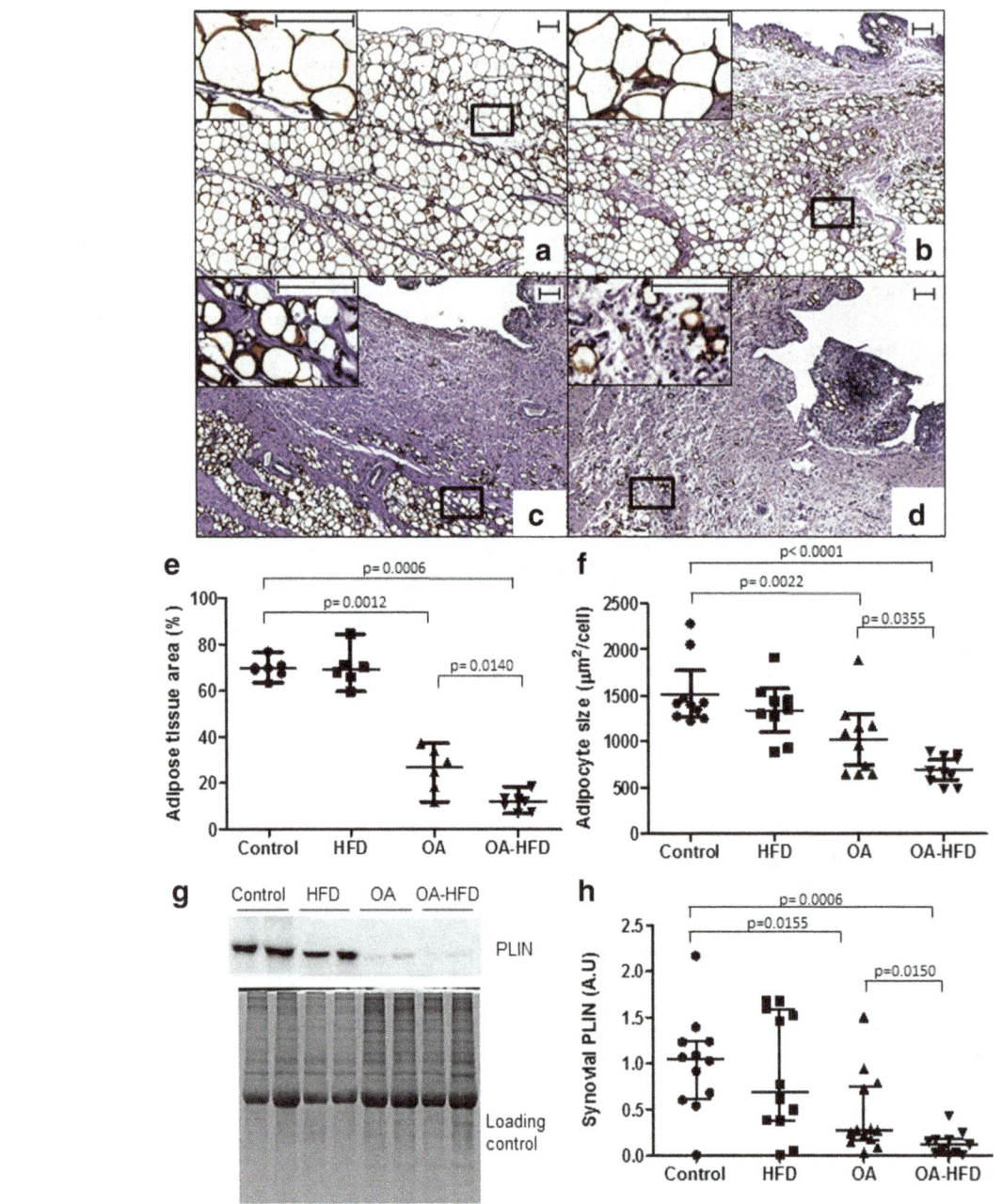

Fig. 4 Characterization of adipose tissue area and adipocyte size. Representative sections of synovial membranes (SM) stained with a monoclonal perilipin 1A (PLIN) antibody. Magnification of the selected area is also shown. **a** Control healthy rabbit; **b** rabbit fed a high-fat diet (HFD); **c** osteoarthritic (OA) rabbit; **d** OA rabbit fed with HFD (OA-HFD); scale bar = 100 μm. **e** Percentage of adipose tissue area in the SM of each group. **f** Mean of the adipocyte size in the SM of each group. **g** Representative western blot of PLIN protein levels expressed in the SM. EZ *blue* staining was used as protein loading control. **h** Densitometric analysis of PLIN measurement by western blot expressed as fold induction. Data from individual measurements and the mean and 95% CI are shown ($n = 9 - 14$ SM per group)

Discussion

In this study, we have shown that HFD aggravated OA synovitis, by inducing severe tissue architecture disorganization of the synovium, along with remarkable intensification of the proinflammatory cytokines IL-1β, IL-6 and TNF, and extensive infiltration of macrophages. However, HFD did not have any effect on the aggravation of the pathologic change in cartilage associated with OA. A relevant histological synovial alteration was the significant loss of synovial adipose tissue content, in correlation with decreased leptin and adiponectin gene expression.

In order to isolate the effect of hyperlipidemia, we employed an experimental model of HFD intake that

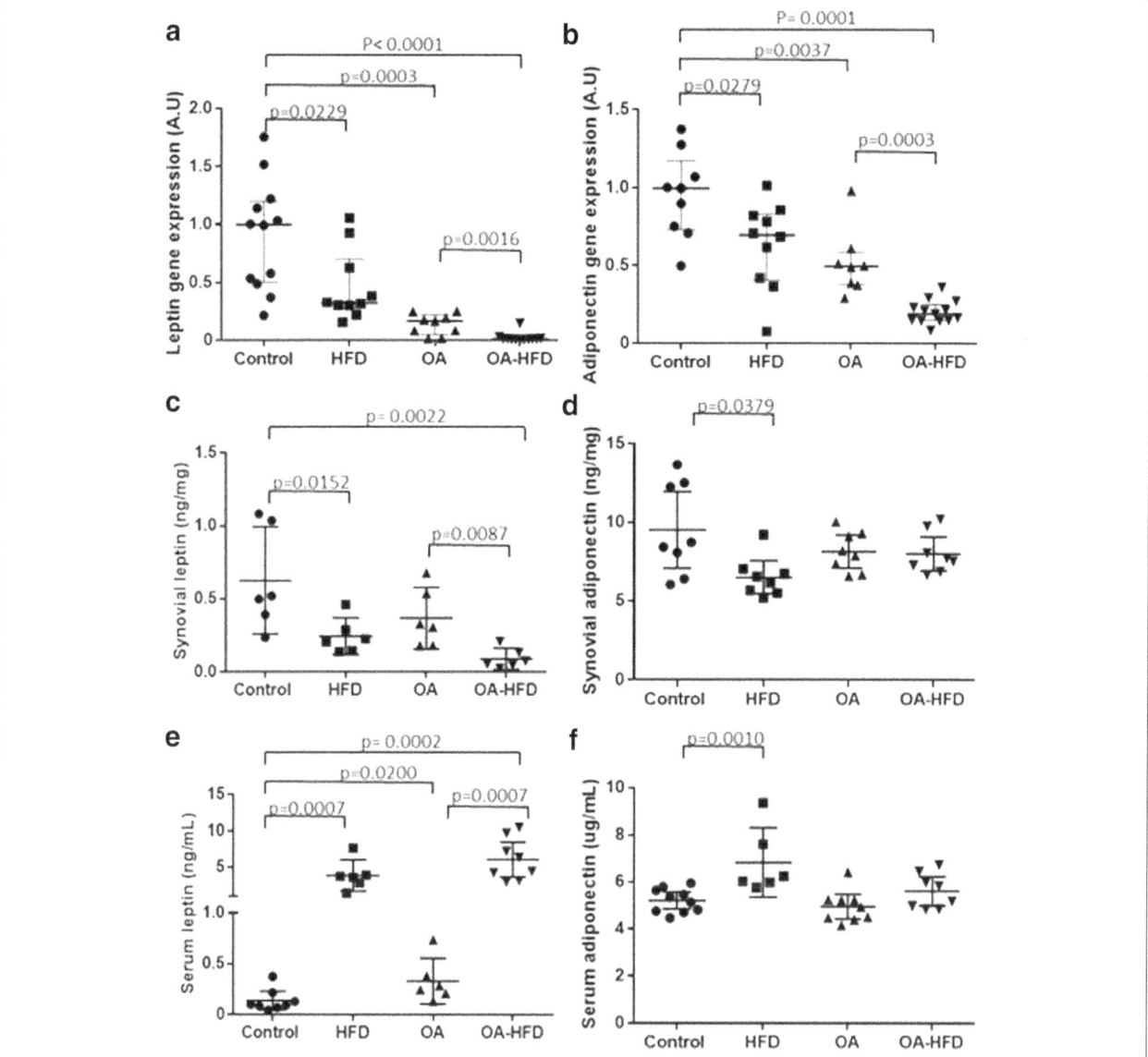

Fig. 5 Adipokine expression profile in the synovial membrane (SM) and serum concentration. **a** Leptin gene expression in rabbit SM measured by quantitative (q)PCR ($n = 10–14$ SM per group). **b** Adiponectin gene expression in rabbit SM measured by qPCR ($n = 10–14$ SM per group). **c** Leptin protein expression in SM membrane measured by ELISA ($n = 6$ SM per group). **d** Adiponectin protein expression in rabbit SM measured by ELISA ($n = 8$ SM per group). **e** Leptin concentration in rabbit serum measured by ELISA ($n = 6–10$ rabbits per group). **f** Adiponectin concentration in rabbit serum measured by ELISA ($n = 6–10$ rabbits per group). Data from individual measurements and mean and 95% CI for each group are shown. HFD, high-fat diet; OA, osteoarthritis

was not associated with weight gain [28]. The lack of significant weight gain in the HFD group has been previously reported and attributed to the animal self-regulation of caloric intake [36]. In fact, animals in both the HFD and OA-HFD groups had a significant decrease in weight gain, which was probably related to the increase in systemic inflammation induced by the diet [28]. Different studies using lipid-rich diets have not been able to adequately apportion the contribution of added mechanical load and hyperlipidemia in OA, a factor that was avoided in our experiments.

Different patterns of synoviopathy have been described in patients with OA, both in late and early disease, such as those with an increased fibrotic component or those essentially characterized by augmented inflammatory parameters [37]. In our rabbits, OA synovitis was associated with a significant increment of fibrotic tissue and partial loss of adipose tissue, and scarce presence of macrophages. A HFD induced both qualitative and quantitative changes in the SM in the rabbits with OA. However, HFD did not significantly aggravate cartilage damage in either the HFD group or the OA-HFD group.

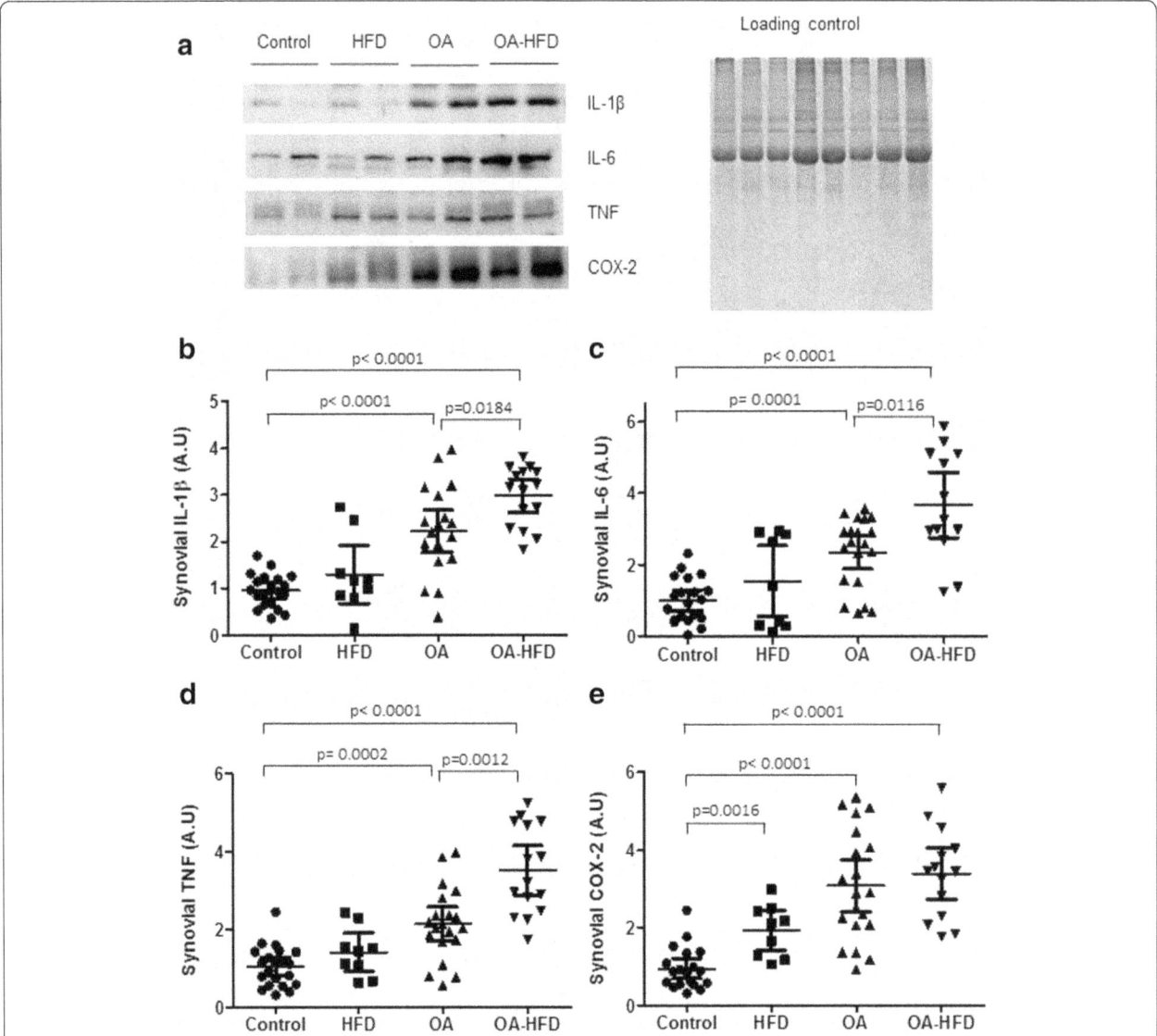

Fig. 6 Proinflammatory mediators in the synovial membrane (SM). **a** Representative western blot of IL-1β, IL-6, TNF and cyclooxygenase-2 (COX-2) protein levels expressed in the SM of the rabbits in each group. EZ *blue* staining was used as protein loading control. **b-e** Densitometric analysis of IL-1β, IL-6, TNF and COX-2 measured by western blot. Data from individual measurements, expressed as fold induction and mean and 95% CI for each group are shown (*n* = 12–20 SM per group). HFD, high-fat diet; OA, osteoarthritis

These data are in line with previously published results [38, 39], and suggest that the aggravation in synovial inflammation induced by HFD is not a secondary event induced by more severe pathological change in the cartilage.

The higher grade of synovial inflammation in the OA-HFD group was characterized by the remodeling of adipose tissue and by adipocyte loss. The remaining adipocytes had heterogeneous morphology and were significantly smaller in comparison to the OA and control groups, confirmed by the decreased presence of PLIN. HFD further increased synovial macrophages, most of them with the appearance of foam cells, whereas the fibrotic component was similar to that observed in the OA group. To our knowledge, this is the first report of correlation between synovial inflammation and loss of adipose tissue in this localization. Contradictory reports have been published on the contribution of the volume or area of the intra-articular fat tissue to joint deterioration and OA symptoms [40–42]. However, the alterations in adipocyte size, morphology, loss of adipose tissue with increased fibrosis and inflammatory content have been well-described in inflamed adipose tissue in other anatomic localizations, and described as lipodystrophy [43, 44]. The study of the synovial fat pad as an independent adipose intra-articular tissue has contributed to its identification as a crucial player in OA progression [45], although lack of recognition of the synovium as a whole, integrated, functional and structural unit hampers the understanding of the mechanisms involved in the synovial alterations in OA. Histologically, synovial lining, adipose sub-lining and synovial fat pad represent a continuum. Sub-lining adipose tissue and the fat pad seem to share a common inflammatory state, both in cell content and cell phenotype, induced by the disease process more than by tissue-specific signals [24, 46].

The mechanisms by which adipose tissue can be replaced by fibrotic tissue in the OA synovium have not been fully elucidated. However, the increase in the hypoxia-associated mediators, induced by biomechanical alterations and proinflammatory cytokines, could be at least partially responsible for this phenomenon. An increase in hypoxia-induced factor-1 (HIF-1)α has been described in the OA synovium, in correlation with greater joint destruction [47, 48]. In adipose tissue, with a similar structure and cellular component to that observed in the stroma of the SM, HIF-1α induces tissue fibrosis and inhibits pre-adipocyte differentiation [49]. Furthermore, in inflamed adipose tissue from mice fed a HFD, HIF-1α-stimulated macrophages form highly hypoxic structures called crown-like structures (CLS), comprising macrophages encircling dead or dying adipocytes [50]. Indeed, we have previously identified CLS in the OA synovium in both human and hypercholesterolemic rabbits with synovial inflammation [5, 28].

Hyperlipidemia in rabbits in the OA group did not seem to enhance the presence of fibrosis-associated proteins, such as col I. However, it evoked a dramatic increase in macrophage infiltration in the synovium and greater decrease in adipose tissue content. Dyslipemia has been directly related to macrophage infiltration and inflammation in the synovium and adipose tissue [51]. In hyperlipidemic mice with OA, the synovial proinflammatory macrophage subset was identified as responsible for an increase in TNF synthesis and extracellular matrix remodeling in the synovial membrane [51]. In line with these data, we identified greater TNF expression in the synovium in the OA-HFD group that paralleled the increased macrophage density in this tissue. Although little is known about the metabolic regulation of synovial macrophages, prolonged lipid exposure could result in failure of the lipid-handling mechanisms, leading to different lipotoxic events, such as those described in obesity-associated insulin resistance, atherosclerosis and other inflammatory diseases related to MetS [52]. Thus, hyperlipidemia could drive M1 macrophage polarization in the OA synovium, resulting in a major presence of proinflammatory cytokines, as has been described in adipose tissue [52, 53]. Furthermore, adipocyte apoptosis and impaired adipogenesis have been also associated with the increased lipolysis induced by over-nutrition or

HFD feeding [52]. Although hyperlipidemia could aggravate OA synovial inflammation, increasing macrophage density and adipose tissue destruction, the presence of hyperlipidemia per se could only have limited effects on SM alterations, as recently reported in HFD-fed mice [54].

Leptin and adiponectin gene expression diminished in the SM in the OA and OA-HFD group in comparison to control animals. These results appear to correlate with the amount of intra-articular adipose tissue rather than with the presence of a proinflammatory milieu. Furthermore, circulating leptin was significantly increased in HDF-fed animals, probably due to the effect of the diet on the extra-articular fat tissue [55]. Our data are in line with previous reports indicating that hyperlipidemia could be an aggravating factor for OA through the stimulation of systemic proinflammatory mediators [56]. In the OA group we also found increased circulating leptin as previously described in human and experimental OA, related to joint damage [19]. Therefore, our data do not support the hypothesis that hyperlipidemia could be an aggravating factor in metabolic OA, stimulating adipokine expression within the intra-articular adipose tissue. Different joint cells, such as chondrocytes or bone cells, could be responsible for adipokine synthesis in response to biomechanical or proinflammatory stimuli [19, 20].

Conclusions

In summary, these data show that HFD aggravates the inflammation in the SM of rabbits with OA by inducing an increase in the infiltrating macrophages in the synovium, together with macrophage and metabolic-mediated remodeling of adipose tissue, and further elevation of proinflammatory cytokines. The lipotoxic effects induced by dyslipemia in adipocytes and macrophages could play a decisive role in the joint deterioration of patients with OA and MetS, supporting the hypothesis of a plausible link between obesity and OA going beyond mechanical loading.

Abbreviations
ATA: Adipose tissue area; CLS: Crown-like structures; Col I: Collagen I; COX-2: Cyclooxygenase-2; CRP: C-reactive protein; ELISA: Enzyme-linked immunosorbent assay; HFD: High fat diet; IL-1β: Interleukin-1β; IL-6: Interleukin-6; MetS: Metabolic syndrome; OA: Osteoarthritis; PLIN: Perilipin-1A; SBP: Systolic blood pressure; SM: Synovial membrane; TNF: Tumor necrosis factor

Funding
This work was supported by research grants from the Instituto de Salud Carlos III [PI12/00144, PI15/00340, PI16/00065]; co-funded by Fondo Europeo de Desarrollo Regional (FEDER).

Authors' contributions
Conception and design: G H-B and RL; acquisition and assembly of data: A L-V; AL, S P-B, I P-P and LP; analysis and interpretation of the data: A L-V; AL, S P-B, G H-B and RL; drafting of the article: A L-V, G H-B and RL; critical revision of the article for important intellectual content: all authors; final approval of the article: all authors.

Competing interests

The authors have declared no competing interests.

Author details

[1]Bone and Joint Research Unit, IIS-Fundación Jiménez Díaz UAM, Avda. Reyes Católicos, 2, Madrid 28040, Spain. [2]Clinical Analysis Department, HU-Fundación Jiménez Díaz, Madrid, Spain.

References

1. Loeser RF, Goldring SR, Scanzello CR, Goldring MB. Osteoarthritis: a disease of the joint as an organ. Arthritis Rheum. 2012;64:1697–707.

2. Ayral X, Pickering EH, Woodworth TG, Mackillop N, Dougados M. Synovitis: a potential predictive factor of structural progression of medial tibiofemoral knee osteoarthritis – results of a 1 year longitudinal arthroscopic study in 422 patients. Osteoarthritis Cartilage. 2005;13:361–7.

3. Scanzello CR, Goldring SR. The role of synovitis in osteoarthritis pathogenesis. Bone. 2012;51:249–57.

4. Haywood L, McWilliams DF, Pearson CI, Gill SE, Ganesan A, Wilson D, et al. Inflammation and angiogenesis in osteoarthritis. Arthritis Rheum. 2003;48:2173–7.

5. Prieto-Potin I, Largo R, Roman-Blas JA, Herrero-Beaumont G, Walsh DA. Characterization of multinucleated giant cells in synovium and subchondral bone in knee osteoarthritis and rheumatoid arthritis. BMC Musculoskelet Disord. 2015;16:226.

6. Van Lent PLEM, Blom AB, van der Kraan P, Holthuysen AEM, Vitters E, Van Rooijen N, et al. Crucial role of synovial lining macrophages in the promotion of transforming growth factor beta-mediated osteophyte formation. Arthritis Rheum. 2004;50:103–11.

7. Aspden R. Obesity punches above its weight in osteoarthritis. Nat Rev Rheumatol. 2010;7:65–8.

8. Zhuo Q, Yang W, Chen J, Wang Y. Metabolic syndrome meets osteoarthritis. Nat Rev Rheumatol. 2012;8:729–37.

9. Grundy SM, Cleeman JI, Daniels SR, Donato KA, Eckel RH, Franklin BA, et al. Diagnosis and management of the metabolic syndrome: an American Heart Association/National Heart, Lung, and Blood Institute scientific statement. Circulation. 2005;112(17):2735–52.

10. Alberti KG, Zimmet P, Shaw J, IDF Epidemiology Task Force Consensus Group. The metabolic syndrome–a new worldwide definition. Lancet (London, England). 2005;366:1059–62.

11. Yoshimura N, Muraki S, Oka H, Tanaka S, Kawaguchi H, Nakamura K, et al. Accumulation of metabolic risk factors such as overweight, hypertension, dyslipidaemia, and impaired glucose tolerance raises the risk of occurrence and progression of knee osteoarthritis: a 3-year follow-up of the ROAD study. Osteoarthritis Cartilage. 2012;20:1217–26.

12. Puenpatom RA, Victor TW. Increased prevalence of metabolic syndrome in individuals with osteoarthritis: an analysis of NHANES III data. Postgrad Med. 2009;121:9–20.

13. Pottie P, Presle N, Terlain B, Netter P, Mainard D, Berenbaum F. Obesity and osteoarthritis: more complex than predicted! Ann Rheum Dis. 2006; 65:1403–5.

14. Niu J, Clancy M, Aliabadi P, Vasan R, Felson DT. Metabolic syndrome, its components, and knee osteoarthritis: The Framingham Osteoarthritis Study. Arthritis Rheum. 2017;69:1194–203.

15. Farnaghi S, Crawford R, Xiao Y, Prasadam I. Cholesterol metabolism in pathogenesis of osteoarthritis disease. Int J Rheum Dis. 2017;20:131–40.

16. de Munter W, Blom AB, Helsen MM, Walgreen B, van der Kraan PM, Joosten LA, et al. Cholesterol accumulation caused by low density lipoprotein receptor deficiency or a cholesterol-rich diet results in ectopic bone formation during experimental osteoarthritis. Arthritis Res Ther. 2013;15:R178.

17. De Munter W, Van der Kraan PM, Van den Berg WB, Van Lent PLEM. High systemic levels of low-density lipoprotein cholesterol: fuel to the flames in inflammatory osteoarthritis? Rheumatol (United Kingdom). 2016;55:16–24.

18. Chung S, Parks JS. Dietary cholesterol effects on adipose tissue inflammation. Curr Opin Lipidol. 2016;27:19–25.

19. Hu P-F, Bao J-P, Wu L-D. The emerging role of adipokines in osteoarthritis: a narrative review. Mol Biol Rep. 2011;38:873–8.

20. Presle N, Pottie P, Dumond H, Guillaume C, Lapicque F, Pallu S, et al. Differential distribution of adipokines between serum and synovial fluid in patients with osteoarthritis. Contribution of joint tissues to their articular production. Osteoarthritis Cartilage. 2006;14:690–5.

21. de Boer TN, van Spil WE, Huisman AM, Polak AA, Bijlsma JWJ, Lafeber FPJG, et al. Serum adipokines in osteoarthritis; comparison with controls and relationship with local parameters of synovial inflammation and cartilage damage. Osteoarthritis Cartilage. 2012;20:846–53.

22. Martínez-Calatrava MJ, Prieto-Potín I, Roman-Blas JA, Tardio L, Largo R, Herrero-Beaumont G. RANKL synthesized by articular chondrocytes contributes to juxta-articular bone loss in chronic arthritis. Arthritis Res Ther. 2012;14:R149.

23. Martel E, Egner B, Brown SA, King JN, Laveissiere A, Champeroux P, et al. Comparison of high-definition oscillometry – a non-invasive technology for arterial blood pressure measurement – with a direct invasive method using radio-telemetry in awake healthy cats. J Feline Med Surg. 2013;15:1104–13.

24. Harasymowicz NS, Clement ND, Azfer A, Burnett R, Salter DM, Simpson AHWR. Regional differences between perisynovial and infrapatellar adipose tissue depots and their response to class II and class III obesity in patients with osteoarthritis. Arthritis Rheum. 2017;69:1396–406.

25. Lugo L, Villalvilla A, Gómez R, Bellido M, Sánchez-Pernaute O, Largo R, et al. Effects of PTH [1-34] on synoviopathy in an experimental model of osteoarthritis preceded by osteoporosis. Osteoarthritis Cartilage. 2012;20:1619–30.

26. Roman-Blas JA, Mediero A, Tardío L, Portal-Nuñez S, Gratal P, Herrero-Beaumont G, et al. The combined therapy with chondroitin sulfate plus glucosamine sulfate or chondroitin sulfate plus glucosamine hydrochloride does not improve joint damage in an experimental model of knee osteoarthritis in rabbits. Eur J Pharmacol. 2017;794:8–14.

27. Largo R, Sánchez-Pernaute O, Marcos ME, Moreno-Rubio J, Aparicio C, Granado R, et al. Chronic arthritis aggravates vascular lesions in rabbits with atherosclerosis: a novel model of atherosclerosis associated with chronic inflammation. Arthritis Rheum. 2008;58:2723–34.

28. Prieto-Potín I, Roman-Blas J, Martínez-Calatrava M, Gómez R, Largo R, Herrero-Beaumont G. Hypercholesterolemia boosts joint destruction in chronic arthritis. An experimental model aggravated by foam macrophage infiltration. Arthritis Res Ther. 2013;15:R81.

29. Alvarez-Soria MA, Largo R, Santillana J, Sánchez-Pernaute O, Calvo E, Hernández M, et al. Long term NSAID treatment inhibits COX-2 synthesis in the knee synovial membrane of patients with osteoarthritis: differential proinflammatory cytokine profile between celecoxib and aceclofenac. Ann Rheum Dis. 2006;65:998–1005.

30. Krenn V, Morawietz L, Häupl T, Neidel J, Petersen I, König A. Grading of chronic synovitis–a histopathological grading system for molecular and diagnostic pathology. Pathol Res Pract. 2002;198:317–25.

31. Tiraloche G, Girard C, Chouinard L, Sampalis J, Moquin L, Ionescu M, et al. Effect of oral glucosamine on cartilage degradation in a rabbit model of osteoarthritis. Arthritis Rheum. 2005;52:1118–28.

32. Ruifrok AC, Johnston DA. Quantification of histochemical staining by color deconvolution. Anal Quant Cytol Histol. 2001;23:291–9.

33. Largo R, Martínez-Calatrava MJ, Sánchez-Pernaute O, Marcos ME, Moreno-Rubio J, Aparicio C, et al. Effect of a high dose of glucosamine on systemic and tissue inflammation in an experimental model of atherosclerosis aggravated by chronic arthritis. Am J Physiol Heart Circ Physiol. 2009;297:H268–76.

34. Blanchette-Mackie EJ, Dwyer NK, Barber T, Coxey RA, Takeda T, Rondinone CM, et al. Perilipin is located on the surface layer of intracellular lipid droplets in adipocytes. J Lipid Res. 1995;36:1211–26.

35. Cinti S, Mitchell G, Barbatelli G, Murano I, Ceresi E, Faloia E, et al. Adipocyte death defines macrophage localization and function in adipose tissue of obese mice and humans. J Lipid Res. 2005;46:2347–55.

36. Brunner AM, Henn CM, Drewniak EI, Lesieur-Brooks A, Machan J, Crisco JJ, et al. High dietary fat and the development of osteoarthritis in a rabbit model. Osteoarthritis Cartilage. 2012;20:584–92.

37. Oehler S, Neureiter D, Meyer-Scholten C, Aigner T. Subtyping of osteoarthritic synoviopathy. Clin Exp Rheumatol. 2002;20:633–40.

38. de Munter W, van den Bosch MH, Slöetjes AW, Croce KJ, Vogl T, Roth J, et al. High LDL levels lead to increased synovial inflammation and accelerated ectopic bone formation during experimental osteoarthritis. Osteoarthritis Cartilage. 2016;24:844–55.

39. Collins KH, Reimer RA, Seerattan RA, Leonard TR, Herzog W. Using diet-induced obesity to understand a metabolic subtype of osteoarthritis in rats. Osteoarthritis Cartilage. 2015;23:957–65.

40. Pan F, Han W, Wang X, Liu Z, Jin X, Antony B, et al. A longitudinal study of the association between infrapatellar fat pad maximal area and changes in knee symptoms and structure in older adults. Ann Rheum Dis. 2015;74:1818–24.
41. Han W, Cai S, Liu Z, Jin X, Wang X, Antony B, et al. Infrapatellar fat pad in the knee: is local fat good or bad for knee osteoarthritis? Arthritis Res Ther. 2014;16:R145.
42. O'Neill TW, Parkes MJM, Maricar N, Marjanovic EJE, Hodgson R, Gait ADA, et al. Synovial tissue volume: a treatment target in knee osteoarthritis (OA). Ann Rheum Dis. 2016;75:84–90.
43. Giralt M, Domingo P, Guallar JP, Rodriguez de la Concepción ML, Alegre M, Domingo JC, et al. HIV-1 infection alters gene expression in adipose tissue, which contributes to HIV-1/HAART-associated lipodystrophy. Antivir Ther. 2006;11:729–40.
44. Gallego-Escuredo JM, Villarroya J, Domingo P, Targarona EM, Alegre M, Domingo JC, et al. Differentially altered molecular signature of visceral adipose tissue in HIV-1-associated lipodystrophy. J Acquir Immune Defic Syndr. 2013;64:142–8.
45. Ioan-Facsinay A, Kloppenburg M. An emerging player in knee osteoarthritis: the infrapatellar fat pad. Arthritis Res Ther. 2013;15:225.
46. Klein-Wieringa IR, de Lange-Brokaar BJE, Yusuf E, Andersen SN, Kwekkeboom JC, Kroon HM, et al. Inflammatory cells in patients with endstage knee osteoarthritis: a comparison between the synovium and the infrapatellar fat pad. J Rheumatol. 2016;43:771–8.
47. Chu H, Xu ZM, Yu H, Zhu KJ, Huang H. Association between hypoxia-inducible factor-1a levels in serum and synovial fluid with the radiographic severity of knee osteoarthritis. Genet Mol Res. 2014;13:10529–36.
48. Giatromanolaki A, Sivridis E, Maltezos E, Athanassou N, Papazoglou D, Gatter KC, et al. Upregulated hypoxia inducible factor-1alpha and -2alpha pathway in rheumatoid arthritis and osteoarthritis. Arthritis Res Ther. 2003;5:R193–201.
49. Buechler C, Krautbauer S, Eisinger K. Adipose tissue fibrosis. World J Diabetes. 2015;6:548–53.
50. Fujisaka S, Usui I, Ikutani M, Aminuddin A, Takikawa A, Tsuneyama K, et al. Adipose tissue hypoxia induces inflammatory M1 polarity of macrophages in an HIF-1a-dependent and HIF-1a-independent manner in obese mice. Diabetologia. 2013;56:1403–12.
51. Uchida K, Satoh M, Inoue G, Onuma K, Miyagi M, Iwabuchi K, et al. CD11c(+) macrophages and levels of TNF-a and MMP-3 are increased in synovial and adipose tissues of osteoarthritic mice with hyperlipidaemia. Clin Exp Immunol. 2015;180:551–9.
52. Prieur X, Rőszer T, Ricote M. Lipotoxicity in macrophages: evidence from diseases associated with the metabolic syndrome. Biochim Biophys Acta. 2010;1801:327–37.
53. Lumeng CN, Bodzin JL, Saltiel AR. Obesity induces a phenotypic switch in adipose tissue macrophage polarization. J Clin Invest. 2007;117:175–84.
54. Barboza E, Hudson J, Chang WP, Kovats S, Towner RA, Silasi-Mansat R, et al. Profibrotic infrapatellar fat pad remodeling without M1 macrophage polarization precedes knee osteoarthritis in mice with diet-induced obesity. Arthritis Rheumatol. 2017;69:1221–32.
55. Unger RH. Longevity, lipotoxicity and leptin: the adipocyte defense against feasting and famine. Biochimie. 2005;87:57–64.
56. Robinson WH, Lepus CM, Wang Q, Raghu H, Mao R, Lindstrom TM, et al. Low-grade inflammation as a key mediator of the pathogenesis of osteoarthritis. Nat Rev Rheumatol. 2016;12:580–92.

2

H3K27me3 demethylases regulate in vitro chondrogenesis and chondrocyte activity in osteoarthritis

Clarence Yapp[1,2], Andrew J. Carr[1], Andrew Price[1], Udo Oppermann[1,2,3] and Sarah J. B. Snelling[1*]

Abstract

Background: Epigenetic changes (i.e., chromatin modifications) occur during chondrogenesis and in osteoarthritis (OA). We investigated the effect of H3K27me3 demethylase inhibition on chondrogenesis and assessed its utility in cartilage tissue engineering and in understanding cartilage destruction in OA.

Methods: We used a high-content screen to assess the effect of epigenetic modifying compounds on collagen output during chondrogenesis of monolayer human mesenchymal stem cells (MSCs). The impact of GSK-J4 on gene expression, glycosaminoglycan output and collagen formation during differentiation of MSCs into cartilage discs was investigated. Expression of lysine (K)-specific demethylase 6A (*UTX*) and Jumonji domain-containing 3 (*JMJD3*), the HEK27Me3 demethylases targeted by GSK-J4, was measured in damaged and undamaged cartilage from patients with OA. The impact of GSK-J4 on ex vivo cartilage destruction and expression of OA-related genes in human articular chondrocytes (HACs) was assessed. H3K27Me3 demethylase regulation of transforming growth factor (TGF)-β-induced gene expression was measured in MSCs and HACs.

Results: Treatment of chondrogenic MSCs with the H3K27me3 demethylase inhibitor GSK-J4, which targets JMJD3 and UTX, inhibited collagen output; expression of chondrogenic genes, including *SOX9* and *COL2A1*; and disrupted glycosaminoglycan and collagen synthesis. *JMJD3* but not *UTX* expression was increased during chondrogenesis and in damaged OA cartilage, suggesting a predominant role of JMJD3 in chondrogenesis and OA. GSK-J4 prevented ex vivo cartilage destruction and expression of the OA-related genes *MMP13* and *PTGS2*. TGF-β is a key regulator of chondrogenesis and articular cartilage homeostasis, and TGF-β-induced gene expression was inhibited by GSK-J4 treatment of both chondrogenic MSCs and HACs.

Conclusions: Overall, we show that H3K27me3 demethylases modulate chondrogenesis and that enhancing this activity may improve production of tissue-engineered cartilage. In contrast, targeted inhibition of H3K27me3 demethylases could provide a novel approach in OA therapeutics.

Keywords: Epigenetics, TGF-β, Osteoarthritis, JMJD3, Histone demethylase

Background

Osteoarthritis (OA) is the most common of the arthritides and is characterized by loss of articular cartilage. Treatments for OA are limited to pain relief, physiotherapy and joint replacement surgery for end-stage disease. To successfully treat cartilage lesions and OA, it is paramount to improve production of tissue-engineered cartilage and to identify disease-modifying therapeutics that can prevent or limit cartilage degradation.

Gene expression and cellular phenotype changes associated with OA and chondrogenesis are increasingly being attributed to altered activity of epigenetic modifying enzymes and consequent epigenetic regulation of target genes [1, 2]. Commonly, epigenetic modifications occur in gene promoters and include regulation of chromatin structure through cytosine methylation of DNA or through modifications such as acetylation and methylation of lysine residues in histone tails. Pharmacological

* Correspondence: sarah.snelling@ndorms.ox.ac.uk
[1]Nuffield Department of Orthopaedics, Rheumatology and Musculoskeletal Sciences, Botnar Research Centre, University of Oxford, Nuffield Orthopaedic Centre, Windmill Road, Headington, OX3 7LD Oxford, UK
Full list of author information is available at the end of the article

intervention points in oncology have been identified by targeting of "readers, writers and erasers" of an "epigenetic code" [3], an avenue with largely unexplored potential in inflammatory and degenerative diseases.

Correct regulation of transforming growth factor (TGF)-β signalling is essential for cartilage development [4]. Dysregulation of TGF-β pathway components leads to impaired skeletogenesis, increased chondrocyte hypertrophy and an OA-like phenotype in murine models [5, 6]. Furthermore a disrupted TGF-β signalling response in both murine and human OA has been reported [7]. Epigenetic regulation of the TGF-β pathway in fibrosis has been reported, and TGF-β itself regulates expression of epigenetic modifying enzymes [8].

We reasoned that specific targeting of epigenetic modifying enzymes could provide valuable insight into the role of epigenetics in chondrogenesis and OA and help identify exploitable targets for therapeutic development. In this work, we identified and investigated the H3K27me3 demethylases as novel targets in cartilage tissue engineering and OA pathogenesis.

Methods

Cell culture and tissue preparation

Primary human bone marrow-derived mesenchymal stem cells (MSCs) were purchased from Lonza (Walkersville, MD, USA) and cultured in MSC expansion media consisting of MesenPRO RS basal media with MesenPRO RS supplement, 2 mM L-glutamine, 100 IU ml^{-1} penicillin and 100 mg ml^{-1} streptomycin (Life Technologies, Carlsbad, CA, USA). MSCs were used for all experiments before passage 7.

Human articular cartilage for gene expression analysis was from damaged and undamaged regions of the medial tibial plateau of individuals undergoing unicompartmental knee replacement for anteromedial OA ($n = 5$ patients). For cell culture, cartilage from the medial tibial plateau of patients undergoing unicompartmental knee replacement for OA was dissected and digested overnight with collagenase. HACs were cultured in basal medium composed of high-glucose DMEM (Lonza) containing 2 mM glutamine and 100 IU ml^{-1} penicillin and 100 mg ml^{-1} streptomycin (Life Technologies).

Ethical approval was granted (09/H0606/11) by the local research ethics committee (Oxford Research Ethics Committee B) for all work on human articular cartilage and chondrocytes, and informed consent was obtained from all patients.

Chondrogenic differentiation

For monolayer chondrogenesis, MSCs in expansion media were seeded at 20,000 cells/well in a 96-well plate and left to adhere overnight. Expansion media were replaced with high-glucose DMEM (Lonza), chondrogenic differentiation media containing 100 μg/ml sodium pyruvate (Lonza), 10 ng/ml TGF-β3 (R&D Systems, Minneapolis, MN, USA), 100 nM dexamethasone, 1× ITS+ premix (BD Biosciences, San Jose, CA, USA), 40 μg/ml proline, and 25 μg/ml ascorbate 2-phosphate (Sigma-Aldrich, St. Louis, MO, USA). Media were refreshed every 2–3 days.

For cartilage disc generation, MSCs were resuspended in chondrogenic medium and 100 μl of MSCs at 5×10^6 cells/ml were pipetted onto 6.5-mm, 0.8-μm pore polycarbonate Transwell filters (Corning Costar, Corning, NY, USA) in a 24-well plate, centrifuged ($200 \times g$, 5 min) before addition of 500 μl of chondrogenic medium to the lower well. Media were refreshed every 2–3 days.

Compound screen

Using a focused library of 31 small-molecule inhibitors against various readers, writers and erasers of chromatin modifications, we assessed chondrogenic differentiation of MSCs. Chondrogenic monolayer MSCs were incubated for 7 days in the presence or absence of epigenetic modifying compounds, where compounds and media were refreshed every 2–3 days. Cell viability was assessed using the alamarBlue assay (Life Technologies) before fixing cells in 4 % formaldehyde and staining with 10 μg/ml Nile Red, which binds nonspecifically to collagens and lipids and allows visualization of chondrogenic nodules [9]. Nile Red staining intensity was assessed using excitation at 485 nm in the BD Pathway (BD Biosciences). Data are presented as Nile Red incorporation relative to cell viability (Additional file 1: Figure S1).

Cytokine and GSK-J4 treatments

Primary HACs were seeded at 6000 cells/well in a 96-well plate and allowed to adhere overnight. HACs were treated with GSK-J4 (10 μM), interleukin (IL)-1β (5 ng/ml), IL-6 (10 ng/ml), oncostatin M (OSM) (10 ng/ml), TGF-β (4 ng/ml) or TGF-β and GSK-J4. Dimethyl sulphoxide (DMSO) alone was added to all wells not containing GSK-J4. MSCs were seeded at 20,000 cells/well of a 96-well plate and allowed to adhere overnight in MSC expansion medium before 1- and 24-h treatment in basal, chondrogenic (plus DMSO carrier) and chondrogenic medium plus GSK-J4. Treated HACs and MSCs were washed twice in PBS, and cells were harvested in cells to complementary DNA (cDNA) lysis buffer (Ambion; Thermo Fisher Scientific, Austin, TX, USA) prior to cDNA synthesis. GSK-J5 (10 μM), the less active enantiomer of GSK-J4, was used as an additional comparator for experiments (Additional file 1: Figure S1 and Additional file 2: Figure S3).

Small interfering RNA

HACs and MSCs were transfected with 5 nM (final concentration) of small interfering (siRNA) against Jumonji domain-containing 3 (*JMJD3*) and lysine (K)-specific demethylase 6A (*UTX*) (QIAGEN, Hilden, Germany) or AllStars non-targeting negative control (QIAGEN) using DharmaFECT reagent (GE Healthcare, Little Chalfont, UK) according to the manufacturer's instructions. MSCs were pre-treated with siRNA for 48 h prior to induction of chondrogenesis. HACs were transfected with siRNA 72 h prior to harvest for gene expression analysis.

Gene expression analysis

Following cytokine treatment of monolayer HACs and MSCs, cell-to-cDNA lysates were treated with DNase and synthesized with cDNA using Moloney murine leukaemia virus (MMLV) reverse transcriptase (Life Technologies) according to the manufacturer's instructions. MSC cartilage discs were harvested in TRIzol reagent (Life Technologies) and ground using disposable plastic pestles and Molecular Grinding Resin (G-Biosciences, St. Louis, MO, USA). Human articular cartilage was snap frozen, crushed and ground in liquid nitrogen using a pestle and mortar before RNA extraction using TRIzol reagent (Life Technologies). Total RNA was converted to cDNA using MMLV reverse transcriptase (Life Technologies) according to the manufacturer's instructions.

Expression of genes of interest was measured by quantitative reverse transcription polymerase chain reaction (RT-qPCR) on an Applied Biosystems ViiA 7 system using SYBR Green (Life Technologies). Relative quantification is expressed as the comparative cycle threshold ($2^{-\Delta Ct}$), where ΔC_t is C_t(gene of interest) – C_t(reference gene *TBP* or *GAPDH*). Samples where the reference gene C_t was greater than ±1.5 C_t from the median were excluded from further analyses.

Immunocytochemistry

MSCs and HACs were seeded in chamber slides and allowed to adhere overnight. MSCs were treated with control medium (DMSO alone) or chondrogenic medium with or without GSK-J4 (10 μM). HACs were treated with control medium (DMSO alone) or TGF-β with or without GSK-J4. After 24-h (MSCs) and 6-h treatment (HAC), cells were fixed in 4 % formaldehyde and stained overnight at 4 °C with anti-H3K27Me3 (5 μg/ml, catalog number ab6002; Abcam, Cambridge, UK) before 1-h incubation at room temperature with rabbit antimouse immunoglobulin G. Nuclei were visualized using 4′,6-diamidino-2-phenylindole stain, and the cell cytoskeleton was visualized with Texas Red-conjugated phalloidin (Life Technologies). Images were obtained using a Zeiss inverted microscope using AxioVision software (Carl Zeiss Microscopy, Thornwood, NY, USA).

Dimethylmethylene blue assay for glycosaminoglycan content

Primary human articular cartilage explants were incubated with 5 ng/ml IL-1 and 10 ng/ml OSM in the presence or absence of GSK-J4 (10 μM) for 7 days, and media were collected and harvested every 2–3 days. Cartilage explants at day 7 and MSC cartilage discs at 14 days of differentiation were digested with papain overnight. Aliquots of media and digested cartilage were mixed with 1,9-dimethylmethylene blue and immediately read at 630 nm (SpectraMax Plus 384; Molecular Devices, Sunnyvale, CA, USA).

Second harmonic generation

Z-stack images were acquired on a Zeiss LSM 710 NLO confocal scanning microscope (Carl Zeiss Microscopy) coupled to a Chameleon Vision II multiphoton laser (Coherent, Santa Clara, CA, USA) tuned to 900 nm. Second harmonic generation (SHG) was confirmed at precisely 450 nm using a spectral detector and detected between 370 and 480 nm using non-descanned detectors through a × 25, 0.8 numerical aperture glycerol immersion objective. The stack thickness was 80–100 μm with a step size of 1.39 μm.

Statistical analysis

Analyses were carried out using Prism 6.0 software (GraphPad, La Jolla, CA, USA). Student's *t* test was used to test differences between two samples. Analysis of variance with Dunnett's post-test was used for multiple comparisons. $p < 0.05$ was considered statistically significant.

Results

Using a focused library of 31 epigenetic inhibitors in chondrogenesis of human MSCs (Fig. 1), we identified and confirmed the molecule GSK-J4 as an inhibitor of collagen output (0.63-fold; $p = 0.0079$) (Fig. 2a). No impact of GSK-J4 treatment on cell viability was detected (data not shown). GSK-J4 inhibits the KDM6 family of H3K27me3 demethylases JMJD3 and UTX. GSK-J4 has also been shown to target the KDM5 family of H3K4me3 demethylases [10].

Histone arginine or lysine residues can be mono-, di- or trimethylated. Histone 3 lysine 27 trimethylation (H3K27me3) is associated with inactive gene promoters, leading to Polycomb-mediated repression. The JMJD3 and UTX demethylases target these trimethyl groups and overcome this repression [11]. Accordingly, inhibition of UTX and JMJD3 by GSK-J4 maintains H3K27me3-driven repression of gene expression.

JMJD3 regulates chondrogenesis

JMJD3 but not *UTX* expression was increased at day 4 (3.0-fold, $p = 0.017$)), day 7 (2.9-fold, $p = 0.014$) and day

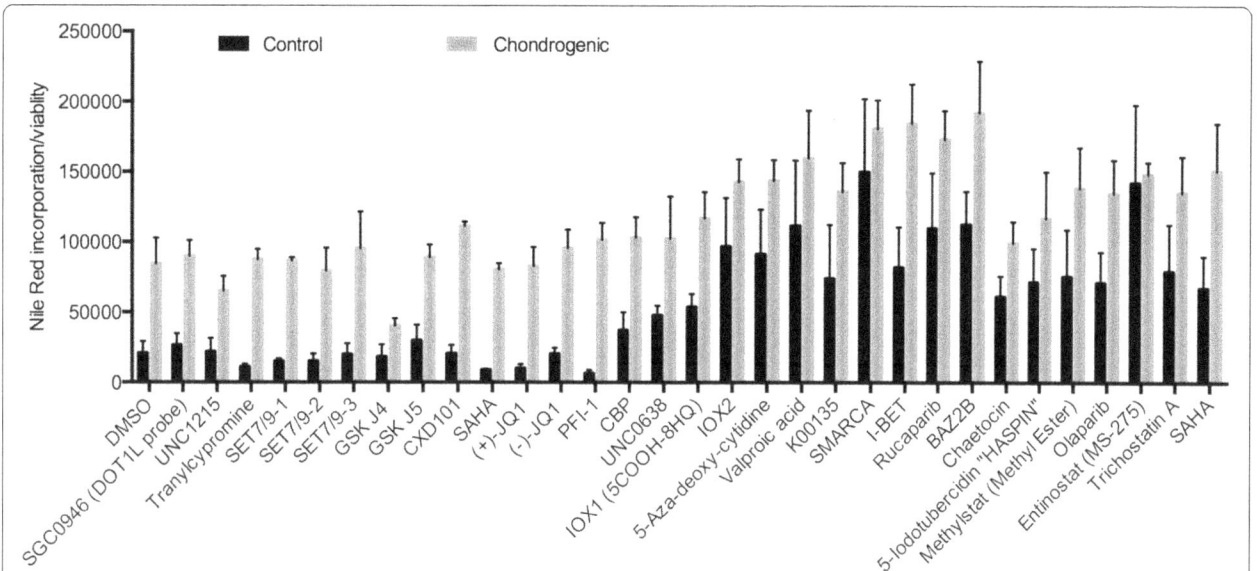

Fig. 1 Screen of epigenetic modifying compounds in chondrogenesis. Mesenchymal stem cells were cultured with epigenetic modifying compounds for 7 days in control and chondrogenic media. Collagen output was assessed via Nile Red incorporation and normalized to viable cells using the alamarBlue assay. *DMSO* dimethyl sulphoxide

14 (2.6-fold, $p = 0.0327$) of chondrogenic differentiation of MSCs into cartilage discs (Fig. 2b). Consequently, the inhibition of JMJD3 and UTX activity was further explored by assessing the expression of chondrogenic markers in MSC-generated cartilage discs.

At days 7 and 14 of chondrogenic differentiation, inhibition of H3K27me3 demethylases led to a reduction in expression of SRY (sex determining region Y)-box 9 (*SOX9*) (0.39-fold, $p < 0.0001$; 0.64-fold, $p = 0.0019$); collagen type II, alpha 1 (*COL2A1*) (0.08-fold, $p < 0.0001$; 0.67-fold, $p = 0.0476$); and collagen type X, alpha 1 (*COL10A1*) (0.36-fold, $p < 0.0001$; 0.50-fold, $p = 0.0002$). Aggrecan (*ACAN*) expression was reduced at day 7 (0.23-fold, $p < 0.0001$) and collagen type I, alpha 1 (*COL1A1*) expression was increased at days 7 and 14 (1.64-fold, $p < 0.0001$; 2.43-fold, $p = 0.0019$) (Fig. 2c–g). To test whether these effects were mediated by JMJD3 and UTX, MSCs were treated with siRNA against JMJD3 and UTX prior to Transwell induction of chondrogenesis. Expression of *ACAN*, *COL2A1*, *COL10A1* and *SOX9* was decreased, whilst expression of *COL1A1* was not altered (Fig. 2h and Additional file 3: Figure S2 show siRNA validation and treatment of MSCs with an additional siRNA against JMJD3 and UTX). Expression of adipogenic and osteogenic genes was not effected by GSK-J4 during chondrogenesis (data not shown). The glycosaminoglycan (GAG) content of cartilage discs was also reduced when GSK-J4 was present in chondrogenic medium (0.83-fold, $p = 0.041$) (Fig. 2i). SHG was used to visualize collagen fibre organization after 14 days of chondrogenic differentiation (Fig. 3). In the presence of

GSK-J4, fibres were disordered and appeared thicker and more sparsely distributed.

We also assessed whether inhibition of H3K27me3 demethylases by GSK-J4 regulated initiation of chondrogenesis and reversion of MSCs to a less stem cell-like phenotype by assessing expression of the MSC-related gene *NANOG*. Induction of chondrogenesis caused a reduction in *NANOG* expression that was inhibited in the presence of GSK-J4 (4.0-fold, $p = 0.0023$) (Fig. 4a). TGF-β initiated MSC condensation and production of healthy cartilage, and expression of the TGF-β target gene *PAI1* by chondrogenic MSCs was inhibited by GSK-J4. Interestingly, *JMJD3* expression was also induced by TGF-β1 and inhibited in the presence of GSK-J4 (Fig. 4b).

To confirm that H3K27me3 levels are regulated in chondrogenesis, we stained chondrogenic MSCs for trimethylated H3K27. MSCs stimulated with chondrogenic medium (containing TGF-β to initiate and drive chondrogenesis) showed a reduction in H3K27me3 staining relative to control basal medium (Fig. 4c). Inhibition of JMJD3 and UTX by addition of GSK-J4 to chondrogenic medium inhibited this reduction in H3K27me3 staining.

OA is postulated to result from reversion of chondrocytes to a more developmental phenotype [12]; thus, we assessed whether there was a role for JMJD3 and UTX in OA. Expression of *JMJD3* (2.16-fold, $p = 0.007$) (Fig. 5a) but not *UTX* was increased in damaged cartilage compared with undamaged cartilage from the tibial plateau of the OA knee. GSK-J4 treatment caused a decrease in gene expression of OA-associated matrix metallopeptidase 13 (*MMP13*) (0.43-fold, $p = 0.0032$), prostaglandin-

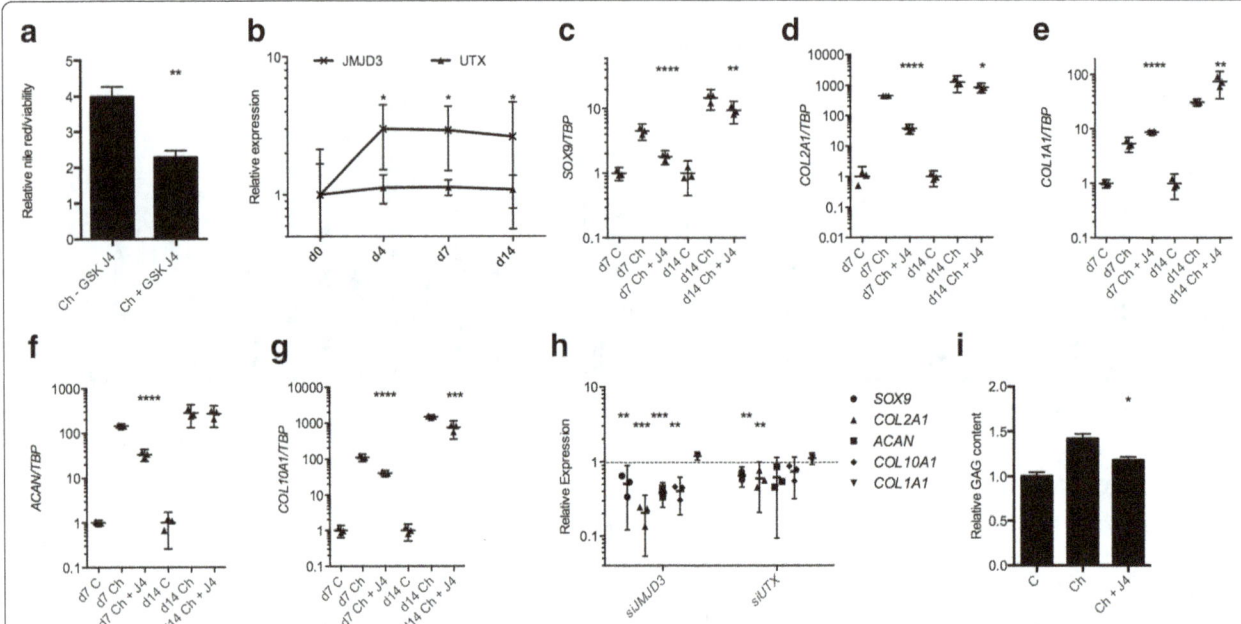

Fig. 2 The impact of trimethylated histone 3 lysine 27 (H3K27me3) inhibition on extracellular matrix production and chondrogenic gene expression. **a** Addition of GSK-J4 to chondrogenic media of human mesenchymal stem cells (MSCs) caused a reduction in collagen production as measured by Nile Red incorporation relative to viable cells (day 7, $n = 3$ individuals, 3 technical replicates per condition). **b** Jumonji domain-containing 3 (*JMJD3*) expression was increased during chondrogenic differentiation of MSCs to form cartilage discs. Assessment of gene expression at days 7 and 14 of chondrogenesis revealed that H3K27me3 inhibition through GSK-J4 addition to chondrogenic media resulted decreased expression of SRY (sex determining region Y)-box 9 (*SOX9*), collagen type II, alpha 1 (*COL2A1*), aggrecan (*ACAN*) and collagen type X, alpha 1 (*COL10A1*) (**c,d,f,g**) and increased expression of collagen type I, alpha 1 (*COL1A1*) (**e**) ($n = 3$ individuals). **h** MSCs were pre-treated with small interfering RNA (siRNA) against *JMJD3*, lysine (K)-specific demethylase 6A (*UTX*) or non-targeting siRNA control prior to chondrogenic induction in Transwell culture. RNA was extracted and cDNA synthesized at day 7 of chondrogenesis, and expression of SOX9, ACAN COL2A1, COL10A1 and COL1A1 was assessed by quantitative reverse transcription polymerase chain reaction ($n = 4$ patients, $n = 2$ technical replicates per patient). *Dashed line* represents expression level following MSC treatment with non-targeting siRNA control. **i** Proteoglycan content at day 14 in cartilage discs generated in Transwell cultures was reduced following addition of GSK-J4 to chondrogenic medium ($n = 3$ individuals). *$p \leq 0.05$, **$p \leq 0.01$, ***$p \leq 0.001$, ****$p \leq 0.0001$. Data are presented as individual data points for biological replicates showing mean ± 95 % CI. **a** and **i** t test, **b–h** analysis of variance with Dunnett's correction for multiple comparisons

endoperoxide synthase 2 (*PTGS2*) (0.49-fold, $p = 0.0480$) and *COL10A1* (0.40-fold, $p = 0.0023$) (Fig. 5b). Expression of *MMP13*, *PTGS2* and *COL10A1* was decreased following treatment of HACs with siRNA against *JMJD3*, but there was no significant decrease in expression of these genes following knockdown of *UTX*. (Fig. 5c and

Additional file 4: Figure S4 show siRNA validation and gene expression in HACs following treatment with an additional siRNA against JMJD3 and UTX.) GSK-J4 inhibited IL-1β/OSM-induced GAG release from human articular cartilage explants (0.73-fold, $p = 0.0015$) (Fig. 5d), while there was no effect of GSK-J4 alone.

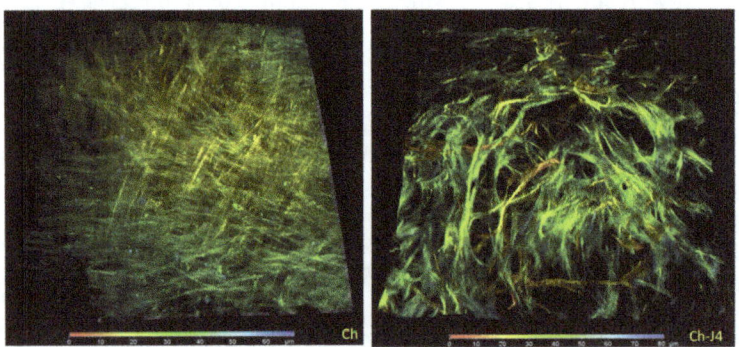

Fig. 3 The impact of trimethylated histone 3 lysine 27 (H3K27me3) inhibition on collagen organization. Collagen organization, as assessed using second harmonic generation, was also disordered in discs generated in the presence of GSK-J4

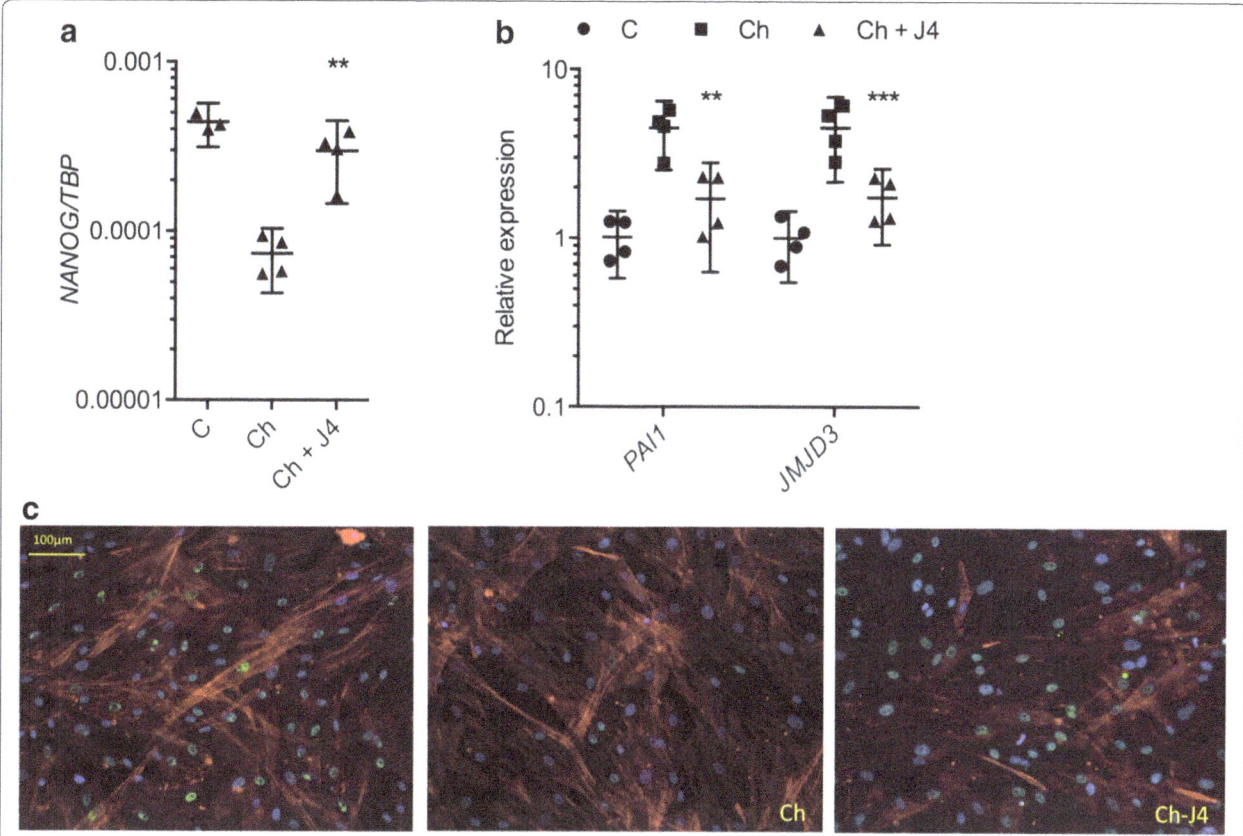

Fig. 4 Impact of trimethylated histone 3 lysine 27 (H3K27me3) demethylase inhibition on mesenchymal stem cell (MSC) behaviour. **a** *NANOG* expression in monolayer MSCs treated for 24 h with GSK-J4 and chondrogenic medium compared with chondrogenic medium alone ($n = 4$ individuals, 4 technical replicates per condition). **b** *PAI1* and *JMJD3* expression were decreased in monolayer MSCs treated for 1 h with GSK-J4 and chondrogenic medium compared with chondrogenic medium alone ($n = 4$ individuals, 4 technical replicates per condition). **c** H3K27me3 staining (*green*) in MSCs cultured for 24 h in control medium, chondrogenic medium or chondrogenic medium plus GSK-J4. Cell cytoskeleton/actin (phalloidin, *red*) and nuclear (4',6-diamidino-2-phenylindole, blue) staining. **$p \leq 0.01$, ***$p \leq 0.001$. Data are presented as individual data points for biological replicates showing mean ± 95 % CI. **a** and **b** Analysis of variance with Dunnett's correction for multiple comparisons

To explore the factors driving *JMJD3* upregulation in damaged OA cartilage, we treated HACs with OA-relevant cytokines. The inflammatory cytokines IL-1β/OSM, which also induce MMP-13 expression, caused a significant increase in *JMJD3* expression (7.56-fold, $p = 0.0085$), as did TGF-β1 (12.97-fold, $p < 0.0001$) (Fig. 5e).

Given the upregulation of *JMJD3* by TGF-β in HACs and the inhibition of TGF-β-driven chondrogenesis and gene expression in MSCs, we postulated that H3K27me3 status may impact the expression of TGF-β target genes in HACs. In the presence of GSK-J4, there was a significant decrease in TGF-β-induced expression of *PAI1* (0.68-fold, $p = 0.0006$), *JMJD3* (0.52-fold, $p = 0.0011$) and *MMP13* (0.42-fold, $p = 0.0023$) (Fig. 5f). Treatment of HACs with TGF-β reduced H3K27me3 staining, and this TGF-β-induced reduction was inhibited in the presence of GSK-J4 (Fig. 6).

Discussion

In this study, we identified the H3K27me3 demethylases as key mediators of both chondrogenesis and OA pathogenesis. We show that inhibition of H3K27me3 demethylase activity by GSK-J4 disrupts in vitro chondrogenic differentiation of human MSCs but inhibits adult human articular cartilage degradation. GSK-J4 inhibited TGF-β-induced gene expression in both MSCs and HACs, implicating H3K27me3 demethylases in TGF-β-led regulation of chondrogenesis and OA. H3K27me3 manipulation may thus improve outcomes in cartilage tissue repair and might be a possible target for OA therapeutics.

Histone arginine or lysine residues can be mono-, di- or trimethylated. H3K27me3 is associated with inactive gene promoters, leading to Polycomb-mediated repression. The JMJD3 and UTX demethylases specifically target these trimethyl groups and overcome this repression of key transcription factors during differentiation [11].

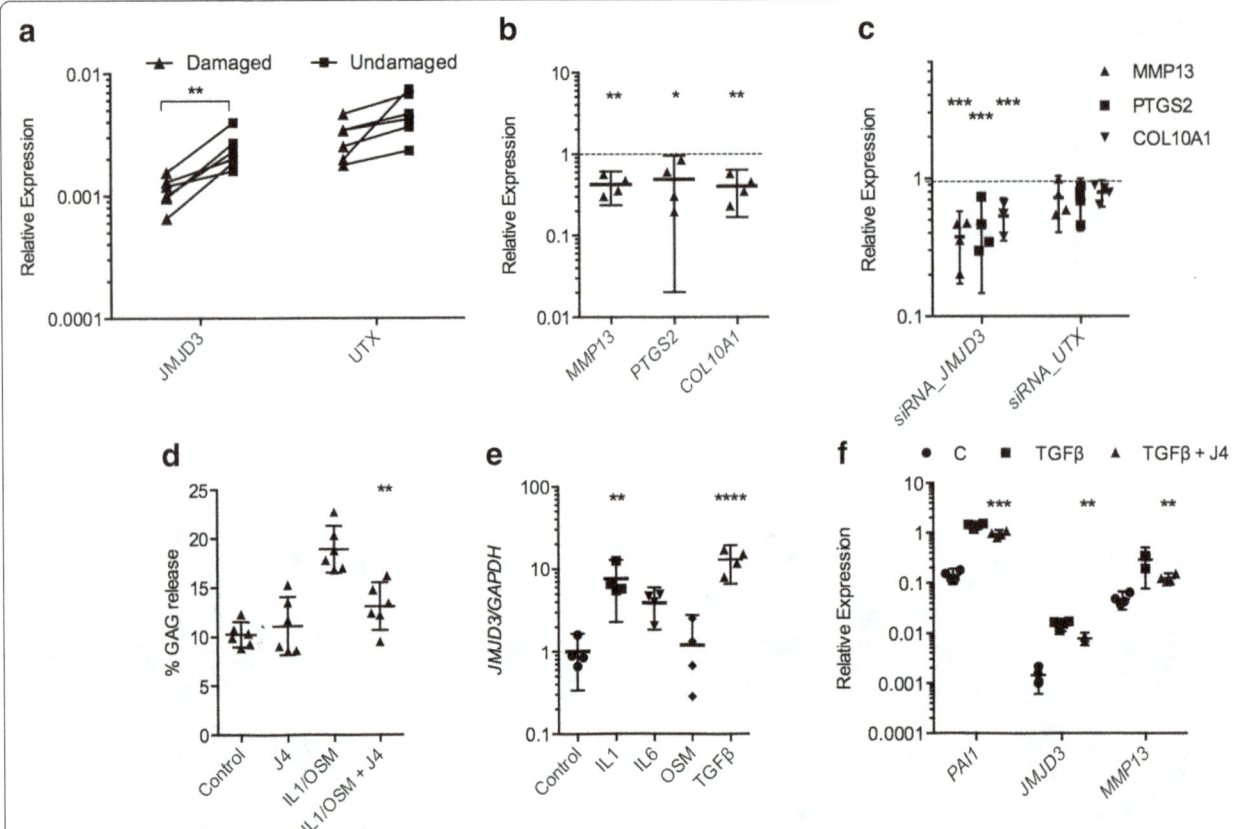

Fig. 5 Regulation of global histone 3 lysine 27 trimethylation (H3K27me3) levels in osteoarthritis (OA) and adult articular cartilage. **a** Jumonji domain-containing 3 (*JMJD3*) was increased in damaged cartilage compared with undamaged cartilage from within the same knees of patients undergoing unicompartmental knee replacement for OA (*n* = 5 patients). **b** Inhibition of H3K27me3 demethylases by treatment of human articular chondrocyte (HACs) with GSK-J4 for 24 h caused a decrease in matrix metallopeptidase 13 (*MMP13*), prostaglandin-endoperoxide synthase 2 (*PTGS2*) and collagen type X, alpha 1 (*COL10A1*) expression (*n* = 4 patients, 4 technical replicates per condition). *Dashed line* shows control expression of each gene. **c** HACs were treated for 72 h with small interfering RNA (siRNA) against JMJD3, lysine (K)-specific demethylase 6A (UTX) and non-targeting siRNA control prior to RNA extraction and complementary DNA synthesis (*n* = 4 patients, *n* = 4 technical replicates per patient). Expression of *MMP13*, *PTGS2* and *COL10A1* was assessed by quantitative reverse transcription polymerase chain reaction. *Dashed line* shows expression level following treatment with non-targeting siRNA control. **d** Interleukin (IL)-1/oncostatin M (OSM)-induced proteoglycan loss from human articular cartilage explants was reduced in the presence of GSK-J4 (*n* = 5 patients, 3 technical replicates per condition). **e** Treatment of HACs with IL-1, IL-6 and transforming growth factor (TGF)-β increased *JMJD3* expression. **f** Expression of *PAI1*, *JMJD3* and *MMP13* following 6-h treatment of HACs with TGF-β with or without GSK-J4 (*n* = 4 patients, 4 technical replicates per condition). *$p \leq 0.05$, **$p \leq 0.01$, ***$p \leq 0.001$, ****$p \leq 0.0001$. Data are presented as individual data points for biological replicates showing mean ± 95 % CI. **a** Paired *t* test, **b–f** Analysis of variance with Dunnett's correction for multiple comparisons. *GAG* glycosaminoglycan

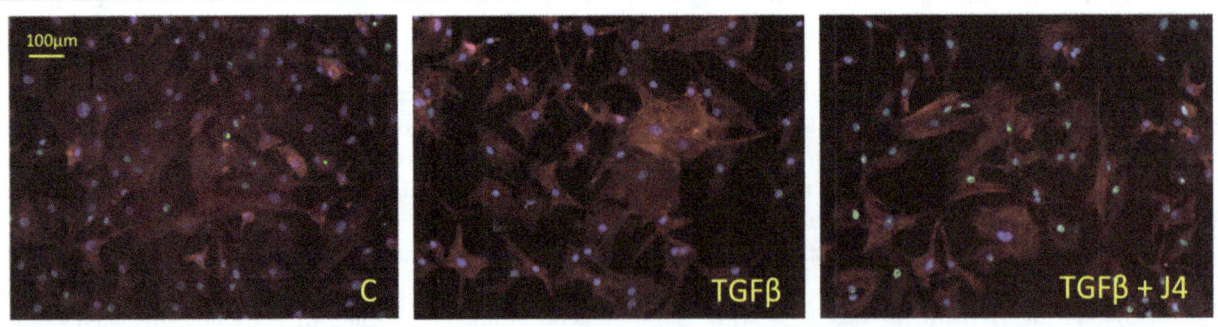

Fig. 6 The impact of transforming growth factor (TGF)-β treatment on histone 3 lysine 27 trimethylation (H3K27me3) levels in human articular chondrocytes (HACs). H3K27me3 staining (*green*) in HACs following 1-h treatment with TGF-β or TGF-β plus GSK-J4. Cell cytoskeleton/actin (phalloidin, *red*) and nuclear (4',6-diamidino-2-phenylindole, *blue*) staining

Accordingly, GSK-J4 inhibits UTX and JMJD3 activity and thus maintains H3K27me3-driven repression of gene expression.

We show that inhibition of JMJD3 and UTX by GSK-J4 results in decreased total collagen and GAG output during chondrogenesis, as well as a reduction in expression of cartilage-associated genes, including *SOX9*. Interestingly, *COL1A1* expression was increased following GSK-J4 treatment, but not following targeted knockdown of JMJD3 and UTX by siRNA. GSK-J4 mediated inhibition of the KDM5 family of demethylases that target the H3K4me3 activating mark may explain the upregulation of *COL1A1* following GSK-J4 treatment but not following specific targeting of JMJD3 and UTX. H3K4me3 and H3K27me3 sites have been identified in collagen genes in other systems [8, 13]. The upregulation of *COL1A1* gene expression following GSK-J4 treatment, in combination with repressed *COL2A1* and *COL10A1*, may reflect the sparser, thicker and more disorganized collagen fibres visualized using SHG. Enhancing H3K27me3 demethylase activity may therefore improve in vitro cartilage tissue generation; this warrants further investigation.

The regulation of *JMJD3* but not *UTX* expression during chondrogenesis suggests that JMJD3 plays the major role, and individually targeting each enzyme using siRNA showed that both regulated chondrogenic gene expression, although UTX knockdown had a lesser effect. A recent study showed that JMJD3 promoted endochondral bone formation in mice via association with Runx2, and also reported that H3K27me3 levels decreased at the *Runx2* promoter during osteogenesis [14]. In combination with our data, this suggests that JMJD3 has multiple roles in differentiation dependent upon the context of its expression. A direct interaction of JMJD3 with *SOX9*, the key transcription factor in regulating chondrogenesis, has not been reported. However, JMJD3 potentially has both direct and indirect effects on SOX9 expression. First, H3K27me3 is present within the *SOX9* promoter in the limb bud mesenchyme and in OA cartilage [1, 15], and *SOX9*, amongst other chondrogenic marker genes, including collagens, has previously been shown to contain H3K27m e3 sites that undergo demethylation during chondrogenesis of human MSCs [16]. Therefore, demethylase activity can directly control *SOX9* expression. Indirectly, demethylation of H3K27me3 at promoter sites of accessory factors such as the *N2RF1* gene can also lead to increased *SOX9* expression via N2RF1 binding to the *SOX9* promoter [17].

To our knowledge, our present study is the first to show H3K27me3 regulation in OA, and the results suggest that upregulation of H3K27me3 demethylase activity may promote OA progression. Inhibition of H3K27me3 demethylases in adult HACs reduced expression of OA- and hypertrophy-associated *MMP13*, *COL10A1* and *PTGS2*. GAG loss from IL-1/OSM-stimulated human cartilage explants was reduced when H3K27me3 demethylase activity was inhibited. Thus, in adult cartilage, increased JMJD3 may enhance chondrocyte hypertrophy and matrix destruction, leading to OA progression. Taken together, this work suggests a protective effect of the H3K27me3 repressive mark on cartilage. The upregulation of *JMJD3* in damaged OA cartilage and by IL-1β/OSM may help drive cartilage destruction partly through upregulating expression of matrix-degrading *MMP13*.

TGF-β-induced gene expression was inhibited in both chondrogenic MSCs and adult HACs following GSK-J4 treatment. TGF-β is a pleiotropic cytokine that is essential for chondrogenesis. The inhibition of chondrogenesis in the presence of GSK-J4 may thus be mediated through its inhibition of TGF-β signalling. In OA pathogenesis, alternate TGF-β signalling pathways are activated and a dysregulated TGF-β response occurs as pathology persists [7, 18]. This dysregulation may be partially driven by direct and indirect effects of JMJD3, which is upregulated in damaged OA cartilage, on H3K27me3 status of TGF-β target genes. We also show that TGF-β increased expression of *JMJD3* itself in both chondrogenic MSCs and HACs, an observation also reported during epithelial-mesenchymal transition [19]. The H3K27me3 status and exact mechanism by which TGF-β signalling is regulated by H3K27me3 demethylases in chondrogenic MSCs and HACs require detailed mechanistic exploration both in vitro and in murine models.

GSK-J4 can target H3K4me3 demethylases of the KDM5 family as well as UTX and JMJD3. A limitation of this study is the impact of these enzymes and sites on chondrogenesis, and we did not assess chondrocyte activity. Targeted inhibition of UTX and JMJD3 by siRNA does, however, support the important role of H3K27me3 demethylases for in vitro cartilage generation and in expression of OA-associated genes, including *MMP13*, by HACs. Future work should characterize H3K4me3 methylation status alongside H3K27me3 in chondrogenesis and in OA and should target the KDM6 and KDM5 demethylases individually.

Conclusions

In the present study, we have shown that GSK-J4 treatment and subsequent maintenance of the H3K27me3 repressive mark decreased total collagen and GAG output during chondrogenesis and reduced expression of cartilage-associated genes. Enhancing H3K27me3 demethylase activity, and thus reducing the H3K27me3 repressive mark, may therefore improve in vitro cartilage tissue generation; this warrants further investigation. In contrast, *JMJD3* was upregulated in damaged OA cartilage and H3K27me3 inhibition prevented ex vivo cartilage degradation and expression of OA-related genes.

Taken together, we provide evidence that correct regulation of H3K27me3 status by demethylases in chondrogenic precursors and chondrocytes is crucial for both chondrogenesis and maintenance of adult articular cartilage. Enhancing H3K27me3 activity, especially that of JMJD3, may improve tissue-engineered cartilage and temporally, and anatomically targeted inhibition could prevent cartilage damage in OA.

Additional files

Additional file 1: Figure S1. The results of treatment with GSK-5, the less active enantiomer of GSK-4, on MSCs undergoing chondrogenesis. (A-E) Assessment of gene expression at days 7 and 14 of MSC chondrogenesis to articular cartilage discs revealed following GSK-J4 and GSK-J5 treatment. (F) *NANOG* expression in monolayer MSCs treated for 24 h with GSK-J4 and GSK-J5. (G) *PAI1* and *JMJD3* expression were decreased in monolayer MSCs treated for 1 h with GSK-J4 and GSK-J5. (H) H3K27Me3 staining (green) in MSCs cultured for 24 h in control, chondrogenic or chondrogenic medium plus GSK-J4 or GSK-J5. Cell cytoskeleton/actin (phalloidin, red), nuclear staining (DAPI, blue). (TIFF 2818 kb)

Additional file 2: Figure S3. The results of treatment with GSK-5, the less active enantiomer of GSK-4, on HACs. A Treatment of HAC with GSK-J5 for 24 h. B IL1/OSM-induced proteoglycan loss from human articular cartilage explants in the presence of GSK-J4 and GSK-J5. C Expression of PAI1, JMJD3 and MMP13 following 6 h treatment of HAC with TGFβ +/- GSK-J4 and GSK-J5. D H3K27me3 staining (green) in HAC following 1 h treatment with TGFβ +/- GSK-J4 or GSK-J5. Cell cytoskeleton/actin (phalloidin, red), nuclear staining (DAPI, blue). (TIFF 1712 kb)

Additional file 3: Figure S2. siRNA validation qPCR on MSCs and validation chondrogenic gene expression following treatment with an additional siRNA against JMJD3 and UTX. MSC were treated with non-targeting siRNA control and two siRNA against JMJD3 (A) and UTX (B) at 2.5, 5 and 10 nM for 48 h. MTC = mock transfection control (no siRNA), NTC = no transfection control. (C) Targeting JMJD3 and UTX with additional siRNA. MSCs were pre-treated with siRNA_2 against JMJD3, UTX or non-targeting siRNA control prior to chondrogenic induction in transwell culture. RNA was extracted and cDNA synthesized at day 7 of chondrogenesis and expression of *SOX9, ACAN COL2A1, COL10A1* and *COL1A1* assessed by RT-qPCR (*n* = 4 patients, *n* =2 technical replicates per patient). Dashed line represents expression level following MSC treatment with non-targeting siRNA control. (TIFF 372 kb)

Additional file 4: Figure S4. siRNA validation qPCR on HAC and validation HAC gene expression following treatment with an additional siRNA against JMJD3 and UTX. HAC were treated with non-targeting siRNA control and two siRNA against JMJD3 (A) and UTX (B) at 2.5, 5 and 10 nM for 48 h. MTC = mock transfection control (no siRNA), NTC = no transfection control. A MSCs were pre-treated with siRNA against JMJD3, UTX or scrambled non-targeting control prior to chondrogenic induction in transwell culture. RNA was extracted and cDNA synthesized at day 7 of chondrogenesis and expression of *SOX9, ACAN COL2A1, COL10A1* and *COL1A1* assessed by RT-qPCR (*n* = 4 patients, *n* = 2 technical replicates per patient). B. HAC were treated for 72 h with siRNA_2 against JMJD3, UTX and scrambled non-targeting control prior to RNA extraction and cDNA synthesis (*n* = 4 patients, *n* = 4 technical replicates per patient). Expression of *MMP13, PTGS2* and *COL10A1* were assessed by RT-qPCR. Dashed line shows expression level following HAC treatment with non-targeting siRNA control. *p**≤0.05, **≤0.01, ***≤0.001, ****≤0.0001. (TIFF 337 kb)

Abbreviations
ACAN, aggrecan; cDNA, complementary DNA; COL1A1, collagen type I, alpha 1; COL2A1, collagen type II, alpha 1; COL10A1, collagen type X, alpha 1; C_t, cycle threshold; DMSO, dimethyl sulphoxide; GAG, glycosaminoglycan; HAC, human articular chondrocyte; H3K27me3, histone 3 lysine 27 trimethylation; IL, interleukin; JMJD3, Jumonji domain-containing 3; MMLV, Moloney murine leukaemia virus; MMP-13, matrix metallopeptidase 13; MSC, mesenchymal stem cell; OA, osteoarthritis; OSM, oncostatin M; PTGS2, prostaglandin-endoperoxide synthase 2; RT-qPCR, quantitative reverse transcription polymerase chain reaction; SHG, second harmonic generation; siRNA, small interfering RNA; SOX9, SRY (sex determining region Y)-box 9; TGF-β, transforming growth factor beta; UTX, lysine (K)-specific demethylase 6A

Acknowledgements
We thank the Oxford Musculoskeletal Biobank, Lucy Roche and Eleanor Mawbrey-Adamson for their help in cartilage collection. We also thank Robert Hedley and Serafim Kiriakidis for their guidance on RNA extraction.

Funding
This study was funded by Arthritis Research UK grants 20087 and 19222 (SJBS), 20522 (UO), the Arthritis Research UK Centre for Osteoarthritis Pathogenesis, the Rosetrees Trust (UO) and the National Institute for Health Research Oxford Musculoskeletal Biomedical Research Unit. The Structural Genomics Consortium is a registered charity (number 1097737) that receives funds from AbbVie, Bayer HealthCare, Boehringer Ingelheim, the Canadian Institutes of Health Research, the Canadian Foundation for Innovation, Eli Lilly and Company, Genome Canada, GlaxoSmithKline, the Ontario Ministry of Economic Development and Innovation, Janssen, the Novartis Research Foundation, Pfizer, Takeda and the Wellcome Trust.

Authors' contributions
SJBS and UO designed the study. SJBS and CY carried out data acquisition. AJC and AP provided patient samples and engaged in discussions on data acquisition. All authors assisted with data interpretation. All authors prepared the manuscript, and all authors read and approved the final manuscript.

Competing interests
The authors declare that they have no competing interests.

Author details
[1]Nuffield Department of Orthopaedics, Rheumatology and Musculoskeletal Sciences, Botnar Research Centre, University of Oxford, Nuffield Orthopaedic Centre, Windmill Road, Headington, OX3 7LD Oxford, UK. [2]Structural Genomics Consortium, University of Oxford, Oxford, UK. [3]Oxford Stem Cell Institute, Oxford, UK.

References
1. Kim KI, Park YS, Im GI. Changes in the epigenetic status of the SOX-9 promoter in human osteoarthritic cartilage. J Bone Miner Res. 2013;28(5):1050–60.
2. Hata K, Takashima R, Amano K, Ono K, Nakanishi M, Yoshida M, Wakabayashi M, Matsuda A, Maeda Y, Suzuki Y, et al. Arid5b facilitates chondrogenesis by recruiting the histone demethylase Phf2 to Sox9-regulated genes. Nat Commun. 2013;4:2850.
3. Dawson MA, Kouzarides T. Cancer epigenetics: from mechanism to therapy. Cell. 2012;150(1):12–27.
4. Leonard CM, Fuld HM, Frenz DA, Downie SA, Massagué J, Newman SA. Role of transforming growth factor-β in chondrogenic pattern formation in the embryonic limb: stimulation of mesenchymal condensation and fibronectin gene expression by exogenous TGF-β and evidence for endogenous TGF-β-like activity. Dev Biol. 1991;145(1):99–109.
5. Yang X, Chen L, Xu X, Li C, Huang C, Deng CX. TGF-β/Smad3 signals repress chondrocyte hypertrophic differentiation and are required for maintaining articular cartilage. J Cell Biol. 2001;153(1):35–46.
6. Shen J, Li J, Wang B, Jin H, Wang M, Zhang Y, Yang Y, Im HJ, O'Keefe R, Chen D. Deletion of the transforming growth factor β receptor type II gene in articular chondrocytes leads to a progressive osteoarthritis-like phenotype in mice. Arthritis Rheum. 2013;65(12):3107–19.
7. Blaney Davidson EN, Remst DF, Vitters EL, van Beuningen HM, Blom AB, Goumans MJ, van den Berg WB, van der Kraan PM. Increase in ALK1/ALK5 ratio as a cause for elevated MMP-13 expression in osteoarthritis in humans and mice. J Immunol. 2009;182(12):7937–45.

8. Sun G, Reddy MA, Yuan H, Lanting L, Kato M, Natarajan R. Epigenetic histone methylation modulates fibrotic gene expression. J Am Soc Nephrol. 2010;21(12):2069–80.

9. Johnson K, Zhu S, Tremblay MS, Payette JN, Wang J, Bouchez LC, Meeusen S, Althage A, Cho CY, Wu X, et al. A stem cell-based approach to cartilage repair. Science. 2012;336(6082):717–21.

10. Heinemann B, Nielsen JM, Hudlebusch HR, Lees MJ, Larsen DV, Boesen T, Labelle M, Gerlach LO, Birk P, Helin K. Inhibition of demethylases by GSK-J1/J4. Nature. 2014;514(7520):E1–2.

11. Hubner MR, Spector DL. Role of H3K27 demethylases Jmjd3 and UTX in transcriptional regulation. Cold Spring Harb Symp Quant Biol. 2010;75:43–9.

12. Saito T, Fukai A, Mabuchi A, Ikeda T, Yano F, Ohba S, Nishida N, Akune T, Yoshimura N, Nakagawa T, et al. Transcriptional regulation of endochondral ossification by HIF-2α during skeletal growth and osteoarthritis development. Nat Med. 2010;16(6):678–86.

13. Chernov AV, Baranovskaya S, Golubkov VS, Wakeman DR, Snyder EY, Williams R, Strongin AY. Microarray-based transcriptional and epigenetic profiling of matrix metalloproteinases, collagens, and related genes in cancer. J Biol Chem. 2010;285(25):19647–59.

14. Zhang F, Xu L, Xu L, Xu Q, Li D, Yang Y, Karsenty G, Chen CD. JMJD3 promotes chondrocyte proliferation and hypertrophy during endochondral bone formation in mice. J Mol Cell Biol. 2015;7(1):23–34.

15. Kumar D, Lassar AB. Fibroblast growth factor maintains chondrogenic potential of limb bud mesenchymal cells by modulating DNMT3A recruitment. Cell Rep. 2014;8(5):1419–31.

16. Herlofsen SR, Bryne JC, Hoiby T, Wang L, Issner R, Zhang X, Coyne MJ, Boyle P, Gu H, Meza-Zepeda LA, et al. Genome-wide map of quantified epigenetic changes during in vitro chondrogenic differentiation of primary human mesenchymal stem cells. BMC Genomics. 2013;14:105.

17. Sosa MS, Parikh F, Maia AG, Estrada Y, Bosch A, Bragado P, Ekpin E, George A, Zheng Y, Lam HM, et al. NR2F1 controls tumour cell dormancy via SOX9- and RARβ-driven quiescence programmes. Nat Commun. 2015;6:6170.

18. van der Kraan PM. Age-related alterations in TGF β signaling as a causal factor of cartilage degeneration in osteoarthritis. Biomed Mater Eng. 2014;24(1 Suppl):75–80.

19. Ramadoss S, Chen X, Wang CY. Histone demethylase KDM6B promotes epithelial-mesenchymal transition. J Biol Chem. 2012;287(53):44508–17.

3

Randomized controlled studies on the efficacy of antiarthritic agents in inhibiting cartilage degeneration and pain associated with progression of osteoarthritis in the rat

Erica M. TenBroek[1][*], Laurie Yunker[1], Mae Foster Nies[1] and Alison M. Bendele[2]

Abstract

Background: As an initial step in the development of a local therapeutic to treat osteoarthritis (OA), a number of agents were tested for their ability to block activation of inflammation through nuclear factor κ-light-chain-enhancer of activated B cells (NF-κB), subchondral bone changes through receptor activator of nuclear factor κB ligand (RANKL)-mediated osteoclastogenesis, and proteolytic degradation through matrix metalloproteinase (MMP)-13 activity. Candidates with low toxicity and predicted efficacy were further examined using either of two widely accepted models of OA joint degeneration in the rat: the monoiodoacetic acid (MIA) model or the medial meniscal tear/medial collateral ligament tear (MMT/MCLT) model.

Methods: Potential therapeutics were assessed for their effects on the activation of nuclear factor (NF)-κB, RANKL-mediated osteoclastogenesis, and MMP-13 activity in vitro using previously established assays. Toxicity was measured using HeLa cells, a synovial cell line, or primary human chondrocytes. Drugs predicted to perform well in vivo were tested either systemically or via intraarticular injection in the MIA or the MMT/MCLT model of OA. Pain behavior was measured by mechanical hyperalgesia using the digital Randall-Selitto test (dRS) or by incapacitance with weight bearing (WB). Joint degeneration was evaluated using micro computed tomography and a comprehensive semiquantitative scoring of cartilage, subchondral bone, and synovial histopathology.

Results: Several agents were effective both in vitro and in vivo. With regard to pain behavior, systemically delivered clonidine was superior in treating MIA-induced changes in WB or dRS, while systemic clonidine, curcumin, tacrolimus, and fluocinolone were all somewhat effective in modifying MMT/MCLT-induced changes in WB. Systemic tacrolimus was the most effective in slowing disease progression as measured by histopathology in the MMT/MCLT model.

Conclusions: All of the agents that demonstrated highest benefit in vivo, excepting clonidine, were found to inhibit MMP-13, NF-κB, and bone matrix remodeling in vitro. The MIA and MMT/MCLT models of OA, previously shown to possess inflammatory characteristics and to display associated pain behavior, were affected to different degrees by the same drugs. Although no therapeutic was remarkable across all measures, the several which showed the most promise in either model merit continued study with alternative dosing and therapeutic strategies.

Keywords: Osteoarthritis, Arthritis, Monoiodoacetic, Meniscal, Therapeutics, Degeneration, Pain, NF-κB, RANKL, Bone remodeling

* Correspondence: tenbre1@comcast.net
[1]Medtronic Inc., 710 Medtronic Parkway, Minneapolis, MN 55432, USA
Full list of author information is available at the end of the article

Background

Osteoarthritis (OA) is a chronic degenerative disease that negatively impacts the lives of more than 27 million individuals in the United States [1]. It has been predicted that OA will be the fourth leading cause of disability by 2020 [2]. The early pain and inflammation of OA are typically treated with oral analgesics or anti-inflammatories, therapies that may be accompanied by significant side effects in a small percentage of patients [3]. As the disease progresses, intraarticular (IA) injections of steroids and hyaluronic acid (HA) offer temporary relief but generally fail to address the underlying degeneration or to consistently block disease progression. In the case of HA, the lack of efficacy may be due at least in part to limited persistence in the joint space [4] and short half-life [5]. Eventually, when the pain and degeneration become intractable, patients have few options other than joint replacement. Further revision or replacement surgeries may be required 15–20 years after the first replacement if the artificial joint fails [6]. Locally delivered therapeutics with the ability to inhibit disease progression and also block chronic pain might significantly delay the need for joint replacement. With the goal of developing an IA therapeutic, agents were chosen on the basis of their predicted ability to inhibit key processes involved in OA disease progression. Several targets were considered, including pivotal points within inflammatory pathways, proteinase production, and osteoclastogenesis.

Complex interactions involving joint inflammation, synovitis, secretion of mediators, cartilage degeneration, and subsequent subchondral bone remodeling have all been identified as playing a role in the development of chronic OA [7–10]. Inflammation is primarily related to activation of the classical nuclear factor κ-light-chain-enhancer of activated B cells (NF-κB) pathway and the synthesis of compounds that amplify the inflammatory process, which then may trigger degradation or remodeling of the cartilaginous matrix [11–13]. Evidence indicates that chemokines and cytokines secreted into the synovial fluid activate chondrocytes and trigger not only the synthesis of extracellular matrix but also additional synthesis of proinflammatory molecules [9]. In preclinical models, the inhibition of NF-κB or active proteinases has been shown to slow joint degeneration [11, 12]. Proteinases include but are not limited to matrix metalloproteinases (MMPs), particularly MMP-13 [14, 15], and aggrecanases, such as a disintegrin and metalloproteinase with thrombospondin motifs 4 and 5 (ADAMTS4 and ADAMTS5, respectively) [12, 16].

Subchondral bone changes associated with OA are driven largely by the nonclassical NF-κB-related receptor activator of nuclear factor κB ligand (RANKL) pathway [17, 18], activation of which may lead to both inflammation [10] and pain [19]. RANKL, a member of the tumor necrosis factor (TNF) superfamily, is produced by synovial tissue and binds to the receptor activator of NF-κB found on immune cells and osteoclasts [20]. Inflammation of synovial tissues within the joint attracts monocytes and macrophages, which, in the presence of RANKL and other signals produced by synovial fibroblasts and activated T cells, become osteoclasts. Such osteoclastogenesis, coupled with the activity of the osteoclasts and other inflammatory cells, may then trigger remodeling of subchondral bone adjacent to the synovium, neurovascular invasion, and formation of potentially painful osteophytes [21]. In addition to the RANKL pathway, increased transforming growth factor (TGF)-β activity in the subchondral bone stimulated by inappropriate mechanical loading may contribute to these boney changes [22].

The following studies were performed in an effort to determine whether the ability of a compound to block activation of NF-κB, synthesis of MMP-13, or activation of RANKL-mediated osteoclastogenesis might predict in vivo efficacy. The toxicity of the compounds was measured in vitro using cartilage, synovial cells, and/or HeLa cells. The most promising candidates were then tested using either of two widely accepted models of OA joint degeneration: the monoiodoacetic acid (MIA) model or the unilateral medial meniscal tear/medial collateral ligament tear (MMT/MCLT) rat model [23, 24]. Both models have been shown by others to recapitulate different aspects of degenerative joint disease [25, 26]. Primary endpoints in these studies included semiquantitative histopathological analysis of the affected joints and quantitative analysis of pain behavior.

Methods
Compound selection

Over 30 compounds either known to have or alleged to have therapeutic effects on any form of arthritis were considered for screening in vitro, with the ultimate goal of developing a local delivery formulation (Table 1 and data not shown). A multifaceted numerical ranking system was used to prioritize compounds, with higher values given to compounds with previously established anti-inflammatory characteristics, the ability to block MMPs associated with cartilage degeneration, and/or the ability to block bone remodeling. Those agents with at least one of these known characteristics and an ability to block a target within a pathway associated with pain were considered particularly attractive. Agents with regulatory approval in at least one country received priority over those not approved for clinical use. Compounds with demonstrated efficacy in clinical trials were ranked more highly than those with only in vitro or animal testing data. A number of agents were screened that are not discussed here, owing to their proprietary nature. The manufacturer, chemical structure, primary effects, published half-lives, and clinical use for the various

Table 1 Therapeutic candidates that were screened in vitro

Therapeutic candidates	MW	Primary effects	Structure	Notes on preclinical or clinical use
Alendronate sodium $C_4H_{12}NaNO_7P_2 \cdot 3H_2O$ Sigma A4978 10 mM stock in H_2O	325.12	Bisphosphonate that targets farnesyl pyrophosphate synthase and inhibits osteoclast activity [68] Used as a positive control for bone changes in osteoclast assays and animal trials $t\frac{1}{2}$ >10 years		Approved for treatment of bone loss in osteoporosis and associated with a reduced prevalence of subchondral bone lesions in knee OA [69]
Ascomycin (FK520) $C_{43}H_{69}NO_{12}$ A3835 (Sigma-Aldrich, St. Louis, MO, USA) 10 mM stock in DMSO	792	Analog of FK506 with strong immunosuppressant properties Acts by binding to immunophilins, especially macrophilin-12 Inhibits production of Th1 (interferon and IL-2) and Th2 (IL-4 and IL-10) Inhibits activation of mast cells [70]		The related compound, Pimicrolimus, is effective for treating atopic dermatitis and may also be effective for treating the same condition in psoriasis [71]
BAY-11-7082 $C_{10}H_9NO_2S$ 196870 (Calbicchem, San Diego, CA, USA) 48 mM stock in DMSO	207.25	Bay 11-7082 is an inhibitor of cytokine-induced IκBα phosphorylation (Calbiochem)		Not clinically approved
BMS-345541 $C_{14}H_{17}N_5$ 401480 (Calbiochem) 3.9 mM stock in DMSO	255.3	Cell-permeable, allosteric site-binding inhibitor of IKK-2 (reported IC_{50} 300 nM) with tenfold higher selectivity for IKK-2 over IKK-1 (IC_{50} = 4 μM) [72, 73] $t\frac{1}{2}$ = 2.2 h		Blocks inflammation and joint destruction in murine arthritis model and blocked MMPs in arthritis model [72, 73] Not clinically approved
Acetyl-11-keto-β-boswellic acid, (*Boswellia serrata*) 110123 (Calbiochem) 9.75 mM stock in DMSO	512.7	Blocked TNF-stimulated MMP expression and protected against experimental arthritis [74] Binds to and inhibits IKKα and IKKβ to inhibit NF-κB signaling [75]		Clinically tested in an Ayurvedic formulation RA-11 (ARTREX, MENDAR; AyurCore, San Jose, CA, USA) with other nutraceuticals [76]
Clonidine $C_9H_9Cl_2N_3 \cdot HCl$ Lot CTM-723 (AAIPharma, Wilmington, NC, USA) 8.69 mM stock (2 mg/ml)	266.55	α2-Receptor agonist and antihypertensive agent Possible induction of iNOS through NF-κB [77] $t_{1/2}$ = 6–20 h		Used clinically to treat hypertension Clinically tested and found to be effective postoperative analgesic for knee arthroscopy [53]

Table 1 Therapeutic candidates that were screened in vitro (Continued)

Compound	MW	Structure	Activity	Clinical note
CORM-2 (tricarbonyldichlororuthenium(II) dimer; CO-releasing molecule) [Ru(CO)₃Cl₂]₂ Aldrich-288144 (Sigma-Aldrich) 10 mM stock in DMSO	512		Decreases oxidative stress in chondrocytes Inhibits IL-1β-induced TNF-α and downregulates NOS-2 and mPGES-1, and COX-2 expression Inhibits p65 NF-κB and HIF-1α DNA-binding activity Reduces IκBα phosphorylation [78] Downregulates MMP-1, MMP-3, MMP-10, MMP-13, and ADAMTS-5 in OA chondrocytes [79]	Not clinically approved
Curcumin Diferuloylmethane (*Curcuma longa*; turmeric) C₂₁H₂₀O₆ C1386 (Sigma-Aldrich) 13.5 mM stock in EtOH	368.4		Reportedly inhibits both NF-κB activation and osteoclastogenesis induced by RANKL [80] Modulates genes involved in oxidative stress, apoptosis, inflammation, regulation of transcription, DNA replication, and cellular morphogenesis [81] $t_{1/2}$ = 10 min intestinal $t_{1/2}$ = 30–50 min plasma	Nutraceutical in clinical trials for treatment of colitis, colorectal cancer, and early Alzheimer's disease Ayurvedic therapeutic and component of RA-11 (nutraceutical mixture) tested in clinical trial for OA [76] Reportedly disease-modifying while blocking pain [76]
Curcumin-14 Curcumin analog EF24 or 3,5-bis(2-flurobenzylidene)piperidin-4-one [82] Synthesized at Medtronic (Minneapolis, MN, USA) 10 mM stock in DMSO	311		Reportedly 10 times more potent than curcumin Inhibits NF-κB by inhibiting IκB kinase (IKK) [82] Potent anticarcinogenic activity inducing death of lung, breast, ovarian, and cervical cancer cells [82]	Novel monoketone analog of curcumin Not yet tested clinically
Diacerein C₁₉H₁₂O₈ Nutraceutical that is enriched in rhubarb Breaks down to active metabolite rhein D9302 (Sigma-Aldrich) 27.15 mM stock in DMSO	368.3		Reportedly reduces IL-1β, caspase-3, inducible nitric oxide synthase (iNOS), and phosphorylation of c-Jun and c-Jun N-terminal kinase (JNK) Enhances expression of TGF-β1 and TGF-β2 [83] Reportedly inhibits osteoclast bone destruction Reportedly increases chondrocyte production of GAGs and collagen in vitro [83, 84]	Claimed disease-modifying OA drug that may slow joint space narrowing [85, 86] Reportedly better than NSAIDs for knee and hip OA with a carryover effect after discontinuation [87] ECHODIAH (3-year placebo-controlled trial on hip OA) showed some positive improvement [85, 86]
Epigallocatechin-3-gallate C₂₂H₁₈O₁₁ 324880 (Calbiochem) 11 mM stock in DMSO	458.4		Catechin inhibitor of osteoclastogenesis and NF-κB found in green tea [88] Potent antioxidant that may inhibit cartilage degradation by suppressing AGE-mediated activation and the catabolic response in human chondrocytes [89, 90] $t_{1/2}$ = 3–5 h	Nutraceutical tested in numerous clinical trials for efficacy in several different diseases [91]

Table 1 Therapeutic candidates that were screened in vitro (Continued)

Compound	MW	Description	Structure	Clinical status
Fluocinolone Acetonide $C_{24}H_{30}F_2O_6$ F3132 (Sigma-Aldrich) 50 mM stock in EtOH	452.5	Corticosteroid (potent) Blocks IL-1 and TNF production and TNF-induced apoptosis [92] $t_{1/2} = 1.3 - 1.7$ h		FDA-approved as sustained-release intraocular implants for the treatment of diabetic macular edema and uveitis [52]
GM6001 (generic names galardin, ilomostat) $C_{20}H_{28}N_4O_4$ 364205 (Calbiochem) 5 mM stock in DMSO	388.5	Cell-permeable, broad-spectrum inhibitor of matrix metalloproteinases (MMPs) Prevents the release of TNF-α and blocks endotoxin-induced death in mice (per Calbiochem)		In clinical testing for eye disease and COPD (Glycomed, San Diego, CA, USA; Arriva Pharmaceuticals, Alameda, CA, USA; Quick-Med Technologies, Gainesville, FL, USA)
IKK-2 inhibitor IV [5-(p-Fluorophenyl)-2-ureido]thiophene-3-carboxamide (TPCA-1) Positive control for IKK-2-mediated inflammation Calbiochem	279.3	Reportedly a potent cell-permeable inhibitor of IKK-2 ($IC_{50} = 18$ nM) with selectivity over IKK-1, JNK, and p38MAPK Inhibits TNF-α in human monocytes ($IC_{50} = 0.15-2.5$ μM) Blocks IL-8 and IL-6 in synovial fibroblasts ($IC_{50} = 100$ nM) [93] Reduced paw edema in rat inflammatory arthritis model (per Calbiochem) (about 100 % at 30 mg/kg)		Not clinically approved Efficacy of TPCA-1 was similar to that of etanercept [93] Inhibitor was tested as potential therapeutic for rheumatoid arthritis (e.g. GSK, London, UK)
NF-κB activation inhibitor IV [resveratrol derivative (E)-2-fluoro-4'-methoxystilbene] 481412 (Calbiochem)	228.1	Experimentally used as an anti-inflammatory but not an antioxidant 130-fold more potent than resveratrol at inhibiting NF-κB [94]		Not clinically approved
IKK-2 inhibitor V IMD-0354 N-(3,5-bis-trifluoromethyl-phenyl)-5-chloro-2-hydroxy-benzamide $C_{15}H_8ClF_6NO_2$ 3.8 mM stock in EtOH 401482 (EMD Millipore, Billerica, MA, USA)	383.7	Cell-permeable IKK-2 inhibitor and established inhibitor of NF-κB pathway Reported $IC_{50} = 250$ nM for block of IκBα phosphorylation [95]		Approved for atopic dermatitis (Institute for Medicinal Molecular Design, Tokyo, Japan)
IKK-2 inhibitor VI (5-Phenyl-2-ureido)thiophene-3-carboxamide $C_{12}H_{11}N_3O_2S$ 401483 (Calbiochem) 3.8 mM stock in DMSO	261.3	Reported cell-permeable, reversible inhibitor of IKK-2 ($IC_{50} = 13-18$ nM) Orally bioavailable		Not clinically approved

Table 1 Therapeutic candidates that were screened in vitro (Continued)

Compound	MW	Description	Structure	Status
IKK-2 inhibitor VIII (ACHP) $C_{21}H_{24}N_4O_2$ 401487 (Calbiochem) 2 mM stock in DMSO	364.4	A cell-permeable piperidinyl-pyridine compound and selective inhibitor of IKK-2 ($IC_{50} = 8.5$ and 250 nM for IKK-2 and IKK-1, respectively) Orally bioavailable in both rats and mice and effectively inhibited arachidonic acid–induced swelling in murine model (per Calbiochem)		Not clinically approved
Meloxicam (Mobic; Boehringer Ingelheim Pharmaceuticals, Ridgefield, CT, USA) $C_{14}H_{13}N_3NaO_4S_2$ M3935 (Sigma-Aldrich) 2 mM stock in DMSO (saline for in vivo)	351.4	Nonsteroidal anti-inflammatory drug (NSAID) that inhibits prostaglandin synthetase (cyclooxygenase) and prostaglandin synthesis Inhibits NF-κB in activated macrophages [96] $t_{1/2} = 15$–20 h		Approved for relief of the symptoms of arthritis, primary dysmenorrhea, and fever and also as an analgesic, especially where there is an inflammatory component
Pimecrolimus $C_{43}H_{68}ClNO_{11}$ S5004 (Selleck Chemicals, Houston, TX, USA) 10 mM stock in DMSO	810.5	Ascomycin macrolactam derivative Like tacrolimus, a calcineurin inhibitor that inhibits release of inflammatory cytokines [97] $t_{1/2} = 30$–100 h		Approved for atopic dermatitis (ELIDEL; Meda Pharma, Luxembourg)
Resveratrol $C_{14}H_{12}O_3$ 554325 (Calbiochem) 50 mM stock in DMSO	228.2	Suppresses IL-1β signaling and IL-1β-stimulated apoptosis in osteoarthritis [98] A natural inhibitor of NF-κB [99] $t_{1/2} = 1$–3 h		Nutraceutical said to protect against neuronal cell death; interferes with the stages of initiation, promotion, and progression of cancer; normalizes blood glucose levels; and acts as an anti-inflammatory The focus of many clinical trials [100]
Rhein (diacerein derivative) $C_{15}H_8O_6$ R7269 (Sigma-Aldrich) 10 mM stock in DMSO	284.2	Anthraquinone-active metabolite of diacerein Reduces proliferation of chondrocytes and synoviocytes; inhibits NF-κB activation in vitro [101] $t_{1/2} = 4.3$ h		Orally administered diacerein is completely converted to rhein before reaching the systemic circulation
SC514 $C_9H_8N_2OS_2$ 401479 (Calbiochem) 2 mM stock in DMSO	224.3	Selective inhibitor of IKK-2 $t_{1/2} = 12$ min		Experimental use only

Table 1 Therapeutic candidates that were screened in vitro (Continued)

Sulfasalazine (Azulfidine; Pfizer, New York, NY, USA) $C_{18}H_{14}N_4O_5S$ S0883 (Sigma-Aldrich) 200 mM stock in DMSO	398.4	NSAID $t_{1/2} = 5 - 10$ h		Approved for use in RA and OA Generic
Sulindac $C_{20}H_{17}FO_3S$ S8139 (Sigma-Aldrich) 70 mM stock in DMSO	356.4	NSAID $t_{1/2} = 7.8$ h		Approved for use in RA and OA Generic
Tacrolimus (FK506) $C_{44}H_{69}NO_{12}$ Anhydrous F4679 (Sigma-Aldrich) or Prograf (Astellas Pharma, Tokyo, Japan) for clinical use 12.4 mM stock in EtOH	804	Immunosuppressant Blocks TNF-α and IL-1β production [64] May be disease-modifying while blocking pain Blocks calcineurin pathway and bone remodeling in RA [65] $t_{1/2} = 11.3$ h		Approved for RA in Japan in 2005 (Astellas Pharma) Approved immunosuppressant in United States (1994) Janus drug-eluting stent (Sorin Biomedica, Milan, Italy) Polymer elution tested in models of uveitis [60]
Tranilast (N-(3',4'-dimethoxycinnamoyl)anthranilic acid; brand name Rizaben) $C_{18}H_{17}NO_5$ Calbiochem 616400 2 mM stock in DMSO (1 % sodium bicarbonate in vivo)	327.3	Anti-inflammatory and analgesic properties in collagen-induced arthritis (RA model) [34]. Suppresses COX-2 and iNOS expression, reduces PGE_2 and iNOS-derived NO production in stimulated macrophages. Diminishes TNF-α and IL-1β production [35]. $T_{1/2} = 7.4$ h		In testing for restenosis (SmithKline Beecham, London, UK; Nuon Therapeutics, San Mateo, CA, USA) Also used and/or tested in Japan (Kissei Pharmaceutical, Matsumoto, Japan) as an antiallergic, antiasthmatic, ophthalmic agent
Triamcinolone acetonide $C_{24}H_{31}FO_6$ T6501 or clinical grade (Sigma-Aldrich) 10 mM stock in EtOH	434.5	Steroid $t_{1/2} = 88$ min		Approved for IA injection in OA

Table 1 Therapeutic candidates that were screened in vitro (Continued)

Triamcinolone hexacetonide $C_{21}H_{27}FO_6$ Aristospan (Sandoz, Princeton, NJ, USA) 37.5 mM stock (20 mg/ml)	532.7	Steroid $t_{1/2} = 88$ min	Approved for IA injection in OA
Withaferin A (withanolide) $C_{28}H_{38}O_6$ ALX-350-153 (Axxora, Farmingdale, NY, USA) 2.125 mM in EtOH	470.6	Reportedly inhibits NF-κB activation by preventing the TNF-α-induced activation of IKK-β (IKK-2) [102] Blocks osteoclastogenesis of bone remodeling [103] $t_{1/2} = 1.36$ h	Medicinal plant derivative (nutraceutical) for RA [104] and other inflammatory disorders, especially in India RA-11 (Ayurvedic therapeutic containing Withaferin A) tested in clinical trial for OA (ARTREX; AyurCore) [76]

ACHP, 2-amino-6-(2-(cyclopropylmethoxy)-6-hydroxyphenyl)-4-(4-piperidinyl)-3-pyridinecarbonitrile; AGE, advanced glycation end product; CORM-2, carbon monoxide-releasing molecule 2; COX-2, cyclooxygenase-2; DMSO, dimethyl sulfoxide; ECHODIAH, Evaluation of the Chondromodulating Effect of Diacerein in Osteoarthritis of the Hip; EGCG, epigallocatechin gallate; FDA, U.S. Food and Drug Administration; FK506, tacrolimus; FK520, ascomycin; GAG, glycosaminoglycan; HIF-1α, hypoxia-inducible factor 1α; IA, intraarticular; IC_{50}, concentration at which the response is reduced by half; IκBα, inhibitor of nuclear factor κB; IKK, inhibitor of nuclear factor κB kinase; IL, interleukin; iNOS, inducible nitric oxide synthase; JNK, c-Jun N-terminal kinase; MAPK, mitogen-activated protein kinase; MMP, matrix metalloproteinase; MW, molecular weight; NF-κB, nuclear factor κ-light-chain-enhancer of activated B cells; NSAID, nonsteroidal anti-inflammatory drug; OA, osteoarthritis; PGE, prostaglandin E; RA, rheumatoid arthritis; RANKL, receptor activator of nuclear factor κB ligand; SC514, selective reversible inhibitor of inhibitor of nuclear factor κB kinase 2; $t_{1/2}$, half-life; TGF-β, transforming growth factor β; Th, helper T immune response-related cell; TNF-α, tumor necrosis factor α; TPCA-1, 5-(p-fluorophenyl)-2-ureido]thiophene-3-carboxamide

Basic information is provided about the source and structure of the chemical, the stock solution, and previous in vitro and in vivo studies [68–104]

compounds evaluated are provided in Table 1. Considerations for testing included cost or availability of the purified compound, stability or shelf life, solubility, required formulation, and the ability to partner or to license the particular compound for clinical use. In some cases, drugs were tested in vitro but were later discovered to be incompatible with delivery formulation for animal studies and so were not tested in vivo.

NF-κB

NF-κB activity was assessed using a previously described dual plasmid reporter system [27]. HeLa cells were transfected with NF-κB luciferase (Stratagene Products Division, Agilent Technologies, La Jolla, CA, USA) and pRLuc-N3 (PerkinElmer, Waltham, MA, USA) at an 8:1 ratio, respectively, in triplicate. After 48 h, drugs were applied with or without TNF-α (20 ng/ml, PH C3016; BioSource, San Diego, CA, USA). NF-κB activity was measured 5 h later with a Dual-Glo Luciferase Assay (Promega, Madison, WI, USA) and an Omni plate reader (BMG Labtech, Cary, NC, USA). The ratio of firefly luciferase luminescence (NF-κB reporter) to Renilla luciferase luminescence (control) was normalized for the number of viable transfected cells. Data are reported as a ratio of activity of viable treated cells over the activity of cells not exposed to TNF-α or drug (fold stimulation above basal untreated levels of activity). The viability of HeLa cells with and without drug was also measured using a CellTiter-Glo luminescent viability assay (Promega). See Additional file 1: Table S3 for results.

Osteoclastogenesis

RAW 264.7 cells (American Type Culture Collection [ATCC], Manassas, VA, USA), a murine monocytic cell line that differentiates in the presence of RANKL, was used for measurements of osteoclastogenesis and osteoclast activity. Cells were amplified on nonadherent culture substratum in high-glucose Dulbecco's modified Eagle's medium (DMEM) containing 10 % fetal bovine serum (FBS) and penicillin-streptomycin in a 37 °C, 5 % CO_2, humidified incubator and were passaged by manual dissociation. Cells were seeded on 16-well osteologic slides (BD BioCoat; BD Biosciences Discovery Labware, Billerica, MA, USA) at 0.125×10^4 cells/0.25 ml/well in triplicate and were allowed to adhere for 24 h, then stimulated to differentiate (30 mg/ml RANKL; PeproTech, Rocky Hill, NJ, USA) with or without drug for 7 days. Plates were subsequently rinsed, bleached, dried, and analyzed for matrix degradation using a Nikon COOL-SCOPE (Nikon Instruments, Melville, NY, USA). Matrix resorption was quantified using EclipseNet (Nikon Instruments)/Visiopharm (Visiopharm, Hørsholm, Denmark) software (see Additional file 1).

MMP-13 activity and toxicity

Differentiated chondrogenic pellets were used both to test the ability of drugs to block MMP-13 activity and to test for drug toxicity. Normal human articular chondrocytes (Clonetics CC-2550, adult male, lot 5 F1452; Lonza, Walkersville, MD, USA) were maintained in complete growth medium (CC-4409, R3-insulin-like growth factor [IGF]-1, human recombinant fibroblast growth factor β, transferrin, insulin, FBS, gentamicin/amphotericin-B and basal medium; Lonza) in a humidified incubator at 37 °C with 5 % CO_2. Cells were trypsinized at approximately 85 % confluence and washed, and $2.2–2.5 \times 10^5$ cells/75 µl were allowed to settle in sterilized, V-bottomed, nonadherent 96-well plates (Thermo Scientific, Waltham, MA, USA). Plates were centrifuged at 600 rpm to form aggregates, and cell pellets were fed into chondrocyte differentiation medium (CC-3225; Lonza) three times per week. By 28 days, the pellets expressed markers of mature cartilage (e.g., type II collagen and aggrecan; data not shown). To mimic osteoarthritic cartilage, pellets were treated with or without TNF-α for 24 h before application of drug with or without TNF for another 24 h. Supernatants were collected and analyzed for MMP-13 using an enzyme-linked immunosorbent assay (GE Healthcare Life Sciences, Little Chalfont, UK). Cytotoxicity to pellets was assessed using CellTiter-Blue (Promega).

Synovial toxicity

SW982 (ATCC HTB-93), a human synovial sarcoma cell line, was grown in low-glucose DMEM with 10 % FBS in a 37 °C, 5 % CO_2, humidified incubator. Cells were trypsinized and plated at $1–2 \times 10^4$ cells/well in Optilux 96-well microtiter plates (BD Falcon; BD Biosciences Discovery Labware) and were exposed to drug for approximately 24 h. Viability was measured with the CellTiter-Glo luminescent viability assay (Promega). A range was first identified in which the drugs might be both effective and nontoxic. To more accurately predict the effects of the drugs on osteoarthritic synovium, cells were tested with or without TNF-α (20 ng/ml; BioSource).

Ethics and compliance

The human chondrocytes used in toxicity and MMP studies were procured from Lonza in accordance with U.S. Food and Drug Administration regulations (21 CFR part 1271: Human Cells, Tissues, and Cellular and Tissue-Based Products) that govern tissue banking. Lonza is registered under the identifier FEI: 0001114298 and holds a permit to operate a tissue bank in the State of Maryland with licenses in tissue banking in the states of New York and California. Records of informed consent were required for all human tissue.

Functional testing

Digital Randall-Selitto test

The digital Randall-Selitto (dRS) test is said to be a reliable and repeatable measure of neuropathic, bone, and inflammatory pain behavior in several different models [28–30], including those of arthritic or joint pain [29, 31, 32]. Baseline and posttreatment values were evaluated using a dRS test device (IITC Life Science, Woodland Hills, CA, USA). Animals were allowed to acclimate to the testing room before all experimentation and for a minimum of 30 minutes before testing. To ensure that their hind limbs were accessible, the animals were gently suspended in a restraint sling. The joint compression threshold was measured once at each time point for the ipsilateral and contralateral knee joints. Pressure was applied gradually over approximately 10 seconds to the medial and lateral aspects of the knee joint. Measurements were taken from the first observed behavior of vocalization, struggle, or withdrawal. A cutoff value of 600 g was used to prevent injury to the animal.

Weight bearing

Weight bearing (WB; incapacitance) was measured five times per day, once per week, using a Linton incapacitance meter (Stoelting Co., Wood Dale, IL, USA). Rats were acclimated to the meter before study initiation, and, similarly, immediately before WB, the animals were placed in the meter and allowed to acclimate for 2–5 minutes. Each hind paw was placed on a separate force plate so that the force exerted by each side could be averaged over a 5-second interval, and the mean of three readings was taken for each data point. Right paw force was compared with that on the left side for each group to confirm that animals were displaying incapacitance and/or pain behavior. Differences in force (left minus right) and right paw force as a percentage of the total force exerted by both paws were determined and compared between groups.

Monosodium iodoacetic acid

Sprague Dawley rats (100–125 g; Harlan Laboratories, Indianapolis, IN, USA) were allowed food and water and maintained on a 12:12-h light/dark schedule. Following isoflurane anesthesia, 50 μl (2 mg) of MIA was injected into the synovial space of the left knee. Animals were randomly assigned to groups, and pain behavior was assessed 7, 14, 21, and 28 days following MIA injection and intervention using WB with the Stoelting incapacitance meter (trial 1) or the dRS test (trials 2 and 3). The dRS test was adopted for the second and third MIA trials after its sensitivity in the MIA model was validated (ALGOS 171.3; 11/16/2008SFN; Algos Therapeutics, St. Paul, MN, USA). Animals received MIA treatment and then saline control or therapeutic. WB or dRS

measurements were done immediately before treatments and at 1, 3, 5, and 24 h posttreatment as described further below. Histopathology was performed at each time point and at study termination. All studies were conducted in accordance with the International Association for the Study of Pain Guidelines and were approved by the Algos Therapeutics, Inc. Institutional Animal Care and Use Committee (IACUC) before initiation. Those running the studies were blind to the treatments. See Additional file 1 for further details.

Medial meniscal tear

Male Lewis rats (260–295 g; Charles River Laboratories, Wilmington, MA, USA) were allowed food and water and maintained on a 12:12-h light/dark schedule. Following isoflurane anesthesia, the medial collateral ligament was transected just below its attachment to the meniscus in the right knee. The meniscus was cut at its narrowest point away from the ossicles so as not to damage the tibial surface and to ensure that the anterior and posterior meniscus halves were freely movable [33]. In trial 1, agents were administered subcutaneously daily for 3 weeks beginning 1 day before surgery. In trial 2, drugs were administered IA weekly beginning 1 week following surgery. Three weeks postsurgery, animals were humanely killed and their right knees were collected for histopathology. All studies were conducted in accordance with the International Association for the Study of Pain Guidelines and were approved by the Bolder BioPATH IACUC (Boulder, CO, USA) in compliance with regulations before study initiation (IACUC protocol BBP03-006). Those running the studies were blinded to the treatments. See Additional file 1 for further details.

Histopathology

Dissected knee joints were fixed in 10 % formaldehyde, decalcified for 2 days in 10 % formic acid, trimmed into two equal frontal halves, and processed and embedded using conventional methods. Sections were stained with either hematoxylin and eosin or toluidine blue stain, or both stains. The histopathologist was blinded to all treatments.

MIA model

Following functional testing in the first and second MIA trials, femurs were fixed in paraformaldehyde, processed, sectioned, stained with hematoxylin and eosin or Safranin O at Premier Laboratory (Longmont, CO, USA), and analyzed by a veterinary pathologist. For MIA trial 1, sections were evaluated for the percentage area of chondrocyte necrosis and/or proteolytic degeneration using a 5-point scale with 0 = none; 1 being <10 %; 2 = 10–30 %; 3 = 30–60 %; 4 = 60–90 %; and 5 being >90 %. Other characteristics of inflammation, proliferation, and integrity of the synovium, subchondral bone, and articular cartilage were scored as normal, minimal, mild, moderate, marked, or increased or decreased when severity was not graded. MIA trial 2 was measured similarly and then cross-checked according to the methods used for MIA trial 3 (see text below).

For MIA trial 3, joints were fixed and toluidine blue–stained sections of the rat knees were comprehensively analyzed from test and control subjects as detailed in Additional file 1. Briefly, a 5-point cartilage matrix score was derived based upon (1) approximate percentage of total loss of articular chondrocytes for each of four articular surfaces, (2) estimated proteoglycan loss (via Safranin O staining), and (3) loss of interstitial matrix. Chondrocyte necrosis and proteolytic degeneration of the femurs were scored on a 5-point scale as in trial 1. A femoral cartilage degeneration score and a three-zone sum of the tibial cartilage degeneration scores (mean of three levels) were also summed to create a total cartilage degeneration score. The mean osteophyte score for each joint was added to this value to create a total joint score with matrix. Other parameters assessed included synovial membrane inflammation and proliferation. Representative images from each group were also collected (see, e.g., Fig. 4 and Additional file 1: Fig. S55, Trial 3).

MMT/MCLT model

For MMT/MCLT rat knee joints, sections were cut in 200-μm steps; stained with toluidine blue (also with a right and left half per section); and similarly analyzed for cartilage degeneration, proteoglycan loss, collagen damage, and osteophyte formation. Results were averaged across the three sections for an overall semiquantitative score. Regional differences across the tibial plateau were taken into consideration by dividing each section into three zones delineated using an ocular micrometer (outside, middle, and inside). Scores were based on the percentage of area affected within the zone.

Cartilage degeneration in the tibia was scored on a 5-point scale as detailed in the Methods section of Additional file 1. The total extent of degeneration of the tibial plateau was measured (in micrometers) and included an analysis of cell loss, proteoglycan loss, and collagen damage. Significant cartilage degeneration reflecting any degeneration extending through more than 50 % of the cartilage thickness was also measured. Collagen damage across the medial tibial plateau (the most severely affected section of the two halves) was also quantified.

Osteophytes and femoral cartilage degeneration were analyzed as detailed in Additional file 1. Scoring of the osteophytes and categorization into small, medium, and large was performed using an ocular micrometer. The actual osteophyte measurement (tidemark to farthest distance point extending toward the synovium) was also recorded. The femoral cartilage degeneration score and the three-zone sum of the tibial cartilage degeneration scores (mean of three levels) were summed to create a total cartilage degeneration score. The mean osteophyte score for each joint was added to this value to create a total joint score.

Overall findings, including synovial health, were also assessed and documented (see, e.g., Additional file 1: Table S1), and representative images were acquired for each animal (see, e.g., Additional file 1: Figs. S57–S59).

μCT

At the end of MIA trial 2, five knees from each group were fixed in formalin and scanned at 55 kV, 145 μA, and 300-ms image acquisition time (μCT40; SCANCO Medical AG, Brüttisellen, Switzerland). Slice thickness was 16 μm with isotropic voxels, and 511 projections were taken for each 360-degree rotation. To correct for beam-hardening artifacts, a μ-law scaling algorithm was applied at a level of 200 mg/cm^3 hydroxyapatite. Scans were reformatted from transverse to sagittal planes before analysis. The tibial plateau was identified, and the slice numbers corresponding to the medial side were recorded. One hundred slices from the middle of the region were selected, and a contour was applied to the subchondral bone that was 50 pixels (800 μm) in diameter. The final size of the region of interest (ROI) was 800 μm × 1600 μm before Gaussian filtering. Care was taken to exclude cortical bone and include only trabecular bone in the ROI. A morphometric analysis on the ROI of each sample was completed, with the same size Gaussian filter and threshold applied throughout the entire study. Every effort was made to minimize variability, including consistently using the same methods and equipment. One specially trained and skilled scientist performed all μCT measurements. The output of this analysis included total volume analyzed, bone volume, trabecular bone measurements, and a structural model index. See Additional file 1 for further details.

Statistics

Statistical analyses were conducted using Prism 5.01 (GraphPad Software, La Jolla, CA, USA) or MS Excel software (Microsoft, Redmond, WA, USA) with the Biobiomedical statistical package designed at Medtronic plugin. For in vitro studies, one- or two-way analysis of variance (ANOVA) was used to look for differences; if significant, then further analysis was done with Dunnett's or pairwise t tests. In general, results of pairwise comparisons with controls using a standard two-tailed t test are shown in the figures with asterisks indicating significance of $p \leq 0.05$. Samples were tested at least in triplicate, and all tests were repeated. Further details are included in the text and figure legends.

The mean and standard error of the mean (SEM) were determined for each animal treatment group. For the MIA dRS studies, one-way ANOVA was used to compare joint compression thresholds of experimental time points with the pretreatment value on any given testing day. OA-related pain in the vehicle group was estimated at each time point on each testing day by comparing ipsilateral (injured) with contralateral (normal) joint compression thresholds using paired t tests. The progression of OA-related pain for other treatments was estimated by comparing pretreatment joint compression thresholds on each testing day with pre-MIA measurements using repeated measures one-way ANOVA and by comparing pretreatment joint compression thresholds with vehicle-treated animals on each testing day using an unpaired t test or one-way ANOVA.

For histopathological comparisons, nonqualitative scales were used for scoring, and a treatment group mean ± SEM for each score and measurement was determined as previously recommended by Gerwin et al. for the Osteoarthritis Research Society International histopathology initiative [25]. Statistical analyses were then performed using parametric ANOVA methods. When several treatment groups were compared, multiple comparison procedures such as the Bonferroni or Tukey correction were used. Dunnett's test was applied for comparisons with vehicle. Scored parameters were analyzed using a Kruskal-Wallis test with Dunn's posttest.

To analyze data from the MMT/MCLT WB studies, a repeated measures one-way ANOVA comparing pre- and posttreatment WB measurements with the vehicle-treated animal or pain behavior control treatment was used as indicated. Similarly, for the MIA WB studies, a repeated measures one-way ANOVA with $p \leq 0.05$ was used, and Dunnett's multiple comparisons post hoc test was performed when appropriate.

For analysis of μCT data, one-way ANOVA was used to look for differences between groups; if $p < 0.05$, then a Bonferroni post hoc test was performed to identify any significant differences between groups.

Results

In vitro studies

Cells typically found in the joint space, such as chondrocytes, synovial cells, and macrophages, proved difficult to transfect with the reporter constructs, so the NF-κB assay was performed in a HeLa cell line previously shown to respond to stimulants of NF-κB in this dual reporter assay [27]. Etanercept (Enbrel; Amgen, Thousand Oaks, CA, USA), a known inhibitor of TNF and NF-κB, was used as a control and inhibited NF-κB at expected concentrations (Fig. 1).

Agents tested in vitro are shown in Table 1. Many of these compounds were found to block NF-κB and MMP-13 activity as well as RANKL-mediated osteoclastogenesis and at a range of concentrations (Figs. 1, 2 and 3, Table 2, and Additional file 1: Figs. S3–S18). The drug IMMD-0354 (Institute for Medicinal Molecular Design, Tokyo, Japan), an inhibitor of nuclear factor κB kinase (IKK)-2 inhibitor, displayed fairly effective inhibition of the three targets and was relatively nontoxic to chondrocytes. However, IMMD-0354 was somewhat toxic to synoviocytes and HeLa cells (Table 3 and Additional file 1: Figs. S19–S28), so it was not prioritized for in vivo testing. Fluocinolone was notably nontoxic and effective in all assays over a broad range of concentrations (Figs. 1, 2 and 3). Curcumin was also relatively nontoxic and effective in all assays (Figs. 1, 2 and 3 and Additional file 1). Tacrolimus inhibited NF-κB and MMP-13 at micromolar concentrations but was more effective in inhibiting the nonclassical (osteologic) NF-κB pathway (2.6 nM). Pimecrolimus and ascomycin, structurally related to tacrolimus, inhibited matrix resorption and NF-κB over a broad and nontoxic range, but they failed to inhibit MMP-13 at the concentrations tested (to 40 μM) (Table 2 and Additional file 1: Fig. S18). Tacrolimus inhibited MMP-13 at 50 μM (Additional file 1: Fig. S10). Triamcinolone acetonide (TA) was more effective in the NF-κB assay than in the bone and MMP-13 assays (Additional file 1: Fig. S4 vs. Figs. S8 and S18). Triamcinolone hexacetonide (TH) was consistently more effective than TA in vitro, possibly because of its formulation (Figs. 1, 2 and 3 and Additional file 1), so this clinical formulation was used in vivo. Withaferin was highly effective in the bone assay (Fig. 2i) and also inhibited NF-κB and MMP-13 at a range of concentrations (Figs. 1 and 3). On the basis of in vitro testing, fluocinolone, curcumin, withaferin, tacrolimus, and TH were chosen for initial testing in the MIA model.

MIA model

The first trial in the MIA model was used to test clonidine, fluocinolone, and morphine as well as to establish the histopathological progression of the model (Table 3; Additional file 1: Figs. S29–S39 and Tables S5–S7). Fluocinolone was found to be the most promising of the three agents in this trial. Not only did it inhibit disease progression, with animals showing a lower percentage of chondrocyte necrosis and proteoglycan degeneration across the tibial and femoral cartilage with minimal bone changes (Table 3; Additional file 1: Tables S5–S7), but it also significantly improved baseline and 1-h WB by 21 days (Additional file 1: Fig. S39). Clonidine, with its known characteristics as an analgesic, was found to be similar in efficacy to morphine when administered systemically daily (Additional file 1: Figs. S30–S37). It was thus used as a control for all subsequent trials.

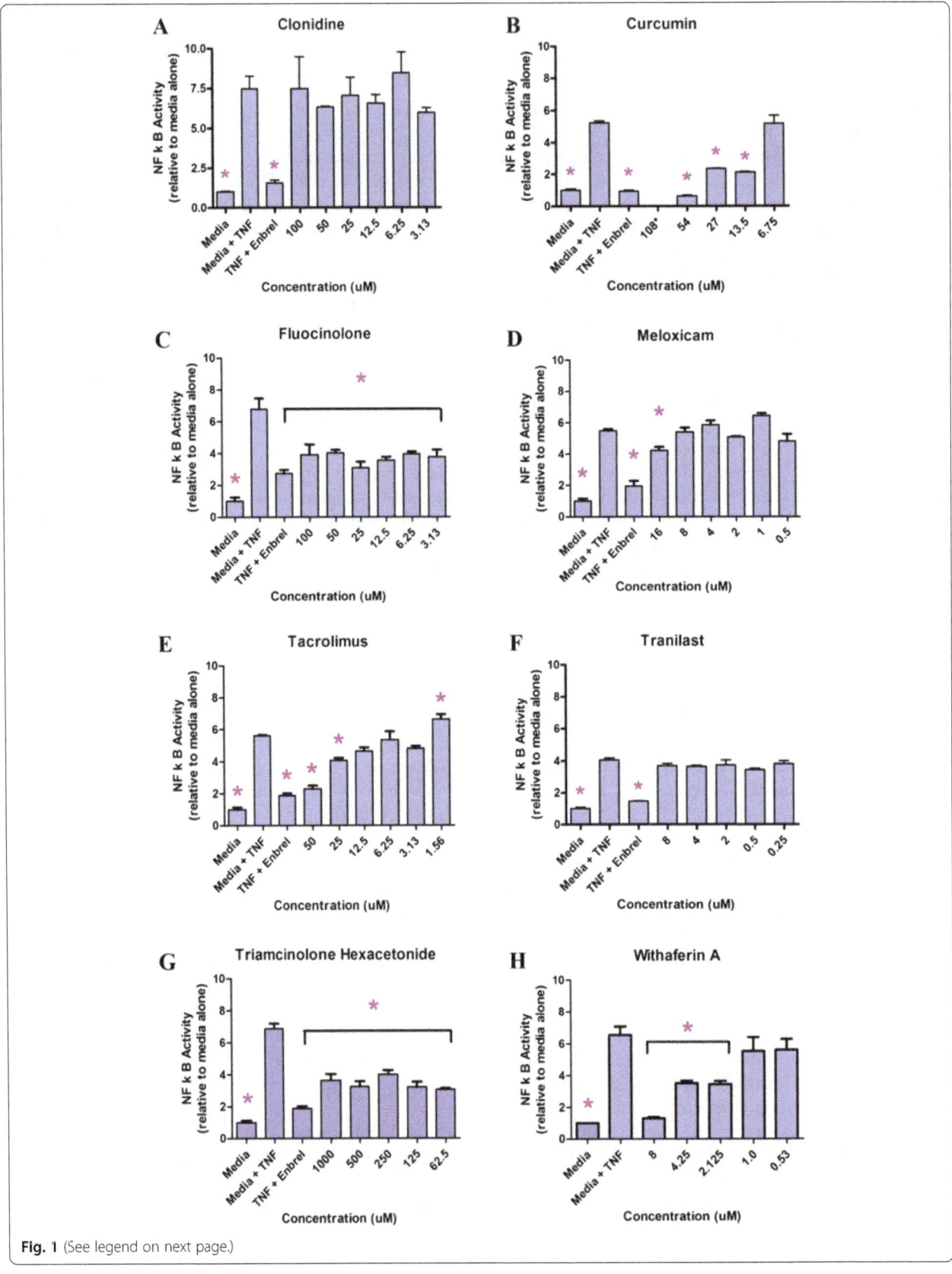

Fig. 1 (See legend on next page.)

(See figure on previous page.)
Fig. 1 a–h Tumor necrosis factor (TNF)-stimulated nuclear factor κ-light-chain-enhancer of activated B cells (NF-κB) activity relative to media alone, with or without drug. The ratio of the NF-κB activity of viable cells to the activity detected without exposure to TNF-α (fold stimulation above basal untreated levels of activity with or without drug). Controls: Media = untreated HeLa cells; Media + TNF = cells treated with TNF-α; Media + Enbrel = cells treated with TNF-α in the presence of Enbrel, a known TNF inhibitor; Test = cells treated with TNF-α in the presence of different concentrations of drug. Shown are resultsFollowing one-way analysis of variance with the drugs tested in vivo (i.e., clonidine, curcumin, fluocinolone, meloxicam, tacrolimus, tranilast, triamcinolone hexacetonide, and withaferin). Following one-way analysis of variance, pairwise comparisons with the media TNF control were made using a standard two-tailed t test. *$p \leq 0.05$. Additional data is provided in Additional file 1

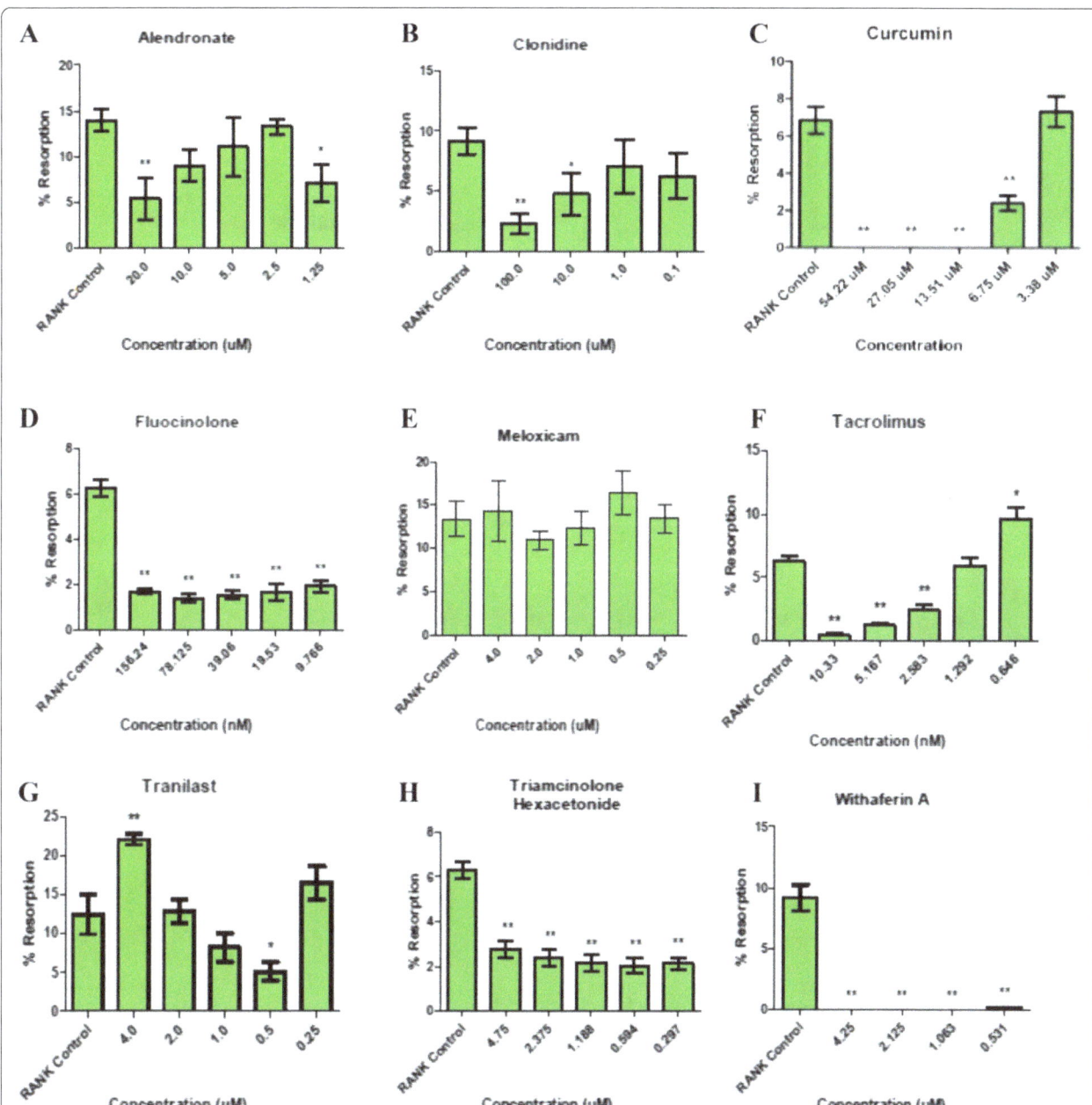

Fig. 2 a–i The effect of tested drugs (alendronate, clonidine, curcumin, fluocinolone, meloxicam, tacrolimus, tranilast, triamcinolone hexacetonide, and withaferin) on osteoclast differentiation and resorption. The lowest concentrations tested are shown; additional data is provided in Additional file 1. Following one-way analysis of variance, pairwise comparisons with the tumor necrosis factor control were made using a standard two-tailed t test. *$p \leq 0.05$, **$p \leq 0.001$. *RANK* receptor activator of NF-κB

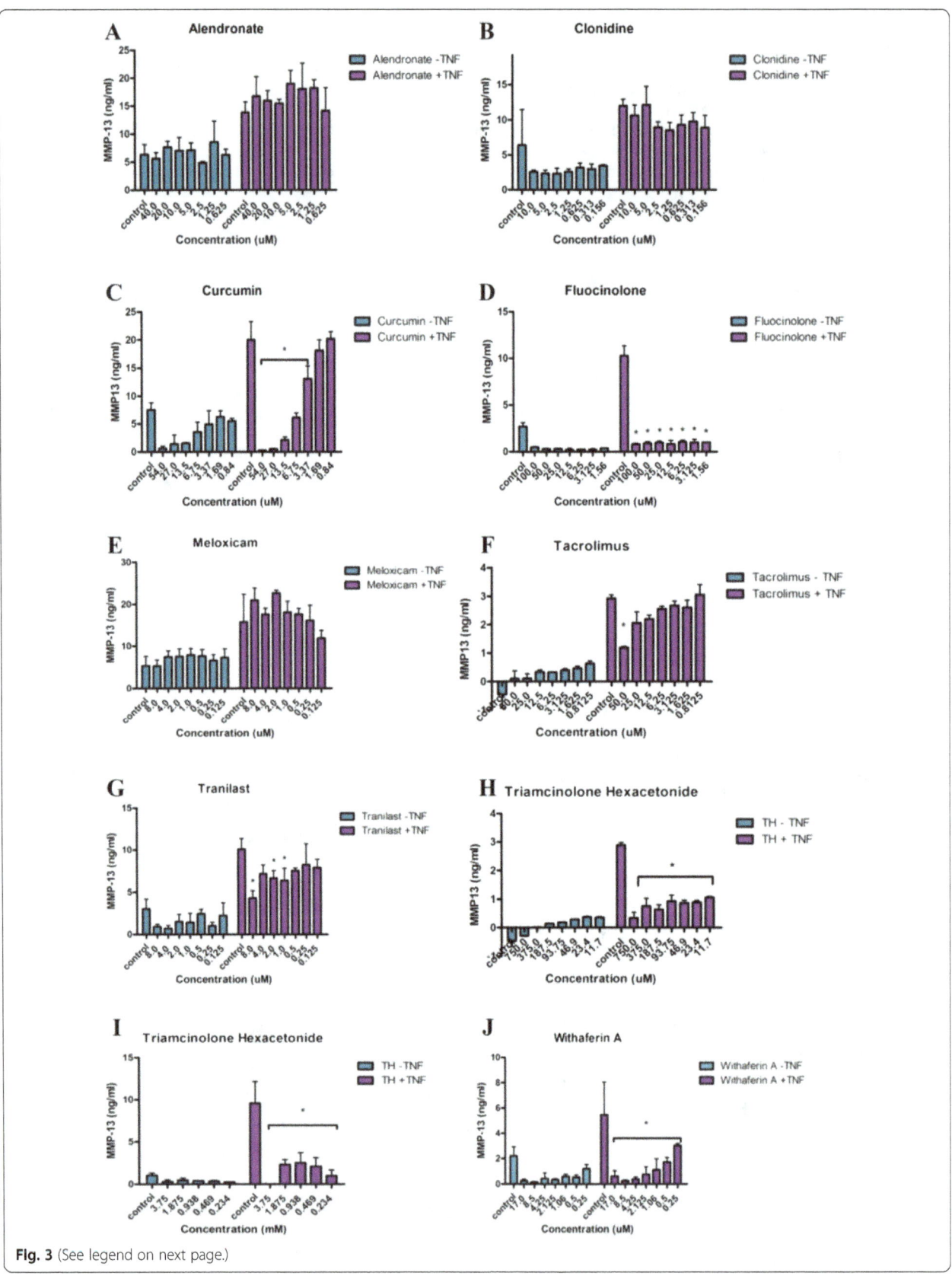

Fig. 3 (See legend on next page.)

Fig. 3 a–d The effect of tested drugs (alendronate, clonidine, curcumin, fluocinolone, meloxicam, tacrolimus, tranilast, triamcinolone hexacetonide, and withaferin) on matrix metalloproteinase (MMP)-13 activity of the chondrogenic pellets. The lowest concentrations tested are shown. Additional data is provided in Additional file 1. Following one-way analysis of variance, pairwise comparisons with the tumor necrosis factor (TNF) control were made using a standard two-tailed t test. *$p \leq 0.05$

In trial 2 (Table 3 and Fig. 4a; Additional file 1: Figs. S41–S49 and Tables S8–S19), fluocinolone was compared with clonidine, tacrolimus, and curcumin and mechanical hyperalgesia was used to measure differences in pain perception. Drug administration began on day 7. Owing to limited oral bioavailability, curcumin was administered by gavage. Unless otherwise noted, the hours shown in Table 3 (dRS column) were those when significant improvement in comparison with baseline was observed. As opposed to trial 1, daily subcutaneous administration of clonidine was better at treating mechanical hyperalgesia, and over a period of at least 5 h (Additional file 1: Figs. S41–S45), in spite of being administered immediately before testing. Clonidine also showed significant effects on the pretreatment joint compression thresholds (Additional file 1: Fig. S41), indicating a persistent effect. Tacrolimus, curcumin, and fluocinolone inconsistently treated mechanical hyperalgesia on days 7, 14, and 21, respectively (Table 3; Additional file 1: Figs. S46–S49). Rats treated with tacrolimus appeared healthy but consistently showed blood in the stool. When all time measures were considered, the cumulative pretreatment effects on pain behavior noted at day 21 for tacrolimus and fluocinolone were not observed on day 28. Histopathological analysis and comparison of total joint scores failed to show significant differences in joint deterioration (Table 3 and Fig. 4b; Additional file 1: Tables S8–S19). However, although cartilage matrix and total joint scores were not found to be significantly different, fluocinolone did block several measures of cartilage degeneration and bone resorption at 0.01 mg/kg ($p < 0.03$) (Additional file 1 Tables S16 and S17), consistent with its effects in vitro.

In the third MIA trial (Table 3 and Fig. 4; Additional file 1: Figs. S50–S54 and Tables S20–S35), IA clonidine, tacrolimus, fluocinolone, meloxicam, tranilast, and TH were compared with systemically delivered clonidine. Tranilast was included because it fared well in two of the in vitro assays and because it was shown to have anti-inflammatory and analgesic properties in a rheumatoid arthritis (RA) model [34]. It was also shown to suppress cyclooxygenase (COX)-2 and inducible nitric oxide synthase (iNOS) expression as well as to reduce prostaglandin E_2 and iNOS-derived NO production in stimulated macrophages [35]. Doses were chosen on the basis of historical data and an estimation of the volume of the bursa–joint space. While none of the agents significantly impacted histopathological progression (Table 3; Additional

file 1: Tables S20–S35), meloxicam, which was included because of its efficacy against NF-κB and approval for treating OA, performed best overall with relatively low cartilage matrix and total joint scores (Table 3 and Fig. 4; Additional file 1: Tables S28 and S29). Meloxicam significantly inhibited mechanical hyperalgesia, both at 7 and 14 days (Table 3; Additional file 1: Figs. S51 and S52). Dosing for meloxicam was based upon previous studies using an IA COX-2 inhibitor, parecoxib, in a rat anterior collateral ligament tear (ACLT) model [36]. Triamcinolone and tranilast also both significantly inhibited pain behavior at 7 and 14 days, but TH was, if anything, negatively effective at 21 and 28 days. Tranilast failed to positively impact histopathological measures (Additional file 1: Tables S30 and S31), so it was not tested in the MMT/MCLT model. Controls showed no to subacute synovitis with generally moderate fibrosis and variable findings following therapy (Additional file 1: Table S21). In this trial, only three animals from each group were analyzed histologically, which likely influenced the ability to discern differences. Representative images from six of the groups are shown in Fig. 4 and are compared with IA delivery in the MMT/MCLT model.

MMT/MCLT model
In MMT/MCLT trial 1 (Table 4 and Fig. 4c; Additional file 1: Fig. S56 and Appendix), several agents were effective when delivered systemically, with morphine and clonidine most positively modifying WB asymmetry. The lower dose of tacrolimus, the highest dose of fluocinolone, and curcumin also significantly alleviated pain behavior (Table 4). Progression in this model has been described previously [25, 33]. Representative images for trial 1 are shown in the Additional file 1: Fig. S57. Tacrolimus (Table 4; Additional file 1: Tables S38 and S39) and fluocinolone (Table 5) both significantly inhibited changes in various measures of cartilage and bone, with tacrolimus demonstrating the most consistent and profound effects across all measures. Tacrolimus unfortunately led to blood in the stool of rats as well as loss of bone trabeculae, effects that could be deleterious with prolonged systemic administration. Both curcumin and withaferin were effective at alleviating WB asymmetry but were without positive effects on joint degeneration. For at least withaferin, this may in part be explained by the cell toxicity noted in the screening.

Several drugs were tested via IA injection in MMT/MCLT trial 2 (Table 4; Additional file 1: Figs. S58–S59, Tables S46–S53). Only systemic clonidine was found to

Table 2 Efficacy of drugs in NF-κB, MMP-13, and bone remodeling assays

Drug	Test range (µM)	Overlapping effective and nontoxic range[a] (µM)	NF-κB	MMP-13	Bone	Tested in vivo
Alendronate	0.625–40	Bone control	N/A	NE	1.25 and 20 µM[b]	MMT/MCLT
Amrinone	0.625–80	80	NE	80	NE	No
Ascomycin	0.01–40	1.25–40	E	NE	E	TBD
BAY-117082	0.188–192	6–192	NE	E	E	Proprietary
BMS-345541	0.24–15.6	0.244	NE	E	E	Proprietary
Boswellic acid	0.61–680	40–680	E	E	E	Purity an issue
Clonidine	0.156–100	10–100	NE	NE	E	MMT/MCLT and MIA
CORM-2	0.625–40	20–40+	N/A	E	E	Proprietary
Curcumin	0.84–108	13.5–54	E	E	E	MMT/MCLT and MIA
Curcumin-14	1.25–80	2.5–10	E	E	NE	TBD
Diacerein	1.5–217	Toxic to chondrocytes	E	E	E	Toxicity and purity issues
EGCG	0.688–44	5.5–44	E	E	NE	Purity an issue
Fluocinolone[c]	0.010–100	3.1–100	E	E	E	MMT/MCLT and MIA
GM6001	0.33–25	NA	NA	25	NE	No
NF-κB activation inhibitor IV	0.156–10	NA	7.7	NE	N/A	No
IKK inhibitor V[d] (IMMD-0354)	0.025–26	1.625–26		E	E	Cost-prohibitive/proprietary
IKK inhibitor VI	0.028–15.2	0.24–15.2	E	E	E	Cost-prohibitive/proprietary
IKK inhibitor VIII (ACHP)	0.25–16	4 (toxicity to synovial cells)	N/A	E	E	Cost-prohibitive/proprietary
Meloxicam	0.125–32	16–32	E	NE	NE	MIA
Pimecrolimus (ELIDEL; Meda Pharma, Luxembourg)	0.625–40	2.5–20	E	NE	E	TBD
Resveratrol	3.125–200	6.25–200	NE	E	E	TBD
Rhein	0.625–40	N/A	NE	E	NE	Lack of potency
SC514	0.125–32	NE in nontoxic range	NE	NE	NE	Proprietary
Sulfasalazine[d]	12.5–1600	150–1600		E	E	Lack of potency
Sulindac	4.35–280	280	E	E	E	Lack of potency
Tacrolimus[e] (FK506)	0.813–100	50	E	E	E	MMT/MCLT and MIA
Tranilast	0.125–8	1–8	NE	E	E	MIA

Table 2 Efficacy of drugs in NF-κB, MMP-13, and bone remodeling assays (Continued)

Triamcinolone acetonide	0.7–2000	250–500	E	E	E	Aristospan (TH) tested instead
Triamcinolone hexacetonide[e]	3.125–3750	62.5–3750	E	E	E	MMT/MCLT and MIA
Withaferin A[f]	0.25–17	4.25–17	E	E	E	MMT/MCLT model

ACHP 2-amino-6-(2-(cyclopropylmethoxy)-6-hydroxyphenyl)-4-(4-piperidinyl)-3-pyridinecarbonitrile, E effective nontoxic concentration that overlaps with other tested agents, EGCG epigallocatechin gallate, FK506 tacrolimus, IKK inhibitor of nuclear factor κB kinase, MIA monoiodoacetic acid, MMP matrix metalloproteinase, MMT/MCLT medial meniscal tear/medial collateral ligament tear, N/A not applicable, NF-κB nuclear factor κ-light-chain-enhancer of activated B cells, NE not effective and nontoxic within the effective/nontoxic range for the other tested drugs, SC514 selective reversible inhibitor of inhibitor of nuclear factor κB kinase 2, TBD to be determined, TH triamcinolone hexacetonide

The overlapping dose range that was effective and nontoxic is also shown. If effective in vitro, it is noted whether in vivo testing occurred and in which models. See Figs. 1, 2 and 3 and Additional file 1 for results in the specific assays

[a] Dose found to inhibit with minimal or no toxicity to synovium or cartilage. Values reflect overlapping range if agent was effective in more than one assay

[b] Used as a bone remodeling control; not tested <1.25 μM in the bone assay

[c] Fluocinolone was effective at much lower doses in both the bone and MMP-13 assays

[d] Effective in the MMP-13 and bone assays; at higher concentrations, this compound blocked NF-κB activity in the HeLa assay but also blocked expression of the Renilla plasmid luciferase. At lower concentrations, it was not effective against NF-κB

[e] Tacrolimus and TH were effective at much lower doses in the bone assay. For TH, lower doses may have been effective in the NF-κB assay but were not tested

[f] Because of the promising results, especially in the bone and MMP-13 assays, and in spite of its slight toxicity in the synovial and chondrocyte assays, Withaferin A was tested in the MMT/MCLT model

Table 3 Summary of the in vivo results using the MIA rat model

Trial 1: systemic delivery

MIA model	Drug (daily)	Dose (s.c.) (mg/kg)	Number of animals	Results — Weight bearing (significant differences; h)				Histopathology (n = 3)[a]	
				7 days	14 days	21 days	28 days	Cartilage	Bone
1	Vehicle saline	5	10				Term	4.7	Severe
2	Clonidine	0.1	10	1, 5, 24	1	1	1, 3	4.7	Severe
3	Fluocinolone	0.002	10	1, 3, 5	1	BL[b], 1	1, 3	3.0	Minimal
4	Morphine	6	10		1	BL, 1, 3	1, 3	N/A	N/A
1H	Vehicle Saline	5 ml/kg	3	Term	N/A	N/A	N/A	4.7	Severe
2H	Vehicle Saline	5 ml/kg	3	N/A	Term	N/A	N/A	5.0	Severe
3H	Vehicle Saline	5 ml/kg	3	N/A	N/A	Term	N/A	4.7	Severe

Trial 2: systemic delivery (n = 10)

	Drug (daily, unless indicated)	Dose (mg/kg)	Route (ml)	Digital Randall-Selitto (significant differences; h)				Histopathology (n = 3 or 4)	
				7 days	14 days	21 days	28 days	Cartilage matrix	Total joints
1	Vehicle saline	N/A	s.c. (5)			1, −5		4.5 ± 0.5	14.3 ± 1.1
2	Clonidine (weekly)[c]	0.1	s.c. (5)	1, 3, 5	1, 3, 5	3	1, 3, 5	3.7 ± 0.3	11.7 ± 0.9
3	Tacrolimus	0.3	i.p. (1)			Pretrt[d]		3.8 ± 0.6	11.5 ± 1.7
4	Tacrolimus	0.6	i.p. (1)			1		3.8 ± 0.6	10.3 ± 2.1
5	Curcumin	50	p.o. (5)	1	5[e]			5.0 ± 0.0	14.5 ± 0.3
6	Fluocinolone	0.01	s.c. (5)			Pretrt[d]		3.3 ± 0.8	9.3 ± 2.5

Trial 3: articular delivery (n = 10)

	Drug (weekly)	Dose (μg)	Route (30 μl for i.a.)	Digital Randall-Selitto test (significant differences; h)				Histopathology (n = 3)	
				7 days	14 days	21 days	28 days	Cartilage matrix	Total joints
1	Vehicle saline	N/A	i.a.					2.7 ± 1.5	5.7 ± 3.8
2	Clonidine	100 μg/kg	s.c.	1, 3, 5	1, 3	1, 3	1, 3	3.7 ± 0.9	10.7 ± 2.8
3	Clonidine	4.5	i.a.	1				3.0 ± 1.1	8.7 ± 3.3
4	Tacrolimus	0.03	i.a.	1				5.0 ± 0.0	13.3 ± 1.7
5	Fluocinolone	0.015	i.a.	1			−24	3.3 ± 1.2	10.3 ± 2.7

Table 3 Summary of the in vivo results using the MIA rat model (*Continued*)

6	Meloxicam	100	i.a.	1	3			1.0 ± 0.0	3.0 ± 1.2
7	Tranilast	0.5	i.a.	1,3	1	1		5.0 ± 0.0	14.3 ± 0.3
8	Triamcinolone H	150	i.a.	3	1	Pretrt[f]	−24	3.3 ± 0.9	8.3 ± 2.6

BL baseline, *i.a.* intraarticular, *i.p.* intraperitoneal, *p.o.* per oral, *s.c.* subcutaneous delivery

The details of the related studies and results are provided in Additional file 1. Shown are hours after drug delivery where a statistically measurable effect ($p \leq 0.05$) was observed on weight bearing or mechanical hyperalgesia compared with the pretreatment baseline of that day, unless noted otherwise. Negative values indicate decreasing of threshold (e.g., −24 = worse at 24 h). "Pretrt" refers to an effect on pain that was measurable before the dosing for that particular day

For histopathology, scores approach 0 with improvement. The femoral cartilage degeneration score and the three-zone sum of the tibial cartilage degeneration scores (mean of three levels) were summed to create a total cartilage degeneration score (shown). The mean osteophyte score for each joint was added to this value to create a total joint score with matrix. Additional measures of tibial cartilage, bone and synovial changes, and details of statistical analysis are provided in Additional file 1

[a] Groups 1–3 necropsy on day 29; group 1H necropsy on day 7, group 2H on day 7, group 2H on day 14, and group 3H on day 21

[b] Significant difference in weight-bearing score on day 21 compared with vehicle control–treated rats

[c] Weekly clonidine showed significant effects on the pretreatment joint compression threshold compared with pretreatment vehicle alone, observed on days 7, 14, 21, and 28

[d] Treatment resulted in a significant increase in pre-treatment joint compression thresholds compared with pretreatment on day 7

[e] Significant decrease in joint compression threshold compared with vehicle controls; no effect compared with day 7 pretreatment baseline

[f] Significant decrease in joint compression threshold compared with day 7 pretreatment baseline

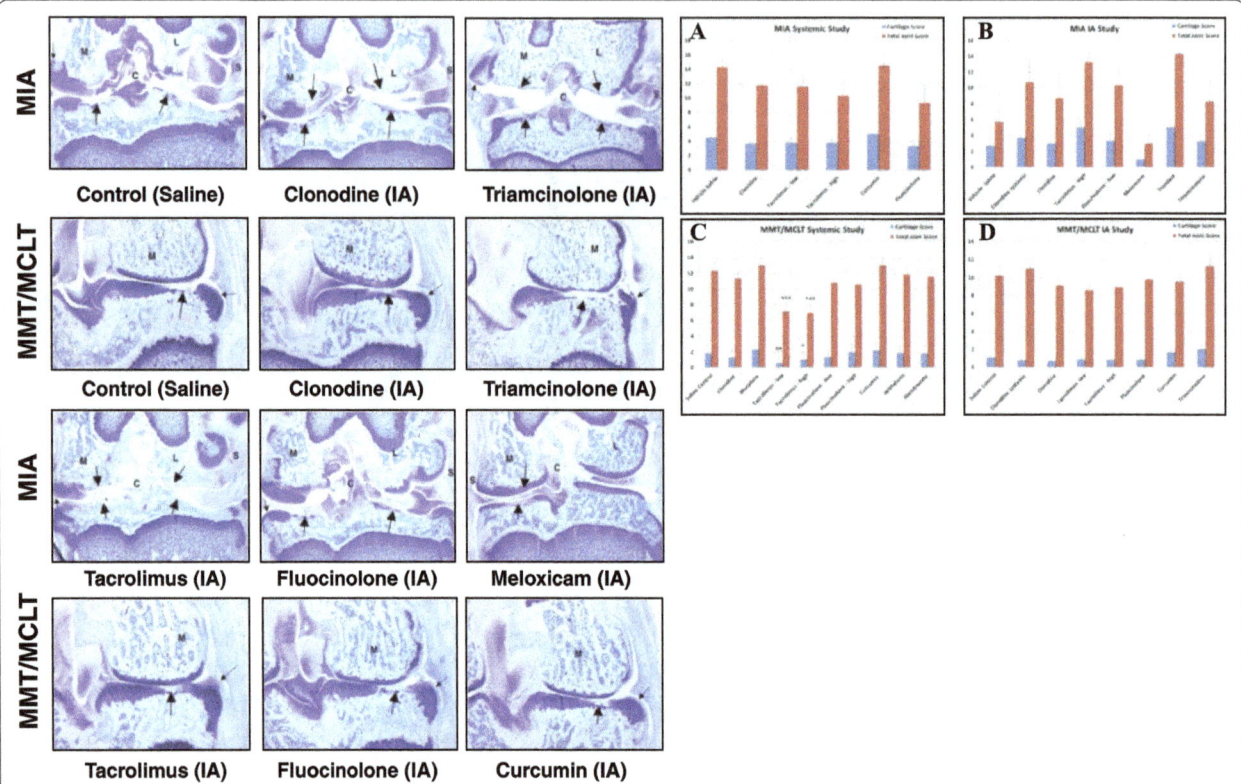

Fig. 4 Representative frontal images from the intraarticular (IA) delivery studies in the monoiodoacetic acid (MIA; original magnification × 16) and medial meniscal tear/medial collateral ligament tear (MMT/MCLT; original magnification × 25) rat models (28 and 21 days postinjury, respectively). Shown are images from animals treated with saline, 4.5 mg of clonidine, 150 mg of triamcinolone, 30 ng of tacrolimus, 15 ng of fluocinolone, 100 mg of meloxicam, or 30 mg of curcumin. MIA: *M* medial, *L* lateral, *S* synovium, *large arrows* affected cartilage surface, *small arrows* osteophyte. MMT/MCLT: *M* marrow, *large arrows* affected cartilage surface, *small arrows* osteophyte. *Top right*: Comparisons of mean cartilage matrix damage and total joint scores with matrix (**a–d**). **a** Trial 2 MIA systemic study (*n* = 10 per group). **b** Trial 3 MIA IA study (*n* = 10 per group). **c** Trial 1 MMT/MCLT systemic study (*n* = 8). **d** Trial 2 MMT/MCLT IA study (*n* = 10). Toluidine blue–stained sections from knees of animals treated with test compounds were analyzed for proteoglycan and cartilage matrix loss, subchondral bone resorption, sclerosis, and osteophyte formation as well as synovitis (see Additional file 1). Femoral and tibial cartilage degeneration scores were summed for total cartilage scores (*blue*). Total joint scores also included osteophyte analysis (*red*)

be effective via WB. Clonidine was also effective at modifying WB when given intraperitoneally (Table 4), but it was not effective as a subcutaneous bolus dosed once weekly before incapacitance testing (s.c.) (Table 4). Similarly, IA administration of 4.5 µg of clonidine once weekly also failed to modify WB asymmetry. In spite of this, histopathological analysis revealed a positive effect on at least one measure of cartilage degeneration (Additional file 1: Fig. S58 and Table S48) with IA clonidine and on medial tibial osteophytes when delivered systemically (Additional file 1: Table S47).

In this same trial with the MMT/MCLT model, tacrolimus and curcumin did not positively affect total joint and cartilage scores, but they had a significantly positive impact on some measures of cartilage degeneration compared with vehicle alone (Additional file 1: Table S50–S51 and S53). For example, animals treated with 15 ng of IA tacrolimus once weekly showed significantly

decreased cartilage degeneration scores for zone 2 of the medial tibia (42 %). The width of total cartilage degeneration was also significantly decreased (12 %). Animals treated with 30 µg of IA curcumin once weekly also had significantly decreased cartilage degeneration scores in zone 2 of the medial tibia (40 %). The depth ratio of any matrix change in zone 2 was similarly significantly decreased (69 %). In contrast, TH-treated animals showed very severe cartilage loss over several measures compared with vehicle alone (Fig. 4). The significantly lower osteophyte scores served to offset this loss, yielding nonsignificant changes in total joint scores (Additional file 1: Table S49). Representative histological images from six of the groups are shown in Fig. 4, and images of the remaining groups are provided in Additional file 1: Fig. S58. The synovium of MMT/MCLT animals at 21 days showed normal fibrous repair with minimal to mild synovitis that consistently improved with TH treatment (Additional file 1: Fig. S59).

Table 4 Summary of in vivo results using the MMT/MCLT rat model

MMT/MCLT model

Trial 1: systemic delivery (n = 8)

	Drug (daily)	Dose	Route (1 ml.)	Weight bearing (significant effects; h; p < 0.05)			Histopathology (n = 8)	
				7 days	14 days	21 days	Cartilage degeneration score	Total joint score
1	Saline control	n.a.	i.p.				1.83 ± 0.31	12.29 ± 0.62
2	Morphine	10 mg/kg	i.p.	1	1,3,5	3,5	2.33 ± 0.66	12.96 ± 0.89
3	Tacrolimus	0.3 mg/kg	i.p.	3	0,1,3,5,24	3	0.5 ± 0.15[a]	7.13 ± 0.69[b]
4	Tacrolimus	0.6 mg/kg	i.p.		1		0.96 ± 0.27[c]	6.96 ± 0.65[b]
5	Fluocinolone	0.005 mg/kg	i.p.	5	1,3	1	1.33 ± 0.14	10.75 ± 0.61
6	Fluocinolone	0.010 mg/kg	i.p.	1, 24	1,3,5,24		1.96 ± 0.77	10.54 ± 0.88
7	Clonidine	0.100 mg/kg	i.p.	1	1,3,5	3,5,24	1.29 ± 0.20	11.33 ± 0.55
8	Alendronate	10 µg/kg	i.p.	5	1		1.79 ± 0.60	11.55 ± 0.72
9	Curcumin	50 mg/kg	p.o.		0,1,3,5,24	0, 3	2.21 ± 0.60	12.96 ± 0.62
10	Withaferin	50 mg/kg	p.o.	1	3		1.83 ± 0.52	11.83 ± 0.61

Trial 2: intraarticular delivery (n = 10)

	Drug (weekly)	Dose	Route (30 µl)	Weight bearing (significant effects)			Histopathology (n = 10)		
				7 days	14 days	21 days	Synovium	Cartilage degeneration score	Total joint score
1	Saline control	n.a.	i.a.				–	1.07 ± 0.24	10.23 ± 0.85
2	Clonidine	100 µg/kg	s.c.	+/–	+/–	+/–	+/–	0.77 ± 0.28	11.03 ± 0.61
3	Clonidine	4.5 µg	i.a.				–	0.67 ± 0.23	9.13 ± 0.54
4	Triamcinolone H	0.15 mg	i.a.				+	2.03 ± 0.52	11.30 ± 1.21
5	Tacrolimus	15 ng	i.a.				–	0.87 ± 0.36	8.60 ± 0.63
6	Tacrolimus	30 ng	i.a.				–	0.8 ± 0.19	8.90 ± 0.66
7	Fluocinolone	15 ng	i.a.				–	0.8 ± 0.25	9.80 ± 0.51
8	Curcumin	30 µg	i.a.				–	1.63 ± 0.61	9.57 ± 0.91

n.a. not applicable, *i.a.* intraarticular, *s.c.* subcutaneous, *MMT/MCLT* medial meniscal tear/medial collateral ligament tear. –24 = worse at 24 h; "Pretrt" refers to an effect on pain that is measurable before dosing

The details of the related studies and results are provided in Additional file 1. In trial 1, drug administration was prophylactic in that test articles were administered subcutaneously daily for 3 weeks beginning 1 day before surgery. In trial 2, drug administration was therapeutic in that drugs were administered weekly beginning 1 week after surgery. For weight bearing, shown are hours after drug delivery when a statistically measurable effect (*p* ≤ 0.05) was observed compared with the pretreatment baseline of that day, unless noted otherwise. With regard to histopathological measurements, medial femur cartilage degeneration and total joint score are noted. The scores approach 0 with improvement. The mean osteophyte score for each joint was added to the total cartilage degeneration score to create a total joint score. Additional measures of tibial cartilage, bone and synovial changes as well as details of statistical analysis are provided in Additional file 1

[a] *p* ≤ 0.005 compared with vehicle alone

[b] *p* ≤ 0.001 compared with vehicle alone

[c] *p* ≤ 0.05 compared with vehicle alone

Table 5 Histological analysis in the MMT/MCLT studies (fluocinolone)

Animal	Knee	Medial tibial cartilage degeneration score[a]				Tibial cartilage degeneration width		Depth ratio, any matrix change[b]		Medial tibial osteophytes		Medial femoral cartilage degeneration score[a]	Bone score	Total joint score without femur	Total joint score
		Three-zone total	Zone 1 (Outside)	Zone 2 (Middle)	Zone 3 (Inside)	Total[c] (μm)	Sig[d] (μm)	Mean	Zone 2	Score[e]	Measure (μm)				
1	R	6.33	4.33	2.00	0.00	1133.33	633.33	0.34	0.05	3.00	413.33	2.00	4.00	9.33	11.33
2	R	4.67	3.33	1.33	0.00	1000.00	433.33	0.28	0.06	1.33	280.00	3.00	1.00	6.00	9.00
3	R	7.00	4.67	2.33	0.00	1133.33	766.67	0.39	0.16	3.00	426.67	2.33	2.00	10.00	12.33
4	R	7.67	4.67	2.67	0.33	1600.00	800.00	0.42	0.31	4.67	586.67	3.00	3.00	12.33	15.33
5	R	5.33	4.00	1.33	0.00	1266.67	566.67	0.33	0.05	3.00	400.00	1.33	3.00	8.33	9.67
6	R	6.00	4.00	2.00	0.00	1100.00	666.67	0.35	0.10	2.67	380.00	2.00	3.00	8.67	10.67
7	R	4.67	3.00	1.67	0.00	1400.00	466.67	0.29	0.13	2.00	333.33	1.00	3.00	6.67	7.67
8	R	5.00	3.00	2.00	0.00	1066.67	433.33	0.32	0.03	2.33	333.33	1.00	2.00	7.33	8.33
Mean		5.83	3.88	1.92	0.04	1212.50	595.83	0.34	0.11	2.75	394.17	1.96	2.63	8.58	10.54
SE		0.39	0.24	0.16	0.04	70.69	51.35	0.02	0.03	0.34	32.50	0.28	0.32	0.71	0.88
t test to G1		0.19	0.23	0.23	1.00	0.27	**0.05**	0.46	0.18	**0.02**	**0.01**	0.77	0.11	**0.04**	0.12
Percentage		0.11	0.10	0.13	0.00	0.08	0.18	0.06	0.41	0.30	0.23	−0.07	0.19	0.18	0.14

SE, standard error; Sig, significant; G1, group 1

Shown are results of the analysis of toluidine-stained sections from three levels within the joints of a group of eight animals treated systemically with 10 μg/kg fluocinolone for 21 days. Note that the cartilage degeneration and total joint scores depicted in Table 4 were not statistically different compared with the control group treated with saline (not shown). Several other measures were significantly different (t test results in boldface type). To view similar data for all the groups in both models, see Additional file 1

[a]Cartilage degeneration score = depth (0–5) for each of three zones, then summed (mean of three-step section)

[b]Mean lesion depth in micrometers versus depth to tidemark in center of zone in the tibial plateau (mean of three-step section)

[c]Width of any cartilage lesion (mean of three-step section)

[d]Width of cartilage degeneration extending >50 % of total thickness (mean of three-step section)

[e]Osteophyte scores 1 = small up to 299 μm, 2 = medium 300–399 μm, 3 = large 400–499 μm, 4 = very large 500–599 μm, 5 = very large >600 μm

μCT analysis

The drug treatments did not significantly affect the parameters analyzed by μCT, although the trends were somewhat consistent with the histopathological findings (Fig. 5) and could potentially prove to be significant in a larger study.

Discussion

Chronic OA is depicted by a self-perpetuating cycle whereby loss of cartilage leads to altered joint biomechanics and an instability that furthers nerve damage, inflammation, boney changes, and resultant pain [10]. The development of pain is strongly correlated with formation of osteophytes, changes in subchondral bone, joint effusion, and inflammation [37, 38]. Both models used in this set of studies showed significant osteophyte formation that likely contributed to pain (Fig. 4, *small arrows*). Although normal articular cartilage is avascular and aneural, sensory nerves found in vascular channels within the cartilage in mild and severe OA may

contribute to tibiofemoral pain [21]. Perivascular and free nerve fibers, as well as nerve trunks, are also observed in subchondral bone and osteophytes [21, 39].

Although it is not clear which targets are most important in OA, NF-κB, bone remodeling, and MMP-13 have been identified to play key roles in progression [11, 40–42], and all continue to be of interest in the pathogenesis of OA [7, 12, 43]. We chose to test existing, well-characterized drugs and nutraceuticals [43] proposed to be potential OA therapeutics (Table 1).

In the relatively severe MIA model, rapid degeneration of joint cartilage and disruption of the underlying subchondral bone ensue from the MIA-induced death of chondrocytes, and cells in the outer margins proliferate, often forming large osteophytes [23, 44]. In the presence of normal load-bearing, there is a progressive loss of proteoglycan, fibrillation, collapse of collagenous matrix, and resorption of subchondral bone [45], with concomitant increases in aggrecanases, MMPs, and inflammatory mediators [46]. IA MIA may also significantly injure

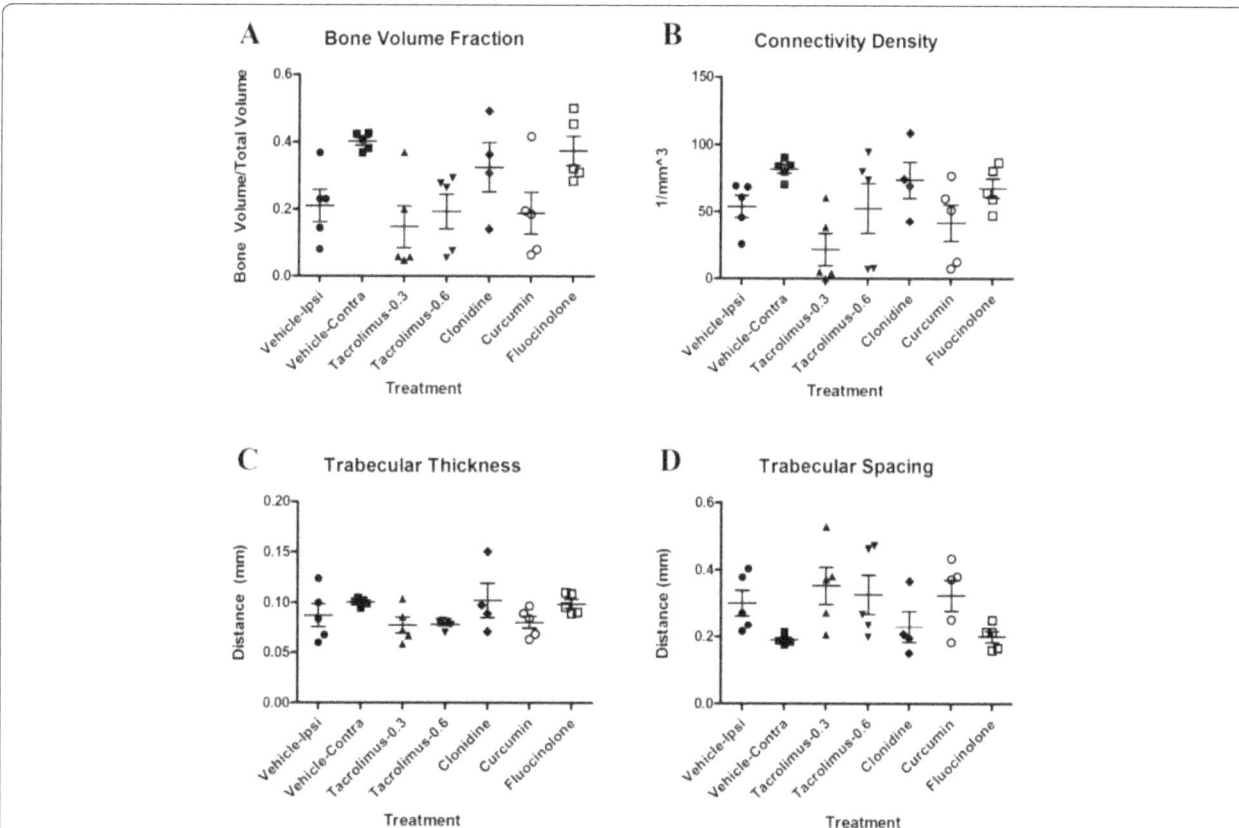

Fig. 5 Micro computed tomographic (μCT) analysis of knee joints from rats treated with monoiodoacetic acid (MIA) in trial 2 (*n* = 5). Vehicle ipsilateral is the injured joint, and vehicle contralateral is the untreated control joint, of the vehicle-treated animal. Comparison of joints analyzed by μCT from five animals of each group in MIA trial 2. Note that only four knees from the clonidine group were analyzed. **a** Relative bone volume fraction (bone volume/total volume). **b** Connectivity density (1/mm³). **c** Trabecular thickness (distance in millimeters). **d** Trabecular spacing (distance in millimeters). One-way analysis of variance was used to look for differences between groups. If *p* ≤ 0.05, then Bonferroni's post hoc test was performed to identify significant differences between groups

dorsal root ganglion cells, including those that innervate targets outside the knee joint, such as hind paw skin [47].

In contrast to the MIA model, transection of the medial collateral ligament and medial meniscus of the femorotibial joint in the MMT/MCLT rat [20] results in rapidly progressive degeneration characterized by chondrocyte and proteoglycan loss, fibrillation, osteophyte formation, and chondrocyte cloning [25, 33, 48]. Damage in this model may best mirror posttraumatic human OA [26]. Its more severe and rapidly progressing phenotype compared with the ACLT model potentially allows for detection of smaller differences between treatments [20]. Broad-spectrum MMP inhibitors are effective in this model [48], which also has relevance to human OA, where MMPs play an active role [49]. While broad-spectrum MMP inhibitors have failed in clinical trials because of their dose-limiting musculoskeletal side effects [50], attention to MMP-13 has been revived by the development of targeted inhibitors [15, 51]. MMP-knockout mice have further demonstrated the importance of MMP-13 in cartilage remodeling [49].

Owing to the complex nature of OA, one model does not fully recapitulate all its characteristics [12, 25, 26]. It seems evident that therapeutics are needed that address such complexity. Indeed, the combination of the selective COX-2 inhibitor meloxicam with pregabalin (a calcium channel $\alpha_2\delta$ ligand developed to manage neuropathic pain) was found to most effectively treat knee pain in patients with OA [19]. The MIA and MMT/MCLT models differ significantly, although both display synovial inflammation, chondropathy, and osteophytosis [26]. Inflammation and osteophyte scores appear to be more pronounced in the MMT/MCLT model [26] (see also Fig. 4). In the MIA model, both inflammatory and protease mediator gene clusters are active, including interleukin (IL)-1β, TNF-α, IL-15, IL-12, chemokines, and NF-κB, and all have also been identified as controlling the progression of cartilage destruction [46]. Upregulation of asporin and downregulation of transforming growth factor β, Sry-related high-mobility group box 9 (SOX-9), IGF, and connective tissue growth factor have been shown to be critical for the suppression of matrix synthesis and chondrocytic anabolic activities, which collectively contribute to the progression of cartilage destruction in the MIA model [46].

Fluocinolone was fairly effective overall, inhibiting all three targets in vitro, mildly retarding degeneration in vivo in both models, and consistently demonstrating positive effects on pain behavior in the MMT/MCLT model. Fluocinolone had a significant impact on several measures of cartilage damage and bone resorption in both MIA trial 2 and MMT/MCLT trial 1, although it did not significantly affect total joint scores (Tables 3 and 4; Additional file 1). Owing to the long-term side effects associated with systemic use in humans, fluocinolone

would have clinical potential only via local delivery similar to that used with intraocular delivery devices [52]. In our initial local delivery studies, with the doses and frequency of dosing used here, fluocinolone did not prove as effective.

Triamcinolone, also a corticosteroid, provides some clinical benefit in OA and other arthritis patients for up to 6 months following IA delivery [53, 54]. TH was more effective than the acetonide at inhibiting NF-κB, but a clear dose–response relationship was not always observed, potentially due to solubility limitations or to an insufficient sensitivity of the assay. In spite of efficacy in humans, IA TH did not result in improvement in WB in the MMT/MCLT model. It is possible that this was related to the dose used. IA TA attenuated WB asymmetry and distal allodynia to control levels in the MMT/MCLT model in a study by Mapp et al. [26] when the treatment was initiated at 14 days; however, the dose per knee was higher than our 150 μg at 1 mg. In contrast, distal allodynia was unaltered in their MIA model [26], while sporadically positive effects on dRS were seen in our MIA studies (Table 3). In our hands, TH negatively affected several of the cartilage and bone scores measured histologically (Additional file 1: Table S49). TH showed efficacy against in vitro targets, so it is possible that these negative findings were due to a block of pain feedback resulting in an increased use of the joint and worsening of the disease (Fig. 4). It is also possible that TH affected joint biology, leading to increased deterioration. This could be further tested by treating control joints with TH. As in our study with TH, TA has been shown to reduce synovial inflammation in both the MIA and MMT/MCLT models [26].

When delivered via IA injection following arthroscopy, clonidine has been found to offer longer-lasting analgesia than morphine [53, 55, 56]. In our studies, systemic clonidine performed as well as, and often better than, morphine in treating pain behavior. Unexpectedly, IA clonidine, similar to IA TH, did not consistently relieve pain behavior in spite of efficacy in humans [29, 37]. IA clonidine in the MIA model had significant effects on dRS at 1 h on day 7 and no significant positive effects in the MMT/MCLT model. However, higher IA concentrations of clonidine may be required to inhibit pain targets in the rat [57]. Because clonidine elicits its antinociceptive effect on the central nervous system, the decreased systemic exposure with local delivery may explain the failure of IA clonidine to inhibit pain in these studies. Although systemically delivered clonidine was effective as an analgesic, it was not consistent in slowing joint degeneration and inhibited only some measures of histological progression in the MMT/MCLT model, including development of osteophytes (see Additional file 1). Clonidine also inhibited osteoclastogenesis in vitro at high concentrations (Fig. 2b).

In the MMT/MCLT model, none of the IA agents significantly affected WB, and all sporadically increased pain behavior compared with the controls. It is possible that the injection itself caused pain, although the average response of dRS and WB of animals that received IA saline did not show this. It has been shown, in fact, that IA saline injections decrease lesion severity in the MMT/MCLT model, and the degree is directly related to frequency and timing of injections postsurgery [58]. (Joint lavage in humans has shown mixed results, however [59].) Doses were chosen on the basis of other studies [52, 60] or were scaled down from concentrations used clinically [53, 55]. For some drugs, such as clonidine, central pain targets exist outside the synovial space [56], and the blood levels associated with IA delivery may not have been sufficient to affect these targets.

In spite of the fact that inhibition of COX-2 has been demonstrated to block TNF activation of NF-κB [61], meloxicam was relatively ineffective in our in vitro assay. This may be the result of NF-κB pathway differences between cell types. In the MIA model, however, IA meloxicam significantly increased joint compression thresholds on days 7 and 14 and had minor, albeit insignificant, positive effects on histopathology (Fig. 4). Several NSAIDs have been shown to block mechanical hyperalgesia in the MIA model (ALGOS 171.3; 11/16/2008SFN), and one of these, rofecoxib, also blocks both nociceptive and neuropathic pain behavior in the MMT/MCLT model [62]. Although not tested in the MMT/MCLT rats, IA meloxicam (0.25 mg) has been shown to inhibit cartilage degeneration and improve nociception in an ACLT model [63]. Interestingly, in a recent clinical study reported by Ohtori et al. [19], IA meloxicam failed to relieve pain unless delivered with pregabalin.

Tacrolimus, a calcineurin inhibitor and RA therapeutic, was tested because of its effects on NF-κB [64] and its ability to inhibit bone remodeling related to RANKL activation of osteoclasts [65]. Tacrolimus was a top inhibitor of bone matrix resorption in vitro and significantly inhibited histological progression in the MMT/MCLT model (Additional file 1: Tables S38 and S39), although there were only minor improvements with IA delivery (Additional file 1: Tables S50 and S51). At the lower dose, tacrolimus also positively influenced WB asymmetry in the MMT/MCLT model. Tacrolimus had a slightly negative impact on bone and cartilage measures in the MIA model when delivered intraarticularly (Additional file 1: Tables S24 and S25), although not on total bone and joint scores, and this was not seen when it was given systemically (Additional file 1: Tables S10–S13). Tacrolimus had minor positive effects on mechanical hyperalgesia in the MIA model when delivered systemically (Additional file 1: Figs. S46 and S47). It remains possible that tacrolimus might be a useful therapeutic in clinical OA. However, the intestinal side effect noted and the immunosuppressive effects previously described clinically [65] suggest that locally delivered tacrolimus might be necessary, possibly with supplementary pain therapy.

Analysis of MIA joints by μCT showed no statistically significant differences between groups, although positive trends were observed with clonidine and fluocinolone (Fig. 5). As noted here, in severe human OA, changes in subchondral bone are observed in the medial tibial compartment, where the relative bone volume and trabecular thickness are less than in controls, and the structural model index and trabecular spacing are greater. These changes typically indicate an increase in bone turnover [66]. Increased subchondral plate thickness, trabecular thickness, and separation have also been documented in the MIA model, with trabecular number decreased compared with control tibiae [67].

Conclusions

Not surprisingly, our results varied between the MIA and the MMT/MCLT models, underscoring differences in mechanisms of degeneration and pain that have been confirmed by others [25, 26]. It is challenging to measure pain in small animals and unclear whether the pain measured is similar to human OA pain. For this reason, histopathological analysis is considered the gold standard for measurement of disease progression [25]. Several agents were at least moderately effective at modifying histopathological progression, including tacrolimus and fluocinolone. Considering pain relief and improved histopathology, systemically delivered tacrolimus performed best in the MMT/MCLT model. Clonidine, used as a pain control in place of morphine, performed fairly effectively in treating pain in both models.

Abbreviations
ACHP: 2-amino-6-(2-(cyclopropylmethoxy)-6-hydroxyphenyl)-4-(4-piperidinyl)-3-pyridinecarbonitrile; ACLT: anterior collateral ligament tear; ADAMTS: a disintegrin and metalloproteinase with thrombospondin motif; AGE: advanced glycation product; ANOVA: analysis of variance; ATCC: American Type Culture Collection; BL: baseline; CORM-2: carbon monoxide-releasing molecule 2; COX-2: cyclooxygenase-2; DMEM: Dulbecco's minimal Eagle's medium; DMSO: dimethyl sulfoxide; dRS: digital Randall-Selitto test; E: effective nontoxic concentration that overlaps with other tested agents; ECHODIAH: Evaluation of the Chondromodulating Effect of Diacerein in Osteoarthritis of the Hip; EGCG: epigallocatechin gallate; FBS: fetal bovine serum; FDA: U.S. Food and Drug Administration; FK520: ascomycin; FK506: tacrolimus; GAG: glycosaminoglycan; HA: hyaluronic acid; HIF-1α: hypoxia-inducible factor 1α; IA: intraarticular; IACUC: Institutional Animal Care and Use Committee; IC_{50}: concentration at which the response is reduced by half; IGF: insulin-like growth factor; IκB-α: inhibitor of nuclear factor κB; IKK: inhibitor of nuclear factor κB kinase; IL: interleukin; iNOS: inducible nitric oxide synthase; i.p.: intraperitoneal; JNK: c-Jun N-terminal kinase; MAPK: mitogen-activated protein kinase; MIA: monoiodoacetic acid; micro-CT or μCT: micro computed tomography; MMP: matrix metalloproteinase; MMT/MCLT: medial meniscal tear/medial collateral ligament tear; M_r: molecular weight; N/A: not applicable; NF-κB:

nuclear factor κ-light-chain-enhancer of activated B cells; NE: not effective and nontoxic within the effective/nontoxic range for the other tested drugs; NSAID: nonsteroidal anti-inflammatory drug; OA: osteoarthritis; PGE: prostaglandin E; Pretrt: pretreatment (measurable before dosing); RA: rheumatoid arthritis; RANK: receptor activator of NF-κB RANKL, receptor activator of nuclear factor κB ligand; ROI: region of interest; SC514: selective reversible inhibitor of inhibitor of nuclear factor κB kinase 2; SEM: standard error of the mean; SOX-9: Sry-related high-mobility group box 9; $t_{1/2}$: half-life; TA: triamcinolone acetonide; TBD: to be determined; TGF-β: transforming growth factor β; TH: triamcinolone hexacetonide; Th1 or Th2: Th, helper T immune response-related cell; TNF-α: tumor necrosis factor α; TPCA: 5-(p-fluorophenyl)-2-ureido]thiophene-3-carboxamide; WB: Weight bearing.

Competing interests

This work was funded in total by Medtronic, Inc. All in vitro studies were conducted at Medtronic. Medtronic did not participate directly in the testing or gathering of data in the animal studies, but it aided in the design, analysis, and facilitation of all studies, in addition to preparing the test agents and performing all μCT. EMT, LY, and MFN were employed by Medtronic when the studies were completed. Bolder BioPATH and AMB were paid to conduct the MMT/MCLT studies but were blinded to the animal groups throughout the interpretation of data and writing of the reports. The authors declare that they have no other competing interests.

Authors' contributions

EMT played a primary role in conceiving all studies presented here, with input from the other authors as well as associated team members. EMT drafted the manuscript; developed or initially tested all in vitro assays; and helped design, manage, and interpret all studies. AMB directed the MMT/MCLT preclinical studies, which were all performed at Bolder BioPATH. AMB carried out the histopathological analyses for MIA trial 3 and all MMT/MCLT studies. AMB participated in the analysis of all MMT/MCLT functional and histopathological data performed at Bolder BioPATH and wrote the initial draft of the associated Results sections of the manuscript. Both LY and MFN helped to draft the Results section of the manuscript. LY played a primary role in overseeing the MIA and MMT/MCLT animal studies and in performing the data analysis for these studies. LY performed all osteologic assays and analyses. MFN helped to design and perform synovial and chondrotoxicity assays as well as the MMP13 assays, and performed the associated statistical analyses. MFN performed all μCT and analyses. All authors read and approved the final manuscript.

Acknowledgments

We appreciate the strong support of Dr. Eric Burright and Dr. Maura Donovan and their efforts to obtain funding for these projects at Medtronic. We also thank Keith Naps for technical help with many of the inflammation assays and Lian Luo for his work in synthesizing curcumin-14. We extend special thanks to Dr. Cheryl Marker at ALGOS Therapeutics, Inc. (St. Paul, MN), who directed testing in the MIA model. We also thank Elizabeth Chipala and her staff at Premier Labs LLC (Longmont, CO, USA) for work in preparing samples from the MIA studies and Dr. Michael Hawes at Charter Preclinical Services (Hudson, MA, USA) for his work in reviewing and scoring histopathological samples from the MIA studies. We thank the employees of Bolder BioPATH (Boulder, CO, USA) for their highly rigorous testing of therapeutics in the MMT/MCLT model and for extensive histopathological analyses. We especially remember Brian Omura (Bolder BioPATH) for all of his help with our studies, and we dedicate this article to his family.

Author details

[1]Medtronic Inc., 710 Medtronic Parkway, Minneapolis, MN 55432, USA.
[2]Bolder BioPATH, Inc., 5541 Central Avenue, Suite 160, Boulder, CO 80301, USA.

References

1. Lawrence RC, Felson DT, Helmick CG, Arnold LM, Choi H, Deyo RA, et al. Estimates of the prevalence of arthritis and other rheumatic conditions in the United States: part II. Arthritis Rheum. 2008;58(1):26–35.
2. Woolf AD, Pfleger B. Burden of major musculoskeletal conditions. Bull World Health Organ. 2003;81(9):646–56.
3. Labianca R, Sarzi-Puttini P, Zuccaro SM, Cherubino P, Vellucci R, Fornasari D. Adverse effects associated with non-opioid and opioid treatment in patients with chronic pain. Clin Drug Investig. 2012;32 Suppl 1:53–63.
4. Singh A, Corvelli M, Unterman SA, Wepasnick KA, McDonnell P, Elisseeff JH. Enhanced lubrication on tissue and biomaterial surfaces through peptide-mediated binding of hyaluronic acid. Nat Mater. 2014;13(10):988–95.
5. Kotz R, Kolarz G. Intra-articular hyaluronic acid: duration of effect and results of repeated treatment cycles. Am J Orthop. 1999;28:5–7.
6. Jarvenpaa J, Kettunen J, Miettinen H, Kroger H. The clinical outcome of revision knee replacement after unicompartmental knee arthroplasty versus primary total knee arthroplasty: 8–17 years follow-up study of 49 patients. Int Orthop. 2010;34(5):649–53.
7. Castañeda S, Roman-Blas JA, Largo R, Herrero-Beaumont G. Subchondral bone as a key target for osteoarthritis treatment. Biochem Pharmacol. 2012;83(3):315–23.
8. Kitaura H, Kimura K, Ishida M, Kohara H, Yoshimatsu M, Takano-Yamamoto T. Immunological reaction in TNF-α-mediated osteoclast formation and bone resorption in vitro and in vivo. Clin Dev Immunol. 2013;2013:181849.
9. Sharma AR, Jagga S, Lee SS, Nam JS. Interplay between cartilage and subchondral bone contributing to pathogenesis of osteoarthritis. Int J Mol Sci. 2013;14(10):19805–30.
10. Sokolove J, Lepus CM. Role of inflammation in the pathogenesis of osteoarthritis: latest findings and interpretations. Ther Adv Musculoskelet Dis. 2013;5(2):77–94.
11. Roman-Blas JA, Jimenez SA. Targeting NF-κB: a promising molecular therapy in inflammatory arthritis. Int Rev Immunol. 2008;27(5):351–74.
12. Pulsatelli L, Addimanda O, Brusi V, Pavloska B, Meliconi R. New findings in osteoarthritis pathogenesis: therapeutic implications. Ther Adv Chronic Dis. 2013;4(1):23–43.
13. Benito MJ, Veale DJ, FitzGerald O, van den Berg WB, Bresnihan B. Synovial tissue inflammation in early and late osteoarthritis. Ann Rheum Dis. 2005;64:1263–7.
14. Baragi VM, Becher G, Bendele AM, Biesinger R, Bluhm H, Boer J, et al. A new class of potent matrix metalloproteinase 13 inhibitors for potential treatment of osteoarthritis: evidence of histologic and clinical efficacy without musculoskeletal toxicity in rat models. Arthritis Rheum. 2009; 60(7):2008–18.
15. Li NG, Shi ZH, Tang YP, Wang ZJ, Song SL, Qian LH, et al. New hope for the treatment of osteoarthritis through selective inhibition of MMP-13. Curr Med Chem. 2011;18(7):977–1001.
16. Wang M, Shen J, Jin H, Im HJ, Sandy J, Chen D. Recent progress in understanding molecular mechanisms of cartilage degeneration during osteoarthritis. Ann N Y Acad Sci. 2011;1240:61–9.
17. Tat SK, Pelletier JP, Lajeunesse D, Fahmi H, Duval N, Martel-Pelletier J. Differential modulation of RANKL isoforms by human osteoarthritic subchondral bone osteoblasts: influence of osteotropic factors. Bone. 2008;43(2):284–91.
18. Zhu S, Chen K, Lan Y, Zhang N, Jiang R, Hu J. Alendronate protects against articular cartilage erosion by inhibiting subchondral bone loss in ovariectomized rats. Bone. 2013;53(2):340–9.
19. Ohtori S, Inoue G, Orita S, Takaso M, Eguchi Y, Ochiai N, et al. Efficacy of combination of meloxicam and pregabalin for pain in knee osteoarthritis. Yonsei Med J. 2013;54(5):1253–8.
20. Gravallese EM. Bone destruction in arthritis. Ann Rheum Dis. 2002;61 Suppl 2:ii84–6.
21. Suri S, Gill SE, Massena de Camin S, Wilson D, McWilliams DF, Walsh DA. Neurovascular invasion at the osteochondral junction and in osteophytes in osteoarthritis. Ann Rheum Dis. 2007;66(11):1423–8.
22. Zhen G, Cao X. Targeting TGFβ signaling in subchondral bone and articular cartilage homeostasis. Trends Pharmacol Sci. 2014;35(5):227–36.
23. Guzman RE, Evans MG, Bove S, Morenko B, Kilgore K. Mono-iodoacetate-induced histologic changes in subchondral bone and articular cartilage of rat femorotibial joints: an animal model of osteoarthritis. Toxicol Pathol. 2003;31(6):619–24.

24. Strassle BW, Mark L, Leventhal L, Piesla MJ, Li XJ, Kennedy JD, et al. Inhibition of osteoclasts prevents cartilage loss and pain in a rat model of degenerative joint disease. Osteoarthritis Cartilage. 2010;18(10):1319–28.

25. Gerwin N, Bendele AM, Glasson S, Carlson CS. The OARSI histopathology initiative: recommendations for histological assessments of osteoarthritis in the rat. Osteoarthritis Cartilage. 2010;18 Suppl 3:S24–34.

26. Mapp PI, Sagar DR, Ashraf S, Burston JJ, Suri S, Chapman V, et al. Differences in structural and pain phenotypes in the sodium monoiodoacetate and meniscal transection models of osteoarthritis. Osteoarthritis Cartilage. 2013; 21(9):1336–45.

27. Gross S, Piwnica-Worms D. Real-time imaging of ligand-induced IKK activation in intact cells and in living mice. Nat Methods. 2005;2(8):607–14.

28. Falk S, Ipsen DH, Appel CK, Ugarak A, Durup D, Dickenson AH, et al. Randall Selitto pressure algometry for assessment of bone-related pain in rats. Eur J Pain. 2015;19(3):305–12.

29. Gainok J, Daniels R, Golembiowski D, Kindred P, Post L, Strickland R, et al. Investigation of the anti-inflammatory, antinociceptive effect of ellagic acid as measured by digital paw pressure via the Randall-Selitto meter in male Sprague–Dawley rats. AANA J. 2011;79(4 Suppl):S28–34.

30. Santos-Nogueira E, Redondo Castro E, Mancuso R, Navarro X. Randall-Selitto test: a new approach for the detection of neuropathic pain after spinal cord injury. J Neurotrauma. 2012;29(5):898–904.

31. Arora R, Kuhad A, Kaur IP, Chopra K. Curcumin loaded solid lipid nanoparticles ameliorate adjuvant-induced arthritis in rats. Eur J Pain. 2015; 19(7):940–52.

32. Prabhavathi K, Chandra US, Soanker R, Rani PU. A randomized, double blind, placebo controlled, cross over study to evaluate the analgesic activity of *Boswellia serrata* in healthy volunteers using mechanical pain model. Indian J Pharm. 2014;46(5):475–9.

33. Bendele AM. Animal models of osteoarthritis. J Musculoskelet Neuronal Interact. 2001;1(4):363–76.

34. Inglis JJ, Criado G, Andrews M, Feldmann M, Williams RO, Selley ML. The anti-allergic drug, *N*-(3',4'-dimethoxycinnamonyl) anthranilic acid, exhibits potent anti-inflammatory and analgesic properties in arthritis. Rheumatology (Oxford). 2007;46(9):1428–32.

35. Pae HO, Jeong SO, Koo BS, Ha HY, Lee KM, Chung HT. Tranilast, an orally active anti-allergic drug, up-regulates the anti-inflammatory heme oxygenase-1 expression but down-regulates the pro-inflammatory cyclooxygenase-2 and inducible nitric oxide synthase expression in RAW264.7 macrophages. Biochem Biophys Res Commun. 2008;371(3):361–5.

36. Jean YH, Wen ZH, Chang YC, Hsieh SP, Tang CC, Wang YH, et al. Intra-articular injection of the cyclooxygenase-2 inhibitor parecoxib attenuates osteoarthritis progression in anterior cruciate ligament-transected knee in rats: role of excitatory amino acids. Osteoarthritis Cartilage. 2007;15(6):638–45.

37. Neogi T, Felson D, Niu J, Nevitt M, Lewis CE, Aliabadi P, et al. Association between radiographic features of knee osteoarthritis and pain: results from two cohort studies. BMJ. 2009;339:b2844.

38. Lo GH, McAlindon TE, Niu J, Zhang Y, Beals C, Dabrowski C, et al. Bone marrow lesions and joint effusion are strongly and independently associated with weight-bearing pain in knee osteoarthritis: data from the osteoarthritis initiative. Osteoarthritis Cartilage. 2009;17(12):1562–9.

39. Mapp PI, Walsh DA. Mechanisms and targets of angiogenesis and nerve growth in osteoarthritis. Nat Rev Rheumatol. 2012;8(7):390–8.

40. Hayami T, Pickarski M, Wesolowski GA, McLane J, Bone A, Destefano J, et al. The role of subchondral bone remodeling in osteoarthritis: reduction of cartilage degeneration and prevention of osteophyte formation by alendronate in the rat anterior cruciate ligament transection model. Arthritis Rheum. 2004;50(4):1193–206.

41. Miller RE, Lu Y, Tortorella MD, Malfait AM. Genetically engineered mouse models reveal the importance of proteases as osteoarthritis drug targets. Curr Rheumatol Rep. 2013;15(8):350.

42. Pickarski M, Hayami T, Zhuo Y, Duong LT. Molecular changes in articular cartilage and subchondral bone in the rat anterior cruciate ligament transection and meniscectomized models of osteoarthritis. BMC Musculoskelet Disord. 2011;12:197.

43. Leong DJ, Choudhury M, Hirsh DM, Hardin JA, Cobelli NJ, Sun HB. Nutraceuticals: potential for chondroprotection and molecular targeting of osteoarthritis. Int J Mol Sci. 2013;14(11):23063–85.

44. Sagar DR, Ashraf S, Xu L, Burston JJ, Menhinick MR, Poulter CL, et al. Osteoprotegerin reduces the development of pain behaviour and joint pathology in a model of osteoarthritis. Ann Rheum Dis. 2014;73(8):1558–65.

45. Bendele AM. Animal models of osteoarthritis in an era of molecular biology. J Musculoskelet Neuronal Interact. 2002;2(6):501–3.

46. Nam J, Perera P, Liu J, Rath B, Deschner J, Gassner R, et al. Sequential alterations in catabolic and anabolic gene expression parallel pathological changes during progression of monoiodoacetate-induced arthritis. PLoS One. 2011;6(9):e24320.

47. Thakur M, Rahman W, Hobbs C, Dickenson AH, Bennett DL. Characterisation of a peripheral neuropathic component of the rat monoiodoacetate model of osteoarthritis. PLoS One. 2012;7(3):e33730.

48. Janusz MJ, Bendele AM, Brown KK, Taiwo YO, Hsieh L, Heitmeyer SA. Induction of osteoarthritis in the rat by surgical tear of the meniscus: inhibition of joint damage by a matrix metalloproteinase inhibitor. Osteoarthritis Cartilage. 2002;10(10):785–91.

49. Takaishi H, Kimura T, Dalal S, Okada Y, D'Armiento J. Joint diseases and matrix metalloproteinases: a role for MMP-13. Curr Pharm Biotechnol. 2008;9(1):47–54.

50. Krzeski P, Buckland-Wright C, Balint G, Cline GA, Stoner K, Lyon R, et al. Development of musculoskeletal toxicity without clear benefit after administration of PG-116800, a matrix metalloproteinase inhibitor, to patients with knee osteoarthritis: a randomized, 12-month, double-blind, placebo-controlled study. Arthritis Res Ther. 2007;9(5):R109.

51. La Pietra V, Marinelli L, Cosconati S, Di Leva FS, Nuti E, Santamaria S, et al. Identification of novel molecular scaffolds for the design of MMP-13 inhibitors: a first round of lead optimization. Eur J Med Chem. 2012;47(1):143–52.

52. Jaffe GJ, Yang CH, Guo H, Denny JP, Lima C, Ashton P. Safety and pharmacokinetics of an intraocular fluocinolone acetonide sustained delivery device. Invest Ophthalmol Vis Sci. 2000;41(11):3569–75.

53. Iqbal J, Wig J, Bhardwaj N, Dhillon MS. Intra-articular clonidine vs. morphine for post-operative analgesia following arthroscopic knee surgery (a comparative evaluation). Knee. 2000;7(2):109–13.

54. Scherer J, Rainsford KD, Kean CA, Kean WF. Pharmacology of intra-articular triamcinolone. Inflammopharmacology. 2014;22(4):201–17.

55. Buerkle H, Huge V, Wolfgart M, Steinbeck J, Mertes N, Van Aken H, et al. Intra-articular clonidine analgesia after knee arthroscopy. Eur J Anaesthesiol. 2000;17(5):295–9.

56. Gentili M, Juhel A, Bonnet F. Peripheral analgesic effect of intra-articular clonidine. Pain. 1996;64(3):593–6.

57. Ansah OB, Pertovaara A. Peripheral suppression of arthritic pain by intraarticular fadolmidine, an α2-adrenoceptor agonist, in the rat. Anesth Analg. 2007;105(1):245–50.

58. Flannery CR, Zollner R, Corcoran C, Jones AR, Root A, Rivera-Bermúdez MA, et al. Prevention of cartilage degeneration in a rat model of osteoarthritis by intraarticular treatment with recombinant lubricin. Arthritis Rheum. 2009;60(3):840–7.

59. Reichenbach S, Rutjes AW, Nüesch E, Trelle S, Jüni P. Joint lavage for osteoarthritis of the knee. Cochrane Database Syst Rev. 2010;5:CD007320.

60. Sakurai E, Nozaki M, Okabe K, Kunou N, Kimura H, Ogura Y. Scleral plug of biodegradable polymers containing tacrolimus (FK506) for experimental uveitis. Invest Ophthalmol Vis Sci. 2003;44(11):4845–52.

61. Shishodia S, Koul D, Aggarwal BB. Cyclooxygenase (COX)-2 inhibitor celecoxib abrogates TNF-induced NF-κB activation through inhibition of activation of IκB α kinase and Akt in human non-small cell lung carcinoma: correlation with suppression of COX-2 synthesis. J Immunol. 2004;173(3):2011–22.

62. Bove SE, Laemont KD, Brooker RM, Osborn MN, Sanchez BM, Guzman RE, et al. Surgically induced osteoarthritis in the rat results in the development of both osteoarthritis-like joint pain and secondary hyperalgesia. Osteoarthritis Cartilage. 2006;14(10):1041–8.

63. Wen ZH, Tang CC, Chang YC, Huang SY, Chen CH, Wu SC, et al. Intra-articular injection of the selective cyclooxygenase-2 inhibitor meloxicam (Mobic) reduces experimental osteoarthritis and nociception in rats. Osteoarthritis Cartilage. 2013;21(12):1976–86.

64. Lan CC, Yu HS, Wu CS, Kuo HY, Chai CY, Chen GS. FK506 inhibits tumour necrosis factor-α secretion in human keratinocytes via regulation of nuclear factor-κB. Br J Dermatol. 2005;153(4):725–32.

65. Miyazaki M, Fujikawa Y, Takita C, Tsumura H. Tacrolimus and cyclosporine A inhibit human osteoclast formation via targeting the calcineurin-dependent

NFAT pathway and an activation pathway for c-Jun or MITF in rheumatoid arthritis. Clin Rheumatol. 2007;26(2):231–9.

66. Patel V, Issever AS, Burghardt A, Laib A, Ries M, Majumdar S. MicroCT evaluation of normal and osteoarthritic bone structure in human knee specimens. J Orthop Res. 2003;21(1):6–13.

67. Mohan G, Perilli E, Kuliwaba JS, Humphries JM, Parkinson IH, Fazzalari NL. Application of in vivo micro-computed tomography in the temporal characterisation of subchondral bone architecture in a rat model of low-dose monosodium iodoacetate-induced osteoarthritis. Arthritis Res Ther. 2011;13(6):R210.

68. Mehlhorn AT, Rechl H, Gradinger R, Stemberger A. Alendronate decreases TRACP 5b activity in osteoarthritic bone. Eur J Med Res. 2008;13(1):21–5.

69. Carbone LD, Nevitt MC, Wildy K, Barrow KD, Harris F, Felson D, et al. The relationship of antiresorptive drug use to structural findings and symptoms of knee osteoarthritis. Arthritis Rheum. 2004;50(11):3516–25.

70. Sierra-Paredes G, Sierra-Marcuño G. Ascomycin and FK506: pharmacology and therapeutic potential as anticonvulsants and neuroprotectants. CNS Neurosci Ther. 2008;14(1):36–46.

71. Grassberger M, Baumruker T, Enz A, Hiestand P, Hultsch T, Kalthoff F, et al. A novel anti-inflammatory drug, SDZ ASM 981, for the treatment of skin diseases: in vitro pharmacology. Br J Dermatol. 1999;141(2):264–73.

72. McIntyre KW, Shuster DJ, Gillooly KM, Dambach DM, Pattoli MA, Lu P, et al. A highly selective inhibitor of IκB kinase, BMS-345541, blocks both joint inflammation and destruction in collagen-induced arthritis in mice. Arthritis Rheum. 2003;48(9):2652–9.

73. Pattoli MA, MacMaster JF, Gregor KR, Burke JR. Collagen and aggrecan degradation is blocked in interleukin-1-treated cartilage explants by an inhibitor of IκB kinase through suppression of metalloproteinase expression. J Pharmacol Exp Ther. 2005;315(1):382–8.

74. Roy S, Khanna S, Krishnaraju AV, Subbaraju GV, Yasmin T, Bagchi D, et al. Regulation of vascular responses to inflammation: inducible matrix metalloproteinase-3 expression in human microvascular endothelial cells is sensitive to antiinflammatory Boswellia. Antioxid Redox Signal. 2006;8(3–4):653–60.

75. Syrovets T, Büchele B, Krauss C, Laumonnier Y, Simmet T. Acetyl-boswellic acids inhibit lipopolysaccharide-mediated TNF-α induction in monocytes by direct interaction with IκB kinases. J Immunol. 2005;174(1):498–506.

76. Chopra A, Lavin P, Patwardhan B, Chitre D. A 32-week randomized, placebo-controlled clinical evaluation of RA-11, an Ayurvedic drug, on osteoarthritis of the knees. J Clin Rheumatol. 2004;10(5):236–45.

77. Su NY, Tsai PS, Huang CJ. Clonidine-induced enhancement of iNOS expression involves NF-κB. J Surg Res. 2008;149(1):131–7.

78. Guillén MI, Megías J, Clérigues V, Gomar F, Alcaraz MJ. The CO-releasing molecule CORM-2 is a novel regulator of the inflammatory process in osteoarthritic chondrocytes. Rheumatology (Oxford). 2008;47(9):1323–8.

79. Megías J, Guillén MI, Bru A, Gomar F, Alcaraz MJ. The carbon monoxide-releasing molecule tricarbonyldichlororuthenium(II) dimer protects human osteoarthritic chondrocytes and cartilage from the catabolic actions of interleukin-1β. J Pharmacol Exp Ther. 2008;325(1):56–61.

80. Bharti AC, Takada Y, Aggarwal BB. Curcumin (diferuloylmethane) inhibits receptor activator of NF-κB ligand-induced NF-κB activation in osteoclast precursors and suppresses osteoclastogenesis. J Immunol. 2004;172(10):5940–7.

81. Panchal HD, Vranizan K, Lee CY, Ho J, Ngai J, Timiras PS. Early anti-oxidative and anti-proliferative curcumin effects on neuroglioma cells suggest therapeutic targets. Neurochem Res. 2008;33(9):1701–10.

82. Kasinski AL, Du Y, Thomas SL, Zhao J, Sun SY, Khuri FR, et al. Inhibition of IκB kinase-nuclear factor-κB signaling pathway by 3,5-bis(2-flurobenzylidene)piperidin-4-one (EF24), a novel monoketone analog of curcumin. Mol Pharmacol. 2008;74(3):654–61.

83. Felisaz N, Boumediene K, Ghayor C, Herrouin JF, Bogdanowicz P, Galerra P, et al. Stimulating effect of diacerein on TGF-β1 and β2 expression in articular chondrocytes cultured with and without interleukin-1. Osteoarthritis Cartilage. 1999;7(3):255–64.

84. Wang L, Mao YJ, Wang WJ. Inhibitory effect of diacerein on osteoclastic bone destruction and its possible mechanism of action [in Chinese]. Yao Xue Xue Bao. 2006;41(6):555–60.

85. Dougados M, Nguyen M, Berdah L, Maziéres B, Vignon E, Lequesne M, et al. Evaluation of the structure-modifying effects of diacerein in hip osteoarthritis: ECHODIAH, a three-year, placebo-controlled trial. Arthritis Rheum. 2001;44(11):2539–47.

86. Maziéres B, Garnero P, Guéguen A, Abbal M, Berdah L, Lequesne M, et al. Molecular markers of cartilage breakdown and synovitis at baseline as predictors of structural progression of hip osteoarthritis: the ECHODIAH Cohort. Ann Rheum Dis. 2006;65(3):354–9.

87. Rintelen B, Neumann K, Leeb BF. A meta-analysis of controlled clinical studies with diacerein in the treatment of osteoarthritis. Arch Intern Med. 2006;166(17):1899–906.

88. Lin RW, Chen CH, Wang YH, Ho ML, Hung SH, Chen IS, et al. (−)-Epigallocatechin gallate inhibition of osteoclastic differentiation via NF-κB. Biochem Biophys Res Commun. 2009;379(4):1033–7.

89. Singh R, Akhtar N, Haqqi TM. Green tea polyphenol epigallocatechin-3-gallate: inflammation and arthritis. Life Sci. 2010;86(25–26):907–18.

90. Rasheed Z, Anbazhagan AN, Akhtar N, Ramamurthy S, Voss FR, Haqqi TM. Green tea polyphenol epigallocatechin-3-gallate inhibits advanced glycation end product-induced expression of tumor necrosis factor-α and matrix metalloproteinase-13 in human chondrocytes. Arthritis Res Ther. 2009;11(3):R71.

91. Mereles D, Hunstein W. Epigallocatechin-3-gallate (EGCG) for clinical trials: more pitfalls than promises? Int J Mol Sci. 2011;12(9):5592–603.

92. Messmer UK, Winkel G, Briner VA, Pfeilschifter J. Glucocorticoids potently block tumour necrosis factor-α- and lipopolysaccharide-induced apoptotic cell death in bovine glomerular endothelial cells upstream of caspase 3 activation. Br J Pharmacol. 1999;127(7):1633–40.

93. Podolin PL, Callahan JF, Bolognese BJ, Li YH, Carlson K, Davis TG, et al. Attenuation of murine collagen-induced arthritis by a novel, potent, selective small molecule inhibitor of IκB kinase 2, TPCA-1 (2-[(aminocarbonyl)amino]-5-(4-fluorophenyl)-3-thiophenecarboxamide), occurs via reduction of proinflammatory cytokines and antigen-induced T cell proliferation. J Pharmacol Exp Ther. 2005;312(1):373–81.

94. Heynekamp JJ, Weber WM, Hunsaker LA, Gonzales AM, Orlando RA, Deck LM, et al. Substituted trans-stilbenes, including analogues of the natural product resveratrol, inhibit the human tumor necrosis factor-α-induced activation of transcription factor nuclear factor κB. J Med Chem. 2006;49(24):7182–9.

95. Sugita A, Ogawa H, Azuma M, Muto S, Honjo A, Yanagawa H, et al. Antiallergic and anti-inflammatory effects of a novel IκB kinase β inhibitor, IMD-0354, in a mouse model of allergic inflammation. Int Arch Allergy Immunol. 2009;148(3):186–98.

96. Hu YF, Guo Y, Cheng GF. Inhibitory effects of indomethacin and meloxicam on NF-κB in mouse peritoneal macrophages [in Chinese]. Yao Xue Xue Bao. 2001;36(3):161–4.

97. Sugita T, Tajima M, Tsubuku H, Tsuboi R, Nishikawa A. A new calcineurin inhibitor, pimecrolimus, inhibits the growth of Malassezia spp. Antimicrob Agents Chemother. 2006;50(8):2897–8.

98. Elmali N, Esenkaya I, Harma A, Ertem K, Turkoz Y, Mizrak B. Effect of resveratrol in experimental osteoarthritis in rabbits. Inflamm Res. 2005;54(4):158–62.

99. Shakibaei M, Csaki C, Nebrich S, Mobasheri A. Resveratrol suppresses interleukin-1β-induced inflammatory signaling and apoptosis in human articular chondrocytes: potential for use as a novel nutraceutical for the treatment of osteoarthritis. Biochem Pharmacol. 2008;76(11):1426–39.

100. Mobasheri A, Henrotin Y, Biesalski HK, Shakibaei M. Scientific evidence and rationale for the development of curcumin and resveratrol as nutraceuticals for joint health. Int J Mol Sci. 2012;13(4):4202–32.

101. Legendre F, Heuze A, Boukerrouche K, Leclercq S, Boumediene K, Galera P, et al. Rhein, the metabolite of diacerhein, reduces the proliferation of osteoarthritic chondrocytes and synoviocytes without inducing apoptosis. Scand J Rheumatol. 2009;38(2):104–11.

102. Kaileh M, Vanden Berghe W, Heyerick A, Horion J, Piette J, Libert C, et al. Withaferin A strongly elicits IκB kinase β hyperphosphorylation concomitant with potent inhibition of its kinase activity. J Biol Chem. 2007;282(7):4253–64.

103. Ichikawa H, Takada Y, Shishodia S, Jayaprakasam B, Nair MG, Aggarwal BB. Withanolides potentiate apoptosis, inhibit invasion, and abolish osteoclastogenesis through suppression of nuclear factor-κB (NF-κB) activation and NF-κB-regulated gene expression. Mol Cancer Ther. 2006;5(6):1434–45.

104. Singh D, Aggarwal A, Maurya R, Naik S. Withania somnifera inhibits NF-κB and AP-1 transcription factors in human peripheral blood and synovial fluid mononuclear cells. Phytother Res. 2007;21(10):905–13.

4

Early blockade of joint inflammation with a fatty acid amide hydrolase inhibitor decreases end-stage osteoarthritis pain and peripheral neuropathy in mice

Jason J. McDougall[1,2]*, Milind M. Muley[1,2], Holly T. Philpott[1,2], Allison Reid[1,2] and Eugene Krustev[1,2]

Abstract

Background: The endocannabinoid system has been shown to reduce inflammatory flares and pain in rodent models of arthritis. A limitation of endocannabinoids is that they are rapidly denatured by hydrolysing enzymes such as fatty acid amide hydrolase (FAAH) which renders them physiologically inert. Osteoarthritis (OA) is primarily a degenerative joint disease; however, it can incorporate mild inflammation and peripheral neuropathy. The aim of this study was to determine whether early blockade of FAAH bioactivity could reduce OA-associated inflammation and joint neuropathy. The ability of this treatment to prevent end-stage OA pain development was also tested.

Methods: Physiological saline or sodium monoiodoacetate (MIA; 0.3 mg) was injected into the right knee of male C57Bl/6 mice (20–42 g) and joint inflammation (oedema, blood flow and leukocyte trafficking) was measured over 14 days. Joint inflammation was also measured in a separate cohort of animals treated on day 1 with either saline or the FAAH inhibitor URB597 (0.03–0.3 mg/kg topical onto the knee joint). In other experiments, von Frey hair tactile sensitivity was determined on days 1 and 14 in MIA-injected mice treated prophylactically with URB597 (0.3 mg/kg s.c. over the knee joint on days 0–3). Saphenous nerve myelination was also assessed in these animals on day 14 by G-ratio analysis.

Results: Intra-articular injection of MIA caused an increase in joint oedema ($P < 0.0001$), blood flow ($P < 0.05$), leukocyte rolling ($P < 0.05$) and adherence ($P < 0.001$) on day 1 after treatment which subsequently resolved over later time points. This acute inflammatory response was ameliorated by local URB597 treatment. Prophylactic local administration of URB597 prevented MIA-induced saphenous nerve demyelination, and chronic joint pain was also attenuated.

Conclusions: These data indicate that local inhibition of FAAH in MIA-injected knees can reduce acute inflammatory changes associated with the model. Prophylactic treatment of OA mice with the endocannabinoid hydrolysis inhibitor URB597 was also shown to be neuroprotective and prevented the development of joint pain at later time points.

Keywords: Endocannabinoids, Fatty acid amide hydrolase, Inflammation, Neuropathy, Osteoarthritis, Pain

* Correspondence: jason.mcdougall@dal.ca
[1]Department of Pharmacology, Dalhousie University, 5850 College Street, Halifax, NS B3H 4R2, Canada
[2]Department of Anaesthesia, Pain Management & Perioperative Medicine, Dalhousie University, 5850 College Street, Halifax, NS B3H 4R2, Canada

Background

Chronic joint pain is a multifaceted process involving a complex interaction between joint neuropathophysiology and psychosocial influences. Patient-reported pain does not match the radiographic severity of joint disease [1] while objective pre-clinical studies have confirmed that nociceptor activity does not correlate with joint damage scores [2, 3]. This disconnect between joint destruction and symptom development makes pain management a complicated proposition for arthritis patients. It is currently thought that the pain associated with osteoarthritis (OA) differs between patients with varying degrees of nociceptive, inflammatory and neuropathic qualities [4]. Despite this mixed pain phenotype in OA, the first-line drug therapies used to treat joint symptoms are the non-steroidal anti-inflammatory drugs (NSAIDs). In general, OA joint pain responds better to NSAIDs than to paracetamol which has no anti-inflammatory properties [5]. As the disease progresses, however, the efficacy of NSAIDs declines and the need for higher doses of drugs exposes the patient to a greater risk of cardiovascular and gastrointestinal complications. Thus, safer approaches to ameliorate any inflammatory component of OA are required for long-term treatments.

Examination of joints harvested from OA patients and animal models reveals that the nerves innervating these joints have an abnormal morphology consistent with a peripheral neuropathy [6, 7]. Dorsal root ganglia (DRG) isolated from OA animals express the nerve injury marker activation transcription factor-3 (ATF-3), suggesting that a portion of the pain described in these animal could be neuropathic in nature [8, 9]. The biochemical pathways involved in joint neuropathy are obscure, although it has been found recently that the lipid mediator lysophosphatidic acid is a promising candidate [10]. This molecule, along with other mediators such as substance P, calcitonin gene-related peptide and tumour necrosis factor alpha, are upregulated during the inflammatory phase of the monoiodoacetate (MIA) model of OA [11]. In addition to causing joint pain and inflammation, these molecules are also capable of damaging neurones [12, 13]. Therefore, we hypothesize that acute inflammatory events in the MIA model will drive joint peripheral neuropathy at later time points leading to OA-related neuropathic pain.

The endocannabinoid system consists of endogenous molecules such as anandamide and 2-arachidonoylglycerol (2-AG) and two G protein-coupled receptors CB_1 and CB_2. Both receptors have been localized in knee synovium, where they are associated with sensory nerves [14, 15]. Pharmacological activation of CB_1 receptors has been shown to reduce OA pain and increase joint blood flow [14, 16]. The role of CB_2 receptors in OA pain modulation is less clear, due to the limitations of the available

pharmacological tools. While the CB2 agonist GW405833 reduced mechanonociception in a normal joint, it actually had a sensitizing effect in OA joints causing an enhanced pain response [15]. Alternatively, intraspinal injection of the CB2 agonist JWH133 reduced the central sensitization associated with OA [17], suggesting different sites of action for CB_2 receptors in the control of OA pain. Endocannabinoids are known to accumulate in OA joints [18]; however, they are rapidly broken down by endogenous hydrolases such as fatty acid amide hydrolase (FAAH). Blockade of FAAH activity has been shown to reduce joint pain and inflammation in rodent models of arthritis, indicating that the endocannabinoid system may be an efficacious way of treating joint disease [19, 20].

The aim of the present investigation was to determine whether FAAH inhibition could reduce the incipient inflammatory phase associated with the onset of MIA-induced OA. Secondly, experiments were performed to test whether interfering with this initial inflammatory episode would improve pain perception at later times in the MIA model. Finally, a potential neuroprotective effect of the FAAH inhibitor was assessed to see whether such a treatment could alleviate MIA-induced neuropathy.

Methods
Animals

A total of 178 male C57BL/6 mice (20–42 g; Charles River, QC, Canada) were used in these experiments. Following arrival at the facility, all animals were allowed at least 1 week to acclimate to their new environment. Mice were housed in ventilated racks at 22 ± 2 °C on a 12:12-hr light:dark cycle (light on from 7:00 to 19:00). Cages were lined with woodchip bedding and animals were provided with environmental enrichment. Standard laboratory chow and water were provided ad libitum. All experimental protocols were approved by the Dalhousie University Committee on Laboratory Animals, which acts in accordance with the standards put forth by the Canadian Council for Animal Care.

Sodium monoiodoacetate-induced osteoarthritis

Animals were deeply anaesthetized (2–4% isoflurane; 100% oxygen at 1 L/min). The right knee joint was shaved and swabbed with 100% ethanol, and then 10 μl of MIA (0.3 mg in saline) was injected into the synovial space. A separate cohort of control sham animals received an intra-articular injection of sterile saline. The knee was then manually extended and flexed for 30 s to disperse the solution throughout the joint. In separate groups of mice, inflammation was assessed on days 1, 3, 7, 10 and 14, while pain and saphenous nerve demyelination were assessed on day 14.

Measurements of inflammation

Joint oedema

Joint oedema was assessed by measuring the distance between the medial and lateral femoral condyles using a digital micrometer (VWR, Friendswood, TX, USA). Measurements were taken immediately before intra-articular injection of MIA, and then again on the day of inflammation assessment. Triplicate measurements were carried out and the average joint diameter was calculated.

Synovial blood flow

Animals were deeply anaesthetized by an intraperitoneal injection of urethane (25% in saline; 0.25–0.4 ml). A longitudinal incision was made in the ventral skin of the neck to expose the trachea which was cannulated to permit unrestricted breathing. The left carotid artery and the left jugular vein were also cannulated with PE-10 tubing filled with heparinized saline (1 U/ml) to allow mean arterial pressure (MAP) monitoring and intravenous (i.v.) access, respectively. The articular microcirculation of the right knee was exposed by surgically removing a small ellipse of overlying skin and the hind limb was immobilized. Physiological buffer (37 °C) was immediately and continuously perfused over the exposed joint.

Laser speckle contrast analysis (LASCA) was used to measure synovial vascular perfusion using a PeriCam PSI System (Perimed Inc., Ardmore, PA, USA). Recordings of the exposed knee joint were taken at a working distance of 10 cm with a frame capture rate of 25 images per second. Using dedicated software (PIMSoft, Version 1.5.4.8078), images were averaged to generate one perfusion image per second and a 1-min LASCA recording was taken at each time point. At the end of the experiment, mice were euthanized and a dead scan of the knee was taken post mortem. This "biological zero" value was subtracted from all measurements to account for any optical noise in the tissue. Images were analysed offline where blood perfusion in a defined region of interest approximating the knee joint was calculated. Because resting MAP was different between animals, vascular conductance was calculated:

$$\text{Conductance} = \frac{\text{blood perfusion}}{\text{mean arterial pressure}}$$

Intravital microscopy

Intravital microscopy (IVM) was used to assess leukocyte–endothelial interactions within the microcirculation of the knee joint, as described previously [21]. After surgical exposure of the joint, the synovial microcirculation was visualized under incident fluorescent light using a Leica DM2500 microscope with an HCX APO L 20× objective and an HC Plan 10× eyepiece with a final magnification of 200×. In-vivo leukocyte staining was achieved by intravenous administration of rhodamine 6G (R6G; 0.05%, 0.05 ml, saline) and fluorescent videos were captured for 1 min by a Leica DFC 3000 camera (Leica Microsystems Inc., ON, Canada). Straight, unbranched, post-capillary venules (15–50 µm in diameter) overlying the knee joint capsule were selected for visualization. Two measures of leukocyte–endothelial interactions were used to assess inflammation: the number of rolling leukocytes and the number of adherent leukocytes. Rolling leukocytes are defined here as R6G-stained cells travelling slower than the surrounding flow of blood in the vessel of interest. The rolling leukocyte measure was obtained by counting the number of rolling leukocytes per minute to pass an arbitrary line perpendicular to the vessel of interest. Adherent leukocytes were defined as R6G-stained cells that remained stationary for a minimum of 30 s. Total leukocyte adhesion was quantified by counting the number of adherent cells within a defined portion of the vessel (100 µm).

Measurement of secondary allodynia

Von Frey hair algesiometry was used as a measure of referred nociception. Animals were placed in elevated Plexiglas chambers (30 cm long × 9 cm wide × 24 cm tall) on metal mesh flooring, which allows access to the plantar surface of the paws. After allowing the animal to acclimate until exploratory behaviour ceased, ipsilateral hind paw mechanosensitivity was assessed using a modification of the Dixon up-down method [22]. A von Frey hair of known bending force was applied perpendicular to the plantar surface of the hind paw (avoiding the toe pads) until it just bent, and then was held in place for 3 s. If there was a positive response (i.e. withdrawal, shake or lick of the hind paw), the next lower strength hair was applied; if there was no response, the next higher strength hair was applied up to a maximum cut-off level which corresponded to a 4-g bending force. After the first difference in response was observed, four further measurements were made. The 50% withdrawal threshold was determined using the formula:

$$10^{[Xf + k\delta]}/10,000$$

where Xf is the value (in log units) of the final von Frey hair used, k is the tabular value for the pattern of the last six positive/negative responses and δ is the mean difference (in log units) between stimuli.

Myelination of saphenous neurones

A small section of saphenous nerve was excised post mortem just proximal to the ipsilateral knee joint and fixed for several days in 2.5% glutaraldehyde diluted with 0.1 M sodium cacodylate buffer. Samples were rinsed three times (10 min each) with 0.1 M sodium cacodylate buffer and fixed for 2 h in 1% osmium tetroxide. Nerves were then rinsed in distilled water, placed in 0.25% uranyl acetate at 4 °C overnight, dehydrated through a series of acetone washes (from 50 to 100%), then embedded in 100% epon araldite resin and placed in a 60 °C oven for 48 h to cure. Thin sections (100 nm) were cut and placed on mesh copper grids and stained as follows: 2% aqueous uranyl acetate (10 min), distilled water (2 × 5 min), lead citrate (4 min) and, finally, a distilled water rinse. Samples were viewed under a JEOL JEM 1230 transmission electron microscope at 80 kV. Representative images of saphenous nerve cross-sections were taken with a Hamamatsu ORCA-HR digital camera. For each nerve, one image containing a majority (50–100) of fibres was analysed. Axonal myelination was calculated by G-ratios using Image J software:

$$\text{G-ratio} = \sqrt{\text{internal axonal area}/\text{entire axonal area}}$$

and values were averaged to give a mean G-ratio for each animal.

Acute URB597 treatment for inflammation experiments

The effect of FAAH inhibition on MIA-induced inflammation was tested in day 1 MIA-injected mice. Following baseline IVM and LASCA measurements, URB597 (0.03–0.3 mg/kg) or vehicle (DMSO:cremophor:saline 1:1:8) was applied topically to the exposed mouse knee as a warm (37 °C) bolus (100 µl). Blood flow and leukocyte trafficking measurements were then carried out 20 min later.

Prophylactic URB597 treatment for pain and nerve damage

Pain

Secondary allodynia was measured at days 1 and 14 in four cohorts of mice as follows: Group 1, intra-articular injection of saline (sham control); Group 2, intra-articular injection of MIA only (OA control); Group 3, MIA mice treated with vehicle once per day on days 0–3 (OA with prophylactic vehicle treatment); and Group 4, MIA mice treated with 0.3 mg/kg URB597 on days 0–3 (OA with prophylactic drug treatment). All vehicle and drug treatments for the pain experiments were administered locally (10 µl s.c.) around the knee joint.

Saphenous nerve myelination

Saphenous nerves were removed from three groups of mice consisting of day 14 saline sham control, day 14 MIA mice treated with local vehicle (10 µl s.c. around

the joint) once per day on days 0–3 (OA with prophylactic vehicle treatment) and day 14 MIA mice treated with 0.3 mg/kg URB597 (10 µl s.c. around the joint) on days 0–3 (OA with prophylactic drug treatment).

Drugs and reagents

URB597 (FAAH inhibitor; (3-(3-carbamoylphenyl)phenyl) N-cyclohexylcarbamate) was obtained from Cayman Chemicals (Ann Arbor, MI, USA). Rhodamine 6G, cremophor, dimethyl sulphoxide (DMSO), urethane and sodium monoiodoacetate were obtained from Sigma Aldrich (St. Louis, MO, USA).

URB597 (0.03, 0.3 and 3.0 mg/kg) was dissolved in vehicle (DMSO:cremophor:saline 1:1:8) on the day of use. MIA was dissolved in saline (0.3 mg/10 µl) on the day of use. Rhodamine 6G (0.05%) was dissolved in saline and stored in the dark at 4 °C. Physiological buffered saline (135 mM NaCl, 20 mM $NaHCO_3$, 5 mM KCl, 1 mM $MgSO_4 \cdot 7H_2O$, pH 7.4) was prepared in-house.

Data presentation and analysis

The Gaussian distribution was assessed for each group using a Kolmogorov–Smirnov test. All data were normally distributed and were therefore analysed using parametric statistics (one-way or two-way ANOVA, Student's t test). All data are presented as the mean ± the standard error of the mean (SEM) for n observations. $P < 0.05$ was considered statistically significant.

Results

Time course of MIA-induced inflammation

When compared with saline-injected controls, intra-articular MIA (0.3 mg) significantly increased the knee joint diameter 1 day ($P < 0.0001$; $n = 14–28$; Fig. 1a) and 3 days ($P < 0.0001$; $n = 6–11$; Fig. 1a) after injection. Joint oedema subsequently returned towards control levels thereafter.

Intra-articular injection of MIA increased synovial vascular conductance on day 1 when compared with saline-injected controls ($P < 0.05$; $n = 5–27$; Fig. 1b). This hyperemic response was transient with blood flow returning to control levels from day 3 onwards.

Leukocyte rolling was significantly different between MIA and saline-injected knees on day 1 after injection ($P < 0.05$; $n = 13–27$; Fig. 1c). At later time points, however, there was no statistical difference between MIA and saline-treated mice ($P > 0.05$; $n = 4–11$). Leukocyte adherence was significantly higher at day 1 in MIA-injected knees compared with saline-injected controls ($P < 0.0001$; $n = 15–27$; Fig. 1d). Leukocyte adherence was not statistically different between control and arthritic joints at subsequent time points ($P > 0.05$; $n = 4–11$; Fig. 1d).

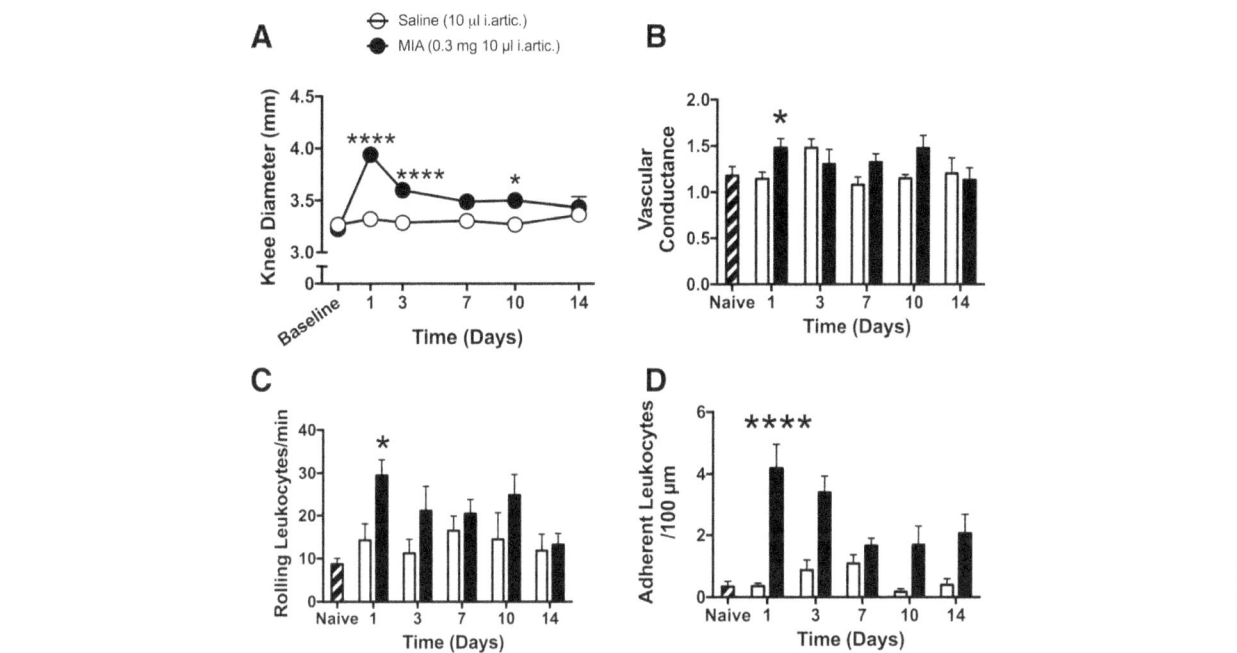

Fig. 1 Early onset of joint inflammation in the MIA model of OA. **a** Knee joint diameter was significantly increased on days 1, 3 and 10 compared with saline control. **b** Joint blood flow increased on day 1, but subsequently was not significantly different from control joints. **c** Leukocyte rolling was augmented on day 1 and then returned to control levels thereafter. **d** Leukocyte adherence within synovial post-capillary venules was significantly increased on day 1, but gradually returned to control over the succeeding days. ****$P < 0.0001$, *$P < 0.05$ two-way ANOVA with Bonferroni post-hoc test; $n = 4$–28. Data presented as mean ± SEM. *i.artic.* intra-articular, *MIA* monoiodoacetate

Effect of URB597 on MIA-induced inflammation
When compared with vehicle control, URB597 had no effect on leukocyte rolling at any of the doses tested ($P > 0.05$; $n = 6$–8; Fig. 2a). With leukocyte adherence, however, only the 0.3 mg/kg dose of URB597 caused a significant decrease ($P < 0.01$; $n = 6$–8; Fig. 2b), while the low and high doses of the drug were ineffective. Treatment of MIA-injected knees with 0.03 and 3.0 mg/kg URB597 had no effect on MIA-induced hyperaemia ($P > 0.05$; $n = 6$–8) whereas the 0.3 mg/kg dose of the drug significantly decreased articular blood flow ($P < 0.05$; $n = 6$–8; Fig. 2c).

Effect of prophylactic URB597 on the chronic development of MIA-induced tactile allodynia
Intra-articular injection of MIA produced secondary allodynia in the ipsilateral hind paw on days 1 and 14 after injection ($P < 0.05$; $n = 8$–15; Fig. 3a, b). On day 1, URB597 had no effect on von Frey hair mechanosensitivity (Fig. 3a). Prophylactic treatment of MIA-injected knees with URB597 on days 0–3, however, completely abolished the development of MIA-induced hypersensitivity during the chronic phase of the disease ($P < 0.05$; $n = 8$–10; Fig. 3b).

Prophylactic effect of URB597 on MIA-induced saphenous nerve demyelination
Fourteen days after injection of intra-articular MIA, ipsilateral saphenous nerve axons showed a significant

loss of myelin thickness, as evidenced by an increase in G-ratio ($P < 0.05$ compared with saline-injected controls; $n = 5$–7; Fig. 4). Repeated treatment of OA joints with URB597 during the acute phase of the model inhibited this end-stage demyelinating effect ($P < 0.05$; $n = 6$–7; Fig. 4).

Discussion
Although OA is primarily a degenerative disease, many other pathophysiological features can contribute to the global symptoms of the disease. Acute inflammatory flares, for example, are associated with burning and aching sensations while chronic neuropathic symptoms tend to be stabbing and like electric shocks. We hypothesize that the acute inflammatory episodes found in OA drive peripheral neuropathy leading to a complex pain syndrome. The results presented here show that intra-articular injection of MIA produces an acute inflammatory response that resolves within 3 days. Thus, in the acute phase of this OA model there is a transient oedema response which is accompanied by an increase in synovial blood flow and leukocyte trafficking. These observations are similar to other reports which showed that intra-articular injection of MIA caused leukocyte infiltration and oedema which gradually resolved within days [23, 24]. This inflammatory response is thought to be mediated by transient receptor potential ankyrin-1

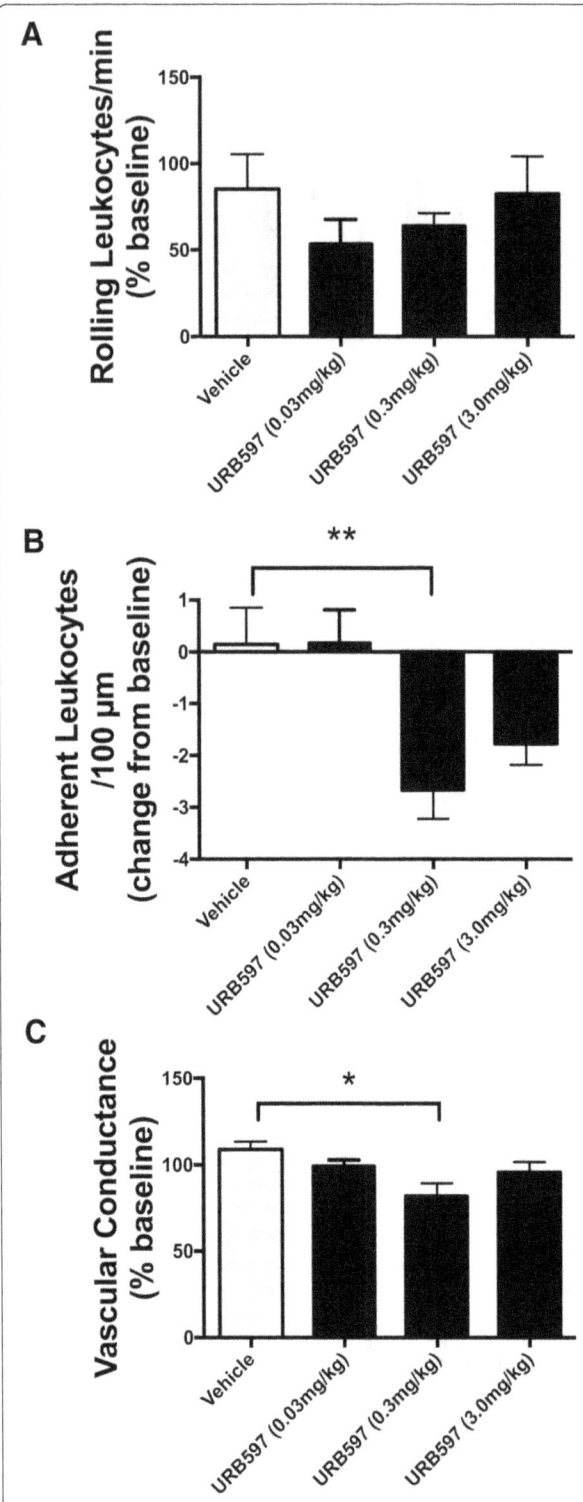

Fig. 2 Local effect of URB597 on day 1 MIA-induced inflammation. **a** URB597 had no significant effect on leukocyte rolling when compared with vehicle. **b** URB597 (0.3 mg/kg) significantly decreased leukocyte adherence when compared with vehicle. **c** URB597 (0.3 mg/kg) significantly decreased knee joint blood flow when compared with vehicle. *******P* < 0.01, ******P* < 0.05 one-way ANOVA with Dunnett's post-hoc test; *n* =5–8. Data presented as mean ± SEM

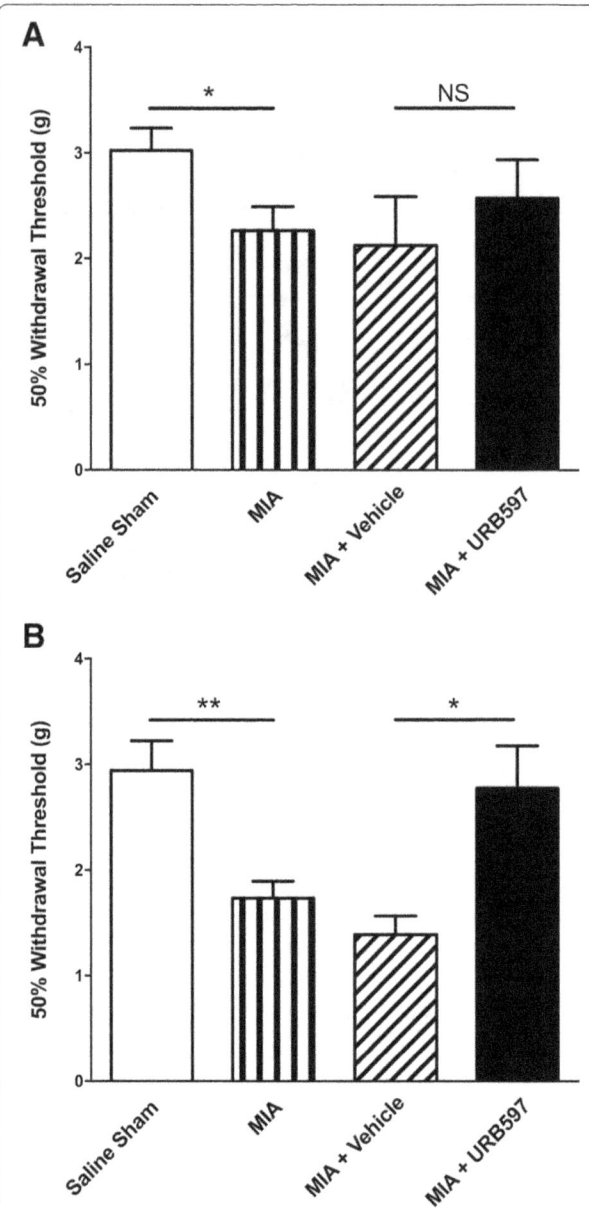

Fig. 3 Effect of prophylactic URB597 treatment on the development of secondary allodynia after MIA injection. Intra-articular injection of MIA significantly reduced von Frey hair withdrawal threshold on day 1 (**a**) and day 14 (**b**) after injection compared with saline-injected knees. Treatment with URB597 (0.3 mg/kg) had no effect on day 1 secondary allodynia while prophylactic URB597 abolished chronic MIA-induced tactile hypersensitivity on day 14 compared with animals treated with a similar regimen of vehicle. **P < 0.01, *P < 0.05 unpaired two-tailed *t* test; *n* = 8–14. Data presented as mean ± SEM. *MIA* monoiodoacetate, *NS* not significant

ion channel opening leading to the subsequent release of neuropeptides and joint neurogenic inflammation [24].

It has been reported previously that the FAAH inhibitor URB597 can reduce acute synovitis and joint neurogenic inflammation in mice [19, 25]. This anti-

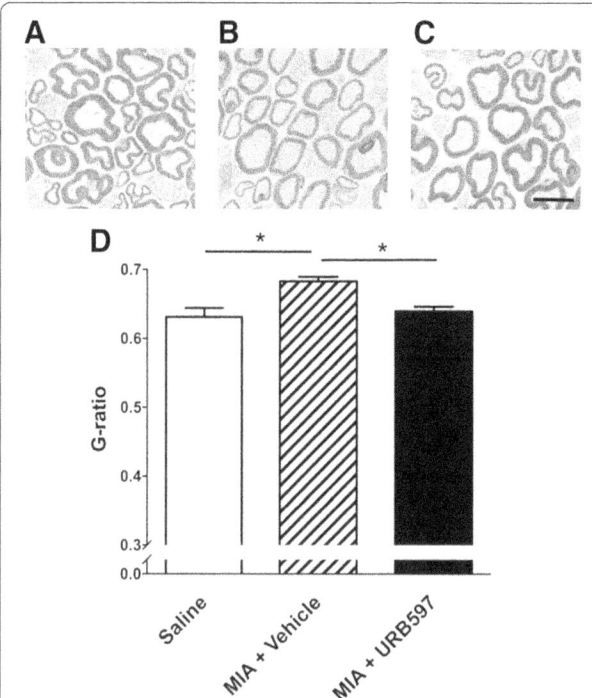

Fig. 4 Prophylactic URB597 inhibits demyelination of joint nerves 14 days after MIA injection. Representative electron micrographs of axons found in saphenous nerves taken at day 14 from animals with a (**a**) saline-injected knee, (**b**) MIA-injected joint treated with vehicle (days 0–3) and (**c**) MIA-injected joint treated with URB597 (0.3 mg/kg, days 0–3). Myelin thickness is noticeably less in OA joint nerves and this demyelination is prevented by prophylactic URB597 treatment. **d** G-ratio calculations showing that MIA causes saphenous axonal demyelination which is prevented by URB597 treatment. *Scale bar* = 6 μm. *$P < 0.05$ one-way ANOVA with Tukey's post-hoc test; $n = 5$–7. Data presented as mean ± SEM. *MIA* monoiodoacetate

net effect of these non-cannabinoid responses would be an attenuation of the anti-inflammatory and analgesic effects seen with the lower dose of URB597.

Local administration of URB597 to MIA-injected knees had no significant effect on the paw withdrawal threshold on day 1, suggesting that this particular FAAH inhibitor does not affect referred pain at the onset of this mouse model. Conversely, treatment of OA joints during the early inflammatory phase of the MIA model prevented the development of secondary allodynia at day 14. The pain generated at this later time point is, in part, due to the joint axonal damage that occurs in the MIA model. Thus, an acute intervention with URB597 during an inflammatory flare has the potential to protect the joint from chronic pain arising at later stages of the disease. Attenuating inflammation at the onset of the model could impede sensory bombardment within the dorsal horn of the spinal cord and avert central sensitization. Previous studies have found that central sensitization occurs in the late stages of the MIA model but not during early stages of the disease [28]. Future studies examining the effect of early URB597 on dorsal horn neuronal excitability in the chronic phase of MIA would help test this hypothesis. Although it is beyond the scope of this pain study, it would be interesting to see whether acute URB597 treatment could alter the course of end-stage joint destruction in OA, because a disease-modifying effect of the drug could also account for the observed prophylactic analgesia described here. While the present study focused on inflammation, pain and joint neuropathy, it would be interesting to see whether acute URB597 treatment could influence joint destruction; however, these histological experiments would be better carried out in a model of OA that more closely mimics the degenerative features of the human disease.

Peripheral neuropathy has been observed in the knees of OA patients [6] and in animal models of joint injury [7]. The present study discovered that MIA-induced OA caused demyelination of the ipsilateral saphenous nerve as evinced by an increase in G-ratio compared with sham control animals. Prophylactic treatment of MIA joints with locally administered URB597 during the inflammatory phase of the model prevented this loss in joint nerve myelination. This finding suggests that promoting endocannabinoids locally in the joint during the onset of OA development can protect the joint from neurodegeneration. Cannabinoids are involved in neurogenesis and are known to be neuroprotective in the nervous system [29, 30]. For example, cannabinoid receptor agonists can inhibit neuronal demyelination in a mouse model of multiple sclerosis by promoting interleukin-6 accumulation which is known to be neuroprotective [31, 32]. In a model of chemical neurotoxicity, the

inflammatory effect of URB597 was reproducible in the current investigation which found that local administration of 0.3 mg/kg URB597 to MIA-injected knees decreased leukocyte adherence and hyperaemia. A lower and higher dose of URB597 failed to alter joint blood flow or leukocyte trafficking and this hormetic response is consistent with a previous finding in a model of acute inflammation [19]. The mechanism by which URB597 loses its efficacy at higher doses has yet to be investigated. One possibility is that the accumulation of endocannabinoids in the joint could trigger cyclooxygenase-2 activity which is known to lead to the production of pro-inflammatory prostamides [26], thereby offsetting any anti-inflammatory effects of FAAH inhibition. An alternative explanation is that high-dose URB597 or the resulting heightened endocannabinoid levels are having off-target effects. In joints, anandamide and the synthetic cannabinoid arachidonyl-2-chloroethylamide can sensitize articular transient receptor potential vanilloid-1 ion channels leading to nociception and hyperaemia [16, 27]. The endocannabinoid hydrolysis inhibitor JZL184 reduced white matter lesions in the spinal cord of affected animals [33]. Interestingly in the same study, URB597 was unable to prevent oligodendrocyte death in vitro; however, the drug was not tested for its neuroprotective potential in vivo using a therapeutic regimen as described here.

Despite the promising data presented here and elsewhere, FAAH inhibition has yet to show a positive clinical effect for treating OA pain in patients. The irreversible FAAH inhibitor PF-04457845 was found to reduce pain in the MIA model [34], but failed to alleviate pain in a heterogeneous population of OA patients [35]. In these preclinical and clinical studies, however, the drug was given systemically, which increases the likelihood of imparting off-target effects in multiple organs. Conversely, the FAAH inhibitor presented here was administered locally around the joint, which would render a more targeted therapy and avoid non-articular side effects. A further limitation of the PF-04457845 clinical trial was that it was carried out on a mixed cohort of OA patients whose disease subtype was undefined. The data described in the present study suggest that FAAH inhibition may be more applicable to OA patients whose pain has a strong neuropathic component.

Conclusion

Inhibition of the endocannabinoid hydrolysis enzyme FAAH results in a reduction in the acute inflammation that occurs at the onset of MIA-induced OA. By blocking this inflammatory response, URB597 reduces OA pain and prevents joint nerve damage during the chronic degenerative phase of the disease. These results suggest that early suppression of an inflammatory flare by articular endocannabinoids may be beneficial in attenuating the development of late-stage OA neuropathic pain.

Abbreviations

2-AG: 2-Arachidonoylglycerol; ATF-3: Activated transcription factor-3; CB: Cannabinoid; DMSO: Dimethylsulphoxide; DRG: Dorsal root ganglia; FAAH: Fatty acid amide hydrolase; IVM: Intravital microscopy; LASCA: Laser speckle contrast analysis; MAP: Mean arterial pressure; MIA: Monoiodoacetate; OA: Osteoarthritis

Acknowledgements
None.

Funding
This work was supported by an operating grant provided by The Arthritis Society.

Authors' contributions
JJM conceived the study, participated in its design, coordinated all experiments, helped analyse data and drafted the manuscript. MMM carried out IVM and LASCA experiments, analysed resulting data and helped draft the manuscript. HTP carried out the G-ratio measurements, analysed the demyelination data and helped draft the revised manuscript. AR conducted the pain behaviour experiments, analysed data and helped draft the manuscript. EK conducted IVM and LASCA experiments, analysed resulting data and helped draft the manuscript. All authors read and approved the final manuscript.

Authors' information
JJM is Professor of Pharmacology and Anaesthesia, Pain Management & Perioperative Medicine, Dalhousie University, Halifax, NS, Canada. MMM, HTP, AR and EK are with the Department of Pharmacology and Department of Anaesthesia, Pain Management & Perioperative Medicine, Dalhousie University, Halifax, NS, Canada.

Competing interests
The authors declare that they have no competing interests.

Consent for publication
Not applicable.

References
1. Hannan MT, Felson DT, Pincus T. Analysis of the discordance between radiographic changes and knee pain in osteoarthritis of the knee. J Rheumatol. 2000;27(6):1513–7.
2. McDougall JJ, Andruski B, Schuelert N, Hallgrimsson B, Matyas JR. Unravelling the relationship between age, nociception and joint destruction in naturally occurring osteoarthritis of Dunkin Hartley guinea pigs. Pain. 2009;141(3):222–32.
3. Kelly S, Dunham JP, Murray F, Read S, Donaldson LF, Lawson SN. Spontaneous firing in C-fibers and increased mechanical sensitivity in A-fibers of knee joint-associated mechanoreceptive primary afferent neurones during MIA-induced osteoarthritis in the rat. Osteoarthr Cartil. 2012;20(4):305–13.
4. Krustev E, Rioux D, McDougall JJ. Mechanisms and mediators that drive arthritis pain. Curr Osteoporos Rep. 2015;13(4):216–24.
5. Wegman A, van der Windt D, van Tulder M, Stalman W, de Vries T. Nonsteroidal antiinflammatory drugs or acetaminophen for osteoarthritis of the hip or knee? A systematic review of evidence and guidelines. J Rheumatol. 2004;31(2):344–54.
6. Grönblad M, Konttinen YT, Korkala O, Liesi P, Hukkanen M, Polak JM. Neuropeptides in the synovium of patients with rheumatoid arthritis and osteoarthritis. J Rheumatol. 1988;15:1807–10.
7. McDougall JJ, Bray RC, Sharkey KA. A morphological and immunohistochemical examination of nerves in normal and injured collateral ligaments of rat, rabbit and human knee joints. Anat Rec. 1997;248:29–39.
8. Ivanavicius SP, Ball AD, Heapy CG, Westwood FR, Murray F, Read SJ. Structural pathology in a rodent model of osteoarthritis is associated with neuropathic pain: increased expression of ATF-3 and pharmacological characterisation. Pain. 2007;128(3):272–82.
9. Thakur M, Rahman W, Hobbs C, Dickenson AH, Bennett DL. Characterisation of a peripheral neuropathic component of the rat monoiodoacetate model of osteoarthritis. PLoS One. 2012;7(3):e33730.
10. McDougall JJ, Albacete S, Schülert N, Mitchell PG, Lin C, Oskins JL, Biu H, Chambers MG. Lysophosphatidic acid provides a missing link between osteoarthritis and joint neuropathic pain. OA Cart. 2017; in press.
11. Orita S, Ishikawa T, Miyagi M, Ochiai N, Inoue G, Eguchi Y, Kamoda H, Arai G, Toyone T, Aoki Y, et al. Pain-related sensory innervation in monoiodoacetate-induced osteoarthritis in rat knees that gradually develops neuronal injury in addition to inflammatory pain. BMC Musculoskelet Disord. 2011;12:134.
12. Milligan ED, Twining C, Chacur M, Biedenkapp J, O'Connor K, Poole S, Tracey K, Martin D, Maier SF, Watkins LR. Spinal glia and proinflammatory cytokines mediate mirror-image neuropathic pain in rats. J Neurosci. 2003;23(3):1026–40.

13. Schafers M, Svensson CI, Sommer C, Sorkin LS. Tumor necrosis factor-alpha induces mechanical allodynia after spinal nerve ligation by activation of p38 MAPK in primary sensory neurons. J Neurosci. 2003;23(7):2517–21.

14. McDougall JJ. Cannabinoids and pain control in the periphery. In: Cairns BE, editor. Peripheral Receptor Targets for Analgesia: Novel Approaches to Pain Management. Hoboken, NJ: John Wiley & Sons Inc.; 2009. p. 325–46.

15. Schuelert N, Zhang C, Mogg AJ, Broad LM, Hepburn DL, Nisenbaum ES, Johnson MP, McDougall JJ. Paradoxical effects of the cannabinoid CB2 receptor agonist GW405833 on rat osteoarthritic knee joint pain. OA Cart. 2010;18(11):1536–43.

16. Baker CL, McDougall JJ. The cannabinomimetic arachidonyl-2-chloroethylamide (ACEA) acts on capsaicin-sensitive TRPV1 receptors but not cannabinoid receptors in rat joints. Br J Pharmacol. 2004;142(8):1361–7.

17. Burston JJ, Sagar DR, Shao P, Bai M, King E, Brailsford L, Turner JM, Hathway GJ, Bennett AJ, Walsh DA, et al. Cannabinoid CB2 receptors regulate central sensitization and pain responses associated with osteoarthritis of the knee joint. PLoS One. 2013;8(11):e80440.

18. Richardson D, Pearson RG, Kurian N, Latif ML, Garle MJ, Barrett DA, Kendall DA, Scammell BE, Reeve AJ, Chapman V. Characterisation of the cannabinoid receptor system in synovial tissue and fluid in patients with osteoarthritis and rheumatoid arthritis. Arthritis Res Ther. 2008;10(2):R43.

19. Krustev E, Reid A, McDougall JJ. Tapping into the endocannabinoid system to ameliorate acute inflammatory flares and associated pain in mouse knee joints. Arthritis Res Ther. 2014;16(5):437.

20. Schuelert N, Johnson MP, Oskins JL, Jassal K, Chambers MG, McDougall JJ. Local application of the endocannabinoid hydrolysis inhibitor URB597 reduces nociception in spontaneous and chemically induced models of osteoarthritis. Pain. 2011;152(5):975–81.

21. Andruski B, McCafferty DM, Ignacy T, Millen B, McDougall JJ. Leukocyte trafficking and pain behavioral responses to a hydrogen sulfide donor in acute monoarthritis. Am J Physiol Regul Integr Comp Physiol. 2008;295(3):R814–20.

22. Chaplan SR, Bach FW, Pogrel JW, Chung JM, Yaksh TL. Quantitative assessment of tactile allodynia in the rat paw. J Neurosci Methods 1994; 53(1):55–63.

23. Bove SE, Calcaterra SL, Brooker RM, Huber CM, Guzman RE, Juneau PL, Schrier DJ, Kilgore KS. Weight bearing as a measure of disease progression and efficacy of anti-inflammatory compounds in a model of monosodium iodoacetate-induced osteoarthritis. OA Cart. 2003;11(11):821–30.

24. Moilanen LJ, Hamalainen M, Nummenmaa E, Ilmarinen P, Vuolteenaho K, Nieminen RM, Lehtimaki L, Moilanen E. Monosodium iodoacetate-induced inflammation and joint pain are reduced in TRPA1 deficient mice—potential role of TRPA1 in osteoarthritis. OA Cart. 2015;23(11):2017–26.

25. Krustev E, Muley MM, McDougall JJ. Endocannabinoids inhibit neurogenic inflammation in murine joints by a non-canonical cannabinoid receptor mechanism. Neuropep. 2017; in press.

26. Alhouayek M, Muccioli GG. COX-2-derived endocannabinoid metabolites as novel inflammatory mediators. Trends Pharmacol Sci. 2014;35(6):284–92.

27. Gauldie SD, McQueen DS, Pertwee R, Chessell IP. Anandamide activates peripheral nociceptors in normal and arthritic rat knee joints. Br J Pharmacol. 2001;132(3):617–21.

28. Kelly S, Dobson KL, Harris J. Spinal nociceptive reflexes are sensitized in the monosodium iodoacetate model of osteoarthritis pain in the rat. OA Cart. 2013;21(9):1327–35.

29. Maccarrone M, Guzman M, Mackie K, Doherty P, Harkany T. Programming of neural cells by (endo)cannabinoids: from physiological rules to emerging therapies. Nat Rev Neurosci. 2014;15(12):786–801.

30. Micale V, Mazzola C, Drago F. Endocannabinoids and neurodegenerative diseases. Pharmacol Res. 2007;56(5):382–92.

31. Arevalo-Martin A, Vela JM, Molina-Holgado E, Borrell J, Guaza C. Therapeutic action of cannabinoids in a murine model of multiple sclerosis. J Neurosci. 2003;23(7):2511–6.

32. Molina-Holgado F, Molina-Holgado E, Guaza C. The endogenous cannabinoid anandamide potentiates interleukin-6 production by astrocytes infected with Theiler's murine encephalomyelitis virus by a receptor-mediated pathway. FEBS Lett. 1998;433(1–2):139–42.

33. Bernal-Chico A, Canedo M, Manterola A, Victoria Sanchez-Gomez M, Perez-Samartin A, Rodriguez-Puertas R, Matute C, Mato S. Blockade of monoacylglycerol lipase inhibits oligodendrocyte excitotoxicity and prevents demyelination in vivo. Glia. 2015;63(1):163–76.

34. Ahn K, Smith SE, Liimatta MB, Beidler D, Sadagopan N, Dudley DT, Young T, Wren P, Zhang Y, Swaney S, et al. Mechanistic and pharmacological characterization of PF-04457845: a highly potent and selective fatty acid amide hydrolase inhibitor that reduces inflammatory and noninflammatory pain. J Pharmacol Exp Ther. 2011;338(1):114–24.

35. Huggins JP, Smart TS, Langman S, Taylor L, Young T. An efficient randomised, placebo-controlled clinical trial with the irreversible fatty acid amide hydrolase-1 inhibitor PF-04457845, which modulates endocannabinoids but fails to induce effective analgesia in patients with pain due to osteoarthritis of the knee. Pain. 2012;153(9):1837–46.

Calcification of the acetabular labrum of the hip: prevalence in the general population and relation to hip articular cartilage and fibrocartilage degeneration

Thelonius Hawellek[1*†], Jan Hubert[1†], Sandra Hischke[2], Matthias Krause[3], Jessica Bertrand[4], Burkhard C. Schmidt[5], Andreas Kronz[5], Klaus Püschel[6], Wolfgang Rüther[1] and Andreas Niemeier[1*]

Abstract

Background: Meniscal calcification is considered to play a relevant role in the pathogenesis of osteoarthritis of the knee. Little is known about the biology of acetabular labral disease and its importance in hip pathology. Here, we analyze for the first time the calcification of the acetabular labrum of the hip (ALH) and its relation to hip cartilage degeneration.

Methods: In this cross-sectional post-mortem study of an unselected sample of the general population, 170 ALH specimens and 170 femoral heads from 85 donors (38 female, 47 male; mean age 62.1 years) were analyzed by high-resolution digital contact radiography (DCR) and histological degeneration grade. The medial menisci (MM) from the same 85 donors served as an intra-individual reference for cartilage calcification (CC). Scanning electron microscopy (SEM), energy dispersive analysis (ED) and Raman spectroscopy were performed for characterization of ALH CC.

Results: The prevalence of CC in the ALH was 100% and that in the articular cartilage of the hip (ACH) was 96.5%. Quantitative analysis revealed that the amount of ALH CC was higher than that in the ACH (factor 3.0, $p < 0.001$) and in the MM (factor 1.3, $p < 0.001$). There was significant correlation between the amount of CC in the fibrocartilage of the left and right ALH ($r = 0.70$, $p < 0.001$). Independent of age, the amount of ALH CC correlated with histological degeneration of the ALH (Krenn score) ($r = 0.55$; $p < 0.001$) and the ACH (Osteoarthritis Research Society International (OARSI), $r = 0.69$; $p < 0.001$). Calcification of the ALH was characterized as calcium pyrophosphate dihydrate deposition.

Conclusion: The finding that ALH fibrocartilage is a strongly calcifying tissue is unexpected and novel. The fact that ALH calcification correlates with cartilage degeneration independent of age is suggestive of an important role of ALH calcification in osteoarthritis of the hip and renders it a potential target for the prevention and treatment of hip joint degeneration.

Keywords: Acetabular labrum, Hip, Chondrocalcinosis, Cartilage calcification, CPPD, Osteoarthritis

* Correspondence: thelonius.hawellek@med.uni-goettingen.de;
niemeier@uke.uni-hamburg.de
†Equal contributors
[1]Department of Orthopaedics, University Medical Center
Hamburg-Eppendorf, Martinistraße 52, 20246 Hamburg, Germany
Full list of author information is available at the end of the article

Background

Osteoarthritis (OA) is a major health problem and represents the most common joint disease in western populations [1]. OA affects the whole joint and therefore involves hyaline cartilage, subchondral bone, the joint capsule, periarticular ligaments and fibrocartilage [2]. Until now the understanding of the molecular events that initiate and maintain OA pathogenesis remain incompletely understood. One factor of interest is cartilage calcification (CC). It is detectable in 100% of the hyaline cartilage of end-stage hip and knee OA [3, 4]. Calcium crystals have the potential to induce a pro-inflammatory intra-articular milieu [5–8] and also to alter the biomechanical properties of the cartilage [9, 10], both of which may finally result in OA [11].

Compared to articular hyaline cartilage, the fibrocartilage of the meniscus of the knee seems to be particularly prone to calcification [12, 13] and meniscal calcification is highly prevalent in knee OA [14, 15]. In addition, meniscal cells calcify more readily in OA than in healthy knees and calcification may alter the biomechanical properties of the meniscus, which may further contribute to OA development [14]. Accordingly, meniscal calcification is considered to play a relevant role in the pathogenesis of knee OA [14–18].

In contrast to the meniscus of the knee, little is known about calcification of the fibrocartilage of the hip, the acetabular labrum (ALH) and its relation to cartilage degeneration. Although the role of the acetabular labrum in hip joint pathology has recently gained much attention [19, 20], knowledge about cellular mechanisms that govern labral function is scarce. It has recently been described that ALH cells appear to have a similar metabolic profile to meniscal cells [21], but to our knowledge there is only one study in which ALH calcification was analyzed in a larger cohort (106 hip joints in 66 individuals) by computed tomography (CT), finding a prevalence of 18% [22]. Of note, CC starts in the nanomicrometer to micrometer range and is therefore hard or almost impossible to detect in the initial stages by standard radiographic methods with low-resolution x-ray, CT or magnetic resonance imaging (MRI). Therefore, little is known about the actual prevalence of early initial crystallization in human joints in general, and in the ALH in particular [23]. The most sensitive method available for the detection of such micro-calcifications is high-resolution digital contact radiography (DCR) [4, 24]. A disadvantage of this method is that DCR can only be applied to tissue samples ex vivo.

The goal of the present study was to describe the prevalence of DCR-detectable ALH calcification in an unselected sample of the general population and to analyze the relationship between the amount of ALH calcification and the degree of fibrocartilage and articular cartilage degeneration in the hip. Since we have recently described that there appears to be a systemic drive for CC [25, 26], here we used both medial menisci (MM) as a reference for the individual propensity to develop CC.

Methods

A total of 170 ALH, femoral heads (FH) and MM were obtained from both hip and knee joints in an unselected sample of 85 individuals (hereafter referred to as "donors") who underwent autopsy at the Department for Legal Medicine [27], University Medical Center Hamburg-Eppendorf. Only donors with bilaterally intact hip and knee joints without any signs of hip and/or knee disease other than OA were included in this study. None of the donors had evidence of previous hip and/or knee surgery. Donors with history of tumors, infections or rheumatic diseases were excluded from the study population. The study was approved by the local ethics committee (reference number PV4570) and is in compliance with the Helsinki Declaration. The mean age was 62.1 years (range 20–93 years); 38 of the donors were female and 47 male. Biometric characteristics of the donors are listed in Table 1. Some of the data on hip articular cartilage calcification in this larger cohort have previously been analyzed and published in another context [25]. First the FH, ALH and MM were resected in toto. Any attached soft tissue was removed from the ALH, FH and MM. For FH analysis, standardized 4 mm bone and cartilage slabs were cut in the central coronal and axial planes, resulting in three standardized (central, anterior and posterior) slabs per sample as published previously [25]. ALH and MM were kept in toto.

Digital contact radiography (DCR)

The ALH, the bone-cartilage slabs of the FH and the MM were washed with physiological solution to remove residual bone debris. Standardized radiographs were taken (25 kV, 3.8 mAs, film focus distance 8 cm) using a

Table 1 Biometric characteristics of the study population ($n = 85$)

Characteristic	Value
Age in years	62.1 ± 19.3
Male	60.1 ± 18.6
Female	64.6 ± 20.0
Height in cm	
Male	176.9 ± 7.1
Female	164.7 ± 7.9
Body weight in kg	
Male	83.2 ± 18.3
Female	72.3 ± 21.0
Body mass index in kg/m^2	26.5 ± 6.0

high-resolution digital radiography device (Faxitron X-Ray, Illinois, USA). Quantitative computerized analysis of the areas of CC of each complete ALH, the three bone-cartilage slabs of the FH and the complete MM was performed with standard software (ImageJ 1.46, National Institutes of Health, Bethesda, USA) as published previously [3, 4, 28]. The percentage of calcification of the ALH and MM was determined by dividing the measured area of calcification by the total fibrocartilage area of the particular anatomical structure. The percentage of CC in each of the three slabs of the FH was determined by dividing the measured area of calcification by the total cartilage area per slab. The mean amount of calcification measured from the three slabs of the FH was regarded to be representative of the entire articular cartilage of the hip (ACH).

Classification of acetabular labrum calcification
Based on previously published soft tissue classifications [29–31], the distribution of ALH calcification was categorized as three different patterns (singular, spotted or streaky) on DCR images (Fig. 1).

Histology
Histological degeneration of the fibrocartilage of the superior-anterior part of each ALH and of the hyaline cartilage of the main load-bearing zone of each FH (central zone, directly adjacent to the central slab plane) was assessed. All specimens were fixed in 4% paraformaldehyde (PFA) for 24 h, dehydrated in 80% alcohol, embedded in paraffin and 4-μm sections were prepared. Sections of the ALH were stained with hematoxylin and eosin (Fig. 2b) and samples of the FH were stained with 1% Safranin-O to evaluate the histological degeneration grade of the tissue sample according

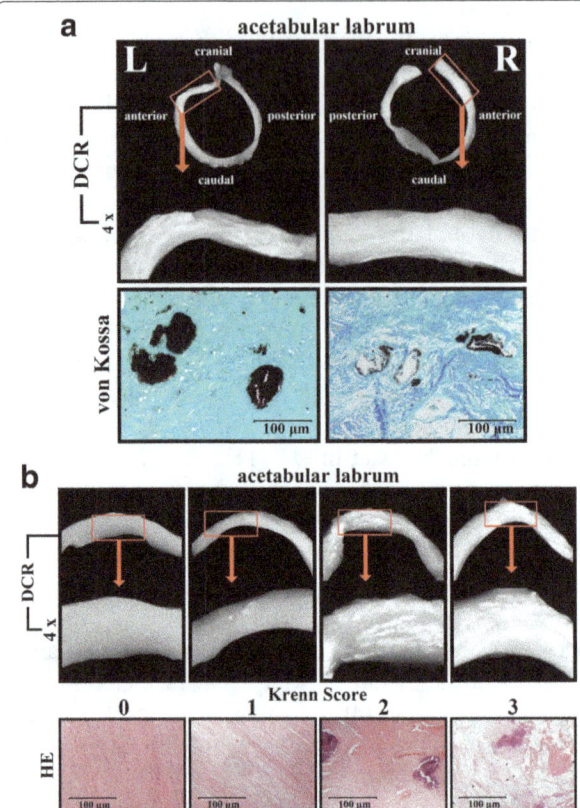

Fig. 2 a Representative digital contrast radiography (DCR) images (presented in original size and × 4 magnification (red boxes)) of the acetabular labrum (L = left, R = right) from one donor showing distinct cartilage calcification and the corresponding histological images in which cartilage calcifications (black) were confirmed histochemically by von Kossa staining. **b** DCR images (presented in original size and × 4 magnification (red boxes)) with increasing cartilage calcifications (from left to the right) of the acetabular labrum from different donors and the corresponding rising histological degeneration grade, which was evaluated by the Krenn score (0–3) on hematoxylin-eosin (HE) staining

to the Krenn-score for fibrocartilage (grade 0–3; Table 2) [32] and the Osteoarthritis Research Society International (OARSI) osteoarthritis cartilage histopathology assessment system for hyaline cartilage (grade 0–6) [33]. Calcifications identified by DCR were confirmed to represent calcium-phosphate crystal deposition by von Kossa staining (Fig. 2a).

Characterization of acetabular labrum calcification
To characterize the physicochemical nature of ALH CC detected by DCR and confirmed by von Kossa staining, 10 randomly selected labral specimens were processed for further analysis.

Scanning electron microscopy
For morphology studies semiquantitative electron probe microanalysis and scanning electron microscopy (SEM) of secondary electrons (SE) were performed on a

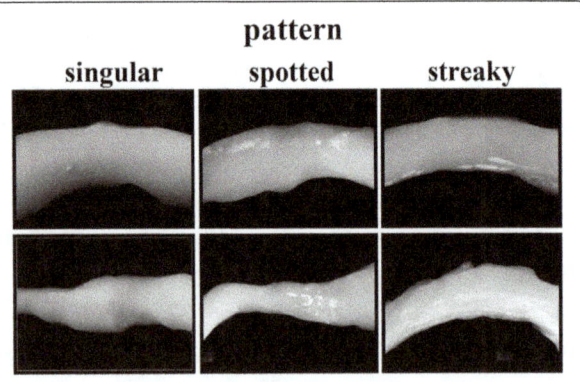

Fig. 1 Exemplary samples of digital contact radiography images of the acetabular labrum from six different donors with distinct cartilage calcification. Cartilage calcification was detected as radiopaque spots within the fibrocartilage of the acetabular labrum. The cartilage calcification was classified into three typical calcification patterns (singular, spotted and streaky)

Table 2 Krenn score – histopathological evaluation of the degeneration grade of the fibrocartilage (0–3)

Grade	Features
0	Normal histological morphology • Isomorphic chondrocytes • Homogeneously eosinophil-stained matrix • Regular cellularity
1	Low-grade degeneration • Low reduction of cellularity (small areas) • Inhomogeneous stained matrix • Small fissures in the matrix
2	Moderate degeneration • Moderate reduction of cellularity (large areas) • Variable size and shape of chondrocytes • Moderate fissures in the matrix
3	High-grade degeneration • Strong reduction of cellularity • Large areas of complete loss of chondrocytes • Reticular/basophilic stained matrix (mucoid degeneration) • Large fissures in the matrix (pseudocysts)

JEOL 8900RL (JEOL, Ltd., Akishima, Japan) to obtain information about the surface of the ALH cartilage and minerals. The accelerating voltage was set to 10 kV and a beam current of 1.5 nA was used for the quantitative analysis. SEM images were performed at 10 kV accelerating voltage and a variable beam current between 0.1 and 0.25 nA.

To determine the chemical elements in the samples and to analyze the qualitative and semiquantitative chemical compositions raw x-ray counts were acquired by a SiriusSD® (SGX Sensortech Ltd.) energy dispersive (ED) silicon drift detector. For calibration a natural apatite crystal $(Ca_5(OH,Cl,F)(PO_4)_3)$ was used for calcium and phosphate and albite $(NaAlSi_3O_8)$ was used for sodium. Prior to the measurement the samples were coated with a thin layer of gold (20 nm).

Raman spectroscopy

Raman spectroscopy was performed on unstained labrum specimens. Raman spectra were obtained using a Horiba Jobin Yvon HR 800 UV Raman spectrometer with an attached Olympus BX41 microscope. The samples were excited using a 488 nm laser line of a Coherent Sapphire solid-state laser, with 50 mW at the laser exit. The use of a holographic grating with 600 lines/mm and a CCD-detector with 1024×256 pixels yielded a spectral dispersion of better than 2.2/cm per pixel. Raman spectra were collected in three spectral windows in the range 200/cm to 4000/cm with an acquisition time of 2×2 s for each spectral window. The Raman spectra were frequency corrected using silicon (Si band at 520.4/cm), which was measured directly after the sample measurement. The collected Raman spectra were compared to reference spectra for hydroxyapatite $(960 \ cm^{-1})$ and calcium pyrophosphate dihydrate $(1050 \ cm^{-1})$ [34].

Statistical analysis

The biometric characteristics of donors are reported as mean values ± standard deviations. For descriptive analysis, mean cartilage calcification values for the hyaline cartilage of the femoral head were used. Data were logarithmically transformed if appropriate. For categorical data Fisher's and McNemar's tests were used. A linear mixed model was used to analyze the difference between the mean amount of cartilage calcification in the ALH, FH and MM considering side and joint as fixed effects. Subject was used as a random effect with a compound symmetry covariance structure. In addition, the mixed model assumptions were checked using residual plots. To report the association between continuous variables Pearson's (r) or Spearman's (r_s) rank correlation coefficient was calculated. To test the correlation between cartilage calcification, histological degeneration and age, the mean value of the left and right femoral head and the mean value of the left and right labrum were calculated for each individual. To avoid spurious correlation, a test of partial correlation was performed adjusting for the respective excluded parameters (cartilage calcification, histological OA grade and age). All statistical analyses were performed with statistical software R [35], version 3.1.1. P values less than 0.05 were considered statistically significant.

Results

Prevalence of cartilage calcification

The prevalence of CC of the ALH was 100% (85/85) (95% CI 0.96, 1.00), of the ACH it was 96.5% (82/85) (95% CI 0.90, 0.99) and of the MM it was 98.8% (84/85) (95% CI 0.94, 1.00) (Table 3). The prevalence of bilateral CC of the ALH was 100% (85/85) (95% CI 0.96, 1.00), of the ACH it was 80.0% (68/85) (95% CI 0.70, 0.88) and of the MM it was 92.9% (79/85) (95% CI 0.85, 0.97) (Table 3). Von Kossa stained histological sections confirmed that DCR-detectable CC actually represents calcium-phosphate crystal depositions at the histological level (Fig. 2a). CC was detected in 100% of the left and right ALH (85/85), in 88.2% of the left and right ACH (75/85), in 94.1% of the left MM (80/85) and in 97.6% of the right MM (83/85). There was no significant preponderance of CC according to left or right side in the ALH $(p = 1.0)$, ACH $(p = 1.0)$ and MM $(p = 0.38)$ (Table 3). There was no significant difference in the prevalence of CC by sex in the ALH $(p = 1.0)$, FH $(p = 0.09)$ and MM $(p = 1.0)$.

Table 3 Prevalence of DCR-detectable cartilage calcification (n = 85)

	Acetabular labrum		Femoral head		Medial meniscus	
	Number	Percentage	Number	Percentage	Number	Percentage
Total calcified cartilage (CC)	85/85	100	82/85	96.5	84/85	98.8
Bilateral CC	85/85	100	68/85	80.0	79/85	92.9
Unilateral CC	0/85	0	14/85	16.5	5/85	5.9
Left CC	85/85	100	75/85	88.2	80/85	94.1
Right CC	85/85	100	75/85	88.2	83/85	97.7

Quantitative analysis of ALH calcification reveals a higher degree of calcification than in articular and meniscal cartilage

There was significant correlation between the amount of CC in the fibrocartilage of the left and right ALH ($r = 0.70$, $p < 0.001$, 95% CI 0.57 0.79) (Fig. 3a) and between the ALH and the MM ($r = 0.66$, $p < 0.001$, 95% CI 0.52 0.76) (Fig. 3b) and the ALH and the ACH ($r = 0.48$, $p < 0.001$, 95% CI 0.30 0.63) (Fig. 3c).

A significant difference was found between the amount of CC in the three distinct cartilage tissues, with the amount of CC in the fibrocartilage in the ALH being significantly higher than that in the ACH by factor 3.0 ($p < 0.001$) and higher than that in the MM by factor 1.3 ($p < 0.001$) per tissue volume unit (Fig. 3d).

Calcification of the ALH correlates with histological hip degeneration independent of age

When adjusted for age there was significant correlation between the amount of CC in the ALH and the histological degeneration grade of the ALH according to the Krenn score ($r = 0.55$, $p < 0.001$) (Figs. 2b and 4a). The distribution of the degeneration grade with detailed data on the donors and according to the mean amount of CC

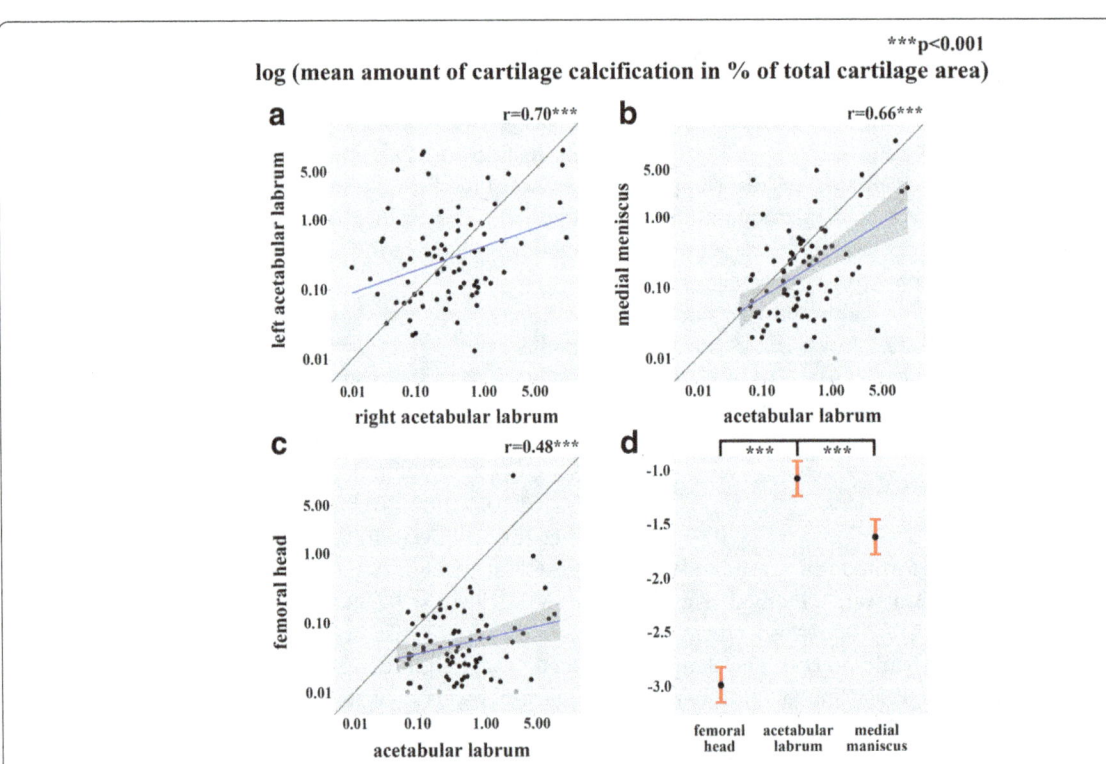

Fig. 3 a–c Logarithmic scatter plots show significant correlation for the mean amount of calcified cartilage (CC) in percentage of total cartilage area between the left and right acetabular labrum ($r = 0.70$, 95% CI 0.57 0.79), $p < 0.001$) (**a**), the medial meniscus and the acetabular labrum ($r = 0.66$, 95% CI 0.52 0.76), $p < 0.001$) (**b**) and the femoral head and the acetabular labrum ($r = 0.48$, 95% CI 0.30 0.63), $p < 0.001$) (**c**). Data points are jittered to avoid over plotting. Logarithmic scatter plots are shown with the blue orthogonal regression line and with the corresponding correlation coefficient (*r*). **d** Logarithmic effect plot of the mean amount of CC in percentage of total cartilage area for the femoral head, the acetabular labrum and the medial meniscus. The amount of CC in the fibrocartilage of the acetabular labrum was significant larger compared to the amount of CC in the medial meniscus (factor of 1.3, $p < 0.001$) and the amount of CC in the acetabular labrum was significant larger compared to the amount of CC in the hyaline cartilage of the femoral head (factor of 3.0, $p < 0.001$)

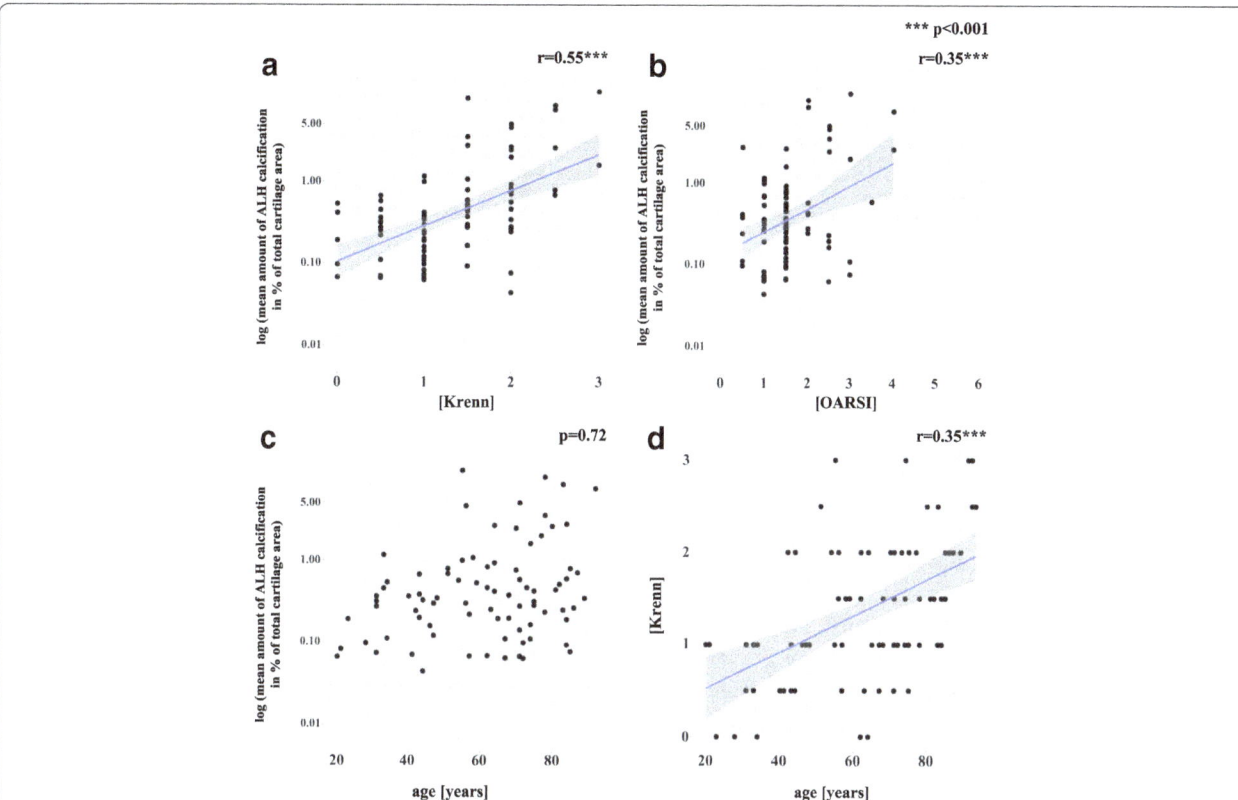

Fig. 4 Logarithmic scatter plots show significant correlation between the mean amount of calcification (percentage of total cartilage area) of the acetabular labrum of the hip (ALH) and the histological degeneration grade (Krenn) of the ALH (*r* = 0.55, *p* < 0.001) after adjustment for age (**a**), the mean amount of ALH calcification (percentage of total cartilage area) and the histological osteoarthritis (OA) grade for the hyaline cartilage (Osteoarthritis Research Society International (OARSI)) of the femoral head (*r* = 0.35, *p* < 0.001) after adjustment for age (**b**) and the histological degeneration grade (Krenn) of the ALH and age (*r* = 0.35, *p* < 0.001) after adjusting for cartilage calcification (**d**). **c** There was no correlation between the mean amount of ALH calcification (percentage of total cartilage area) and age (*p* = 0.72) after adjusting for the histological degeneration grade. Data points are jittered to avoid over plotting. Logarithmic scatter plots are shown with the blue orthogonal regression line and with the corresponding correlation coefficient (*r*)

in the ALH is shown in Table 4. Moreover, there was significant correlation between the amount of CC in the ALH and the histological OA grade of the ACH (OARSI) after adjustment for age ($r = 0.35$, $p < 0.001$) (Fig. 4b). There was significant correlation between the amount of CC in the ALH and age ($r_s = 0.32$, $p = 0.003$), which was no longer significant after adjustment for the histological ALH degeneration grade ($r_s = 0.04$, $p = 0.72$) (Fig. 4c). There was significant correlation between the histological degeneration grade of the ALH and age ($r = 0.50$, $p < 0.001$), which persisted after adjustment for CC ($r = 0.35$, $p < 0.001$) (Fig. 4d).

Classification of acetabular labrum calcification
In 56.5% of all analyzed samples calcification could be classified as a singular calcification pattern. In 28.8% and 14.7% of the samples, respectively, a spotted or a streaky calcification pattern was detected (Fig. 1). In samples with a singular calcification pattern the mean amount of calcification was 0.38% (SD ±0.68) and the mean histological degeneration grade was 1.1 (SD ±0.8). In samples with a spotted or a streaky calcification pattern, respectively, the mean amount of calcification was 0.91% (SD ±1.54) and 10.01% (SD ±12.2) and the mean histological degeneration grade was 1.5 (SD ±0.9) and 2.0 (SD ±1.0) (Table 5).

Table 4 Distribution of the degeneration grade of the acetabular labrum (n = 170)

Grade	Number	Percentage	Male	Percentage	Female	Percentage	Mean amount of calcified cartilage
0	26/170	15.3	17/94	18.1	9/76	11.8	0.25 (SD ±0.31)
1	79/170	46.5	37/94	39.4	42/76	55.3	0.37 (SD ±0.77)
2	44/170	25.9	28/94	29.8	16/76	21.1	1.69 (SD ±4.40)
3	19/170	11.2	10/94	10.6	9/76	11.8	11.70 (SD ±12.25)

Table 5 Calcification pattern of the acetabular labrum (n = 170) with the corresponding mean histological degeneration grade (Krenn score) and the mean amount of cartilage calcification

Pattern			Krenn Score		Mean calcified cartilage	
	Number	Percentage	Mean	SD	Percentage	SD
Singular	96/170	56.5%	1.1	±0.8	0.38	±0.68
Spotted	49/170	28.8	1.5	±0.9	0.91	±1.54
Streaky	25/170	14.7	2.0	±1.0	10.01	±12.2

Characterization of acetabular labrum calcification

Well-developed crystals of prismatic and rhomboid habit, the typical form of calcium pyrophosphate dihydrate (CPPD) crystals, were detected by SEM imaging (Fig. 5a). Using energy dispersive qualitative element analysis (ED) oxygen, phosphorous, calcium and small amounts of sodium were detected. The mean calcium/phosphate (Ca/P) molar ratio was approximately 1.0 in all samples, indicating the presence of CPPD crystals. By Raman spectroscopy only spectra could be detected, which can be assigned to triclinic calcium pyrophosphate dihydrate (t-CPPD, $Ca_2P_2O_7 \cdot 2H_2O$) (Fig. 5b). In conclusion, when assessed by SEM, ED and Raman spectroscopy, only CPPD crystals were detected in the ALH samples. We did not find evidence of the appearance of basic calcium phosphate crystals in the analyzed samples.

Discussion

Here we demonstrated that fibrocartilage calcification of the ALH is highly prevalent in an unselected sample of the general population, including in histologically healthy tissue. The amount of ALH calcification correlates significantly with fibrocartilage and articular cartilage degeneration of the hip independent of age.

These data are entirely novel and shed new and unexpected light on the potential clinical relevance of ALH calcification. Given that in the existing literature the prevalence of ALH calcification is estimated to be smaller than 20% [22], the prevalence of 100% reported here was highly unexpected. This first-sight discrepancy is likely to be explained by the unequalled sensitivity of CC detection by DCR as compared to native CT [24]. Taking this into account, it was still striking to observe that both the prevalence and the amount of CC per unit of tissue volume were significantly higher in the ALH than in the ACH or the MM within the same individuals (Fig. 3d). Most interestingly in this context, we observed CC in histologically healthy labral tissue. Thus, labral calcification cannot just be a result or byproduct of degenerative tissue changes, but rather seems to precede the degeneration. In light of the correlation between the amount of CC in the ALH and histological degeneration of both the labrum and the articular cartilage independent of age (Fig. 4), these data open the possibility (although speculative at the present time) that the calcification crystals may be involved as a causative factor. We have previously reported that articular cartilage calcification can be looked at as the result of a systemically driven process [25, 26], which was reconfirmed by the present data, exemplified by correlation between the amount of CC in the ALH and that in the MM and the contralateral ALH in this unselected cohort of donors (Fig. 3a, b).

The results of this study support the idea that if the degree of CC in the ALH even in young individuals exceeds some yet to be defined threshold, this may trigger labral and subsequently total hip joint pathologic change. Further research will be needed to support this concept, in particular in regard to the underlying cellular and molecular mechanisms and in regard to the

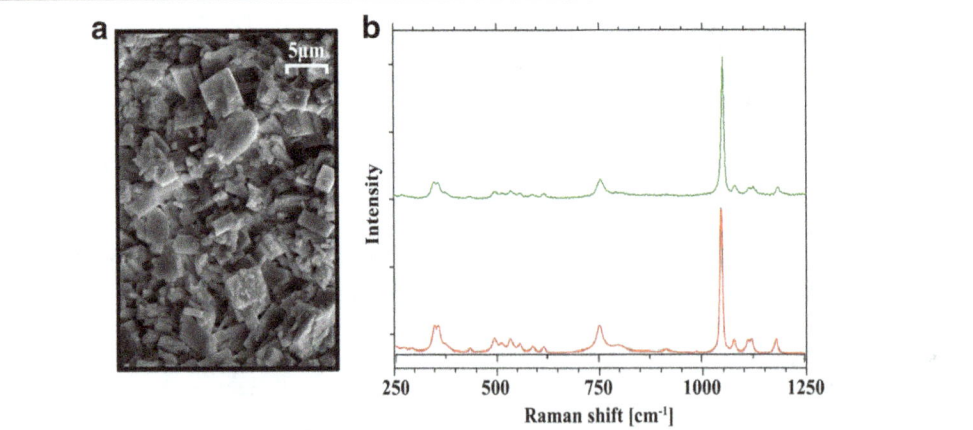

Fig. 5 a Exemplary sample of scanning electron microscopy (SEM) imaging of the acetabular labrum of the hip (ALH) fibrocartilage showing well-developed rhomboid and prismatic crystals in various sizes and spatial arrangements, indicating the presence of calcium pyrophosphate dihydrate (CPPD) crystals. **b** Corresponding sample of measured Raman spectra (green line) with a peak count at 1050 cm^{-1} confirming the presence of CPPD crystals in comparison to the reference spectra of t-CPPD (red line)

epidemiology of the degree of CC in early symptomatic labral tissue in young adults without the presence of advanced OA.

To further analyze the ALH calcification we developed a classification referring to previously published classifications of other types of soft tissue calcification [29–31]. By using three calcification patterns (single, spotted and streaky), we observed that streaky calcification is the pattern in ALH calcification with the highest mean amount of CC. Samples with a singular calcification pattern had the lowest mean amount of CC in ALH calcification. Samples with a spotted calcification pattern had a mean amount of CC that was between the other two patterns. Interestingly ALH samples with a streaky calcification pattern had more histological evidence of degeneration and samples with a singular calcification pattern had less degeneration on average. Moreover, samples with a spotted calcification pattern displayed moderate degeneration. To further characterize ALH calcification we performed scanning electron microscopy, energy dispersive analysis and Raman spectroscopy. By these analyses we found evidence for the deposition of calcium pyrophosphate dihydrate (CPPD) crystals only, but not of basic calcium phosphate (BCP). Several studies have characterized the calcification of hyaline articular cartilage in the hip [3] and knee [4, 36–39] joints. In these studies the detection of BCP and CPPD crystals was reported. To our knowledge there are only few studies in which calcification in the meniscus has been characterized [39, 40] and there are no studies available that have characterized calcification in the ALH. Using Fourier transform infrared (FTIR) spectroscopy, Dessombz et al. detected CPPD crystals in one human meniscus (fibrocartilage) while CPPD crystals and carbonated apatite were detectable at the same time in the other meniscus that was analyzed [39]. Kiraly et al. analyzed the type of crystals in 10 menisci by histological examination [40]. They reported that 80% of the calcified meniscal tissue contained CPPD crystals and 20% BCP crystals. They noticed that both crystal types can be found in the meniscal tissue but the large amount of crystals within the fibrocartilage of the knee appeared to be CPPD crystals. Currently, it remains speculative whether BCP crystals can be found in ALH calcification. In our ALH samples that underwent detailed physico-chemical crystal characterization (n = 10), we found only CPPD and no BCP crystals. We conclude that calcification of the ALH seems to appear mainly by CPPD deposition, but this need to be confirmed in future studies.

Limitations of the present study include limited available information on the medical history of the donors. Moreover there was no information about clinical symptoms of hip or knee pain and function. The standardized slab specimens of the FH reflect representative standardized planes, but only a small part of the articulating surface of the joint in absolute terms, which, theoretically, opens up the possibility of sampling error. None of the mentioned limitations is likely to have had any profound impact on the major new findings and conclusions that we draw from the present study.

Conclusions

Calcification of the acetabular labrum of the hip is unexpectedly highly prevalent and occurs even in healthy labral tissue, but the amount of labral calcification significantly correlates with overall hip joint degeneration independent of age. Calcification of the acetabular labrum can be classified into three typical patterns (singular, spotted and streaky) and is mainly induced by calcium pyrophosphate dihydrate deposition. We propose that acetabular labral calcification deserves further detailed study as a potentially causative factor in labral pathological change and early osteoarthritis of the hip.

Abbreviations

ACH: Articular cartilage of the hip; ALH: Acetabular labrum of the hip; BCP: Basic calcium phosphate; CC: Cartilage calcification; CT: Computed tomography; CPPD: Calcium pyrophosphate dihydrate; DCR: High-resolution digital contact radiography; ED: Energy dispersive analysis; FH: Femoral head; MM: Medial meniscus; OA: Osteoarthritis; OARSI: Osteoarthritis Research Society International; SEM: Scanning electron microscopy

Acknowledgements

We like to thank Prof. Michael Amling, IOBM University Medical Center Hamburg, Germany, for helpful discussions and support in this project. Moreover we would like to thank Elke Leicht for expert technical assistance.

Funding

This project was supported by Deutsche Arthrose-Hilfe e.V. Grant-Nr.: P336-A117-Rüther-EP5-hawe2-schulter-pr-III-10 k-2016-16.

Authors' contributions

TH and JH contributed to the conception and design of the study, acquisition of data, analysis and interpretation of data and drafting and revision of the manuscript. SH was responsible for statistical analysis and interpretation of the data. MK contributed to DCR and histological analysis and interpretation of the data. JB contributed to the conception and design of the study and interpretation. BCS and AK contributed to analysis and interpretation of calcification analysis and revision of the manuscript. KP contributed to the acquisition of data. WR contributed to the conception and design of the study. AN contributed to the conception and design of the study, analysis and interpretation of data and drafting and revision of the manuscript. All authors read and approved the final manuscript.

Competing interests

The authors declare that they have no competing interests.

Author details

[1]Department of Orthopaedics, University Medical Center Hamburg-Eppendorf, Martinistraße 52, 20246 Hamburg, Germany.

[2]Department of Medical Biometry and Epidemiology, University Medical Center Hamburg-Eppendorf, Hamburg, Germany. [3]Department of Osteology and Biomechanics, University Medical Center Hamburg-Eppendorf, Hamburg, Germany. [4]Department of Orthopaedic Surgery, Otto-von-Guerricke-University Magdeburg, Magdeburg, Germany. [5]Centrum of Geoscience, Georg-August-University Göttingen, Göttingen, Germany. [6]Department of Legal Medicine, University Medical Center Hamburg-Eppendorf, Hamburg, Germany.

References

1. Glyn-Jones S, Palmer AJ, Agricola R, Price AJ, Vincent TL, Weinans H, Carr AJ. Osteoarthritis. Lancet. 2015;386(9991):376–87.
2. Loeser RF, Goldring SR, Scanzello CR, Goldring MB. Osteoarthritis: a disease of the joint as an organ. Arthritis Rheum. 2012;64(6):1697–707.
3. Fuerst M, Niggemeyer O, Lammers L, Schäfer F, Lohmann C, Rüther W. Articular cartilage mineralization in osteoarthritis of the hip. BMC Musculoskelet Disord. 2009;10:166.
4. Fuerst M, Bertrand J, Lammers L, Dreier R, Echtermeyer F, Nitschke Y, Rutsch F, Schäfer FK, Niggemeyer O, Steinhagen J, Lohmann CH, Pap T, Rüther W. Calcification of articular cartilage in human osteoarthritis. Arthritis Rheum. 2009;60(9):2694–703.
5. McCarthy GM, Westfall PR, Masuda I, Christopherson PA, Cheung HS, Mitchell PG. Basic calcium phosphate crystals activate human osteoarthritic synovial fibroblasts and induce matrix metalloproteinase-13 (collagenase-3) in adult porcine articular chondrocytes. Ann Rheum Dis. 2001;60(4):399–406.
6. Morgan MP, Whelan LC, Sallis JD, McCarthy CJ, Fitzgerald DJ, McCarthy GM. Basic calcium phosphate crystal-induced prostaglandin E2 production in human fibroblasts: role of cyclooxygenase 1, cyclooxygenase 2, and interleukin-1beta. Arthritis Rheum. 2004;50(5):1642–9.
7. Ea HK, Uzan B, Rey C, Lioté F. Octacalcium phosphate crystals directly stimulate expression of inducible nitric oxide synthase through p38 and JNK mitogen-activated protein kinases in articular chondrocytes. Arthritis Res Ther. 2005;7(5):R915–26.
8. Nasi S, So A, Combes C, Daudon M, Busso N. Interleukin-6 and chondrocyte mineralisation act in tandem to promote experimental osteoarthritis. Ann Rheum Dis. 2016; https://doi.org/10.1136/annrheumdis-2015-207487.
9. Roemhildt ML, Beynnon BD, Gardner-Morse M. Mineralization of articular cartilage in the Sprague-Dawley rat: characterization and mechanical analysis. Osteoarthr Cartil. 2012;20(7):796–800.
10. Roemhildt ML, Gardner-Morse MG, Morgan CF, Beynnon BD, Badger GJ. Calcium phosphate particulates increase friction in the rat knee joint. Osteoarthr Cartil. 2014;22(5):706–9.
11. Ea HK, Nguyen C, Bazin D, Bianchi A, Guicheux J, Reboul P, Daudon M, Lioté F. Articular cartilage calcification in osteoarthritis: insights into crystal-induced stress. Arthritis Rheum. 2011;63(1):10–8.
12. Crema MD, Guermazi A, Li L, Nogueira-Barbosa MH, Marra MD, Roemer FW, Eckstein F, Le Graverand MP, Wyman BT, Hunter DJ. The association of prevalent medial meniscal pathology with cartilage loss in the medial tibiofemoral compartment over a 2-year period. Osteoarthr Cartil. 2010;18(3):336–43.
13. Hunter DJ, Zhang YQ, Niu JB, Tu X, Amin S, Clancy M, Guermazi A, Grigorian M, Gale D, Felson DT. The association of meniscal pathologic changes with cartilage loss in symptomatic knee osteoarthritis. Arthritis Rheum. 2006;54(3):795–801.
14. Sun Y, Mauerhan DR, Honeycutt PR, Kneisl JS, Norton HJ, Zinchenko N, Hanley EN Jr, Gruber HE. Calcium deposition in osteoarthritic meniscus and meniscal cell culture. Arthritis Res Ther. 2010;12(2):R56.
15. Pauli C, Grogan SP, Patil S, Otsuki S, Hasegawa A, Koziol J, Lotz MK, D'Lima DD. Macroscopic and histopathologic analysis of human knee menisci in aging and osteoarthritis. Osteoarthr Cartil. 2011;19(9):1132–41.
16. Sun Y, Mauerhan DR. Meniscal calcification, pathogenesis and implications. Curr Opin Rheumatol. 2012;24(2):152–7.
17. MacMullan PA, McCarthy GM. The meniscus, calcification and osteoarthritis: a pathologic team. Arthritis Res Ther. 2010;12(3):116.
18. Stone AV, Vanderman KS, Willey JS, Long DL, Register TC, Shively CA, Stehle JR Jr, Loeser RF, Ferguson CM. Osteoarthritic changes in vervet monkey knees correlate with meniscus degradation and increased matrix metalloproteinase and cytokine secretion. Osteoarthr Cartil. 2015;23(10):1780–9.
19. Bsat S, Frei H, Beaulé PE. The acetabular labrum: a review of its function. Bone Joint J. 2016;98-B(6):730–5.
20. Rankin AT, Bleakley CM, Cullen M. Hip joint pathology as a leading cause of groin pain in the sporting population: a 6-year review of 894 cases. Am J Sports Med. 2015;43(7):1698–703.
21. Dhollander AA, Lambrecht S, Verdonk PC, Audenaert EA, Almqvist KF, Pattyn C, Verdonk R, Elewaut D, Verbruggen G. First insights into human acetabular labrum cell metabolism. Osteoarthr Cartil. 2012;20(7):670–7.
22. Cooke WR, Gill HS, Murray DW, Ostlere SJ. Discrete mineralisation of the acetabular labrum: a novel marker of femoroacetabular impingement? Br J Radiol. 2013;86(1021):20120182.
23. Lioté F, Ea HK. Clinical implications of pathogenic calcium crystals. Curr Opin Rheumatol. 2014;26(2):192–6.
24. Abreu M, Johnson K, Chung CB, De Lima JE Jr, Trudell D, Terkeltaub R, Pe S, Resnick D. Calcification in calcium pyrophosphate dihydrate (CPPD) crystalline deposits in the knee: anatomic, radiographic, MR imaging, and histologic study in cadavers. Skelet Radiol. 2004;33(7):392–8.
25. Hawellek T, Hubert J, Hischke S, Krause M, Bertrand J, Pap T, Püschel K, Rüther W, Niemeier A. Articular cartilage calcification of the hip and knee is highly prevalent, independent of age but associated with histological osteoarthritis: evidence for a systemic disorder. Osteoarthritis Cart. 2016;24(12):2092-9.
26. Hawellek T, Hubert J, Hischke S, Vettorazzi E, Wegscheider K, Bertrand J, Pap T, Krause M, Püschel K, Rüther W, Niemeier A. Articular cartilage calcification of the humeral head is highly prevalent and associated with osteoarthritis in the general population. J Orthop Res. 2016;34(11):1984-90.
27. Püschel K. Teaching and research on corpses. Mortui vivos docent. Rechtsmedizin. 2016;26(2):115–9. https://doi.org/10.1007/s00194-016-0087-0.
28. Mitsuyama H, Healey RM, Terkeltaub RA, Coutts RD, Amiel D. Calcification of human articular knee cartilage is primarily an effect of aging rather than osteoarthritis. Osteoarthr Cartil. 2007;15(5):559–65.
29. Mazzone PJ, Stoller JK. The pulmonologist's perspective regarding the solitary pulmonary nodule. Semin Thorac Cardiovasc Surg. 2002;14(3):250–60.
30. Yu MH, Kim YJ, Park HS, Jung SI, Jeon HJ. Imaging patterns of intratumoral calcification in the abdominopelvic cavity. Korean J Radiol. 2017;18(2):323–35. https://doi.org/10.3348/kjr.2017.18.2.323. Epub 2017 Feb 7
31. Kaltenbach B, Brandenbusch V, Möbus V, Mall G, Falk S, van den Bergh M, Chevalier F, Müller-Schimpfle M. A matrix of morphology and distribution of calcifications in the breast: analysis of 849 vacuum-assisted biopsies. Eur J Radiol. 2017;86:221–6. https://doi.org/10.1016/j.ejrad.2016.11.022. Epub 2016 Nov 23
32. Krenn V, Knöss P, Rüther W, Jakobs M, Otto M, Krukemeyer MG, Heine A, Möllenhoff G, Kurz B. Meniscal degeneration score and NITEGE expression : immunohistochemical detection of NITEGE in advanced meniscal degeneration. Orthopade. 2010;39(5):475–85.
33. Pritzker KP, Gay S, Jimenez SA, Ostergaard K, Pelletier JP, Revell PA, Salter D, van den Berg WB. Osteoarthritis cartilage histopathology: grading and staging. Osteoarthr Cartil. 2006;14(1):13–29.
34. Gras P, Rey C, Marsan O, Sarda S, Combes C. Synthesis and characterisation of hydrated calcium pyrophosphate phases of biological interest. Eur J Inorg Chem. 2013;34:5886–95.
35. R Core Team. R: A language and environment for statistical computing. Vienna: R Foundation for Statistical Computing; 2014. http://www.R-project.org/
36. Nguyen C, Ea HK, Thiaudiere D, Reguer S, Hannouche D, Daudon M, Lioté F, Bazin D. Calcifications in human osteoarthritic articular cartilage: ex vivo assessment of calcium compounds using XANES spectroscopy. J Synchrotron Radiat. 2011;18(Pt 3):475–80.
37. Nguyen C, Bazin D, Daudon M, Chatron-Colliet A, Hannouche D, Bianchi A, Côme D, So A, Busso N, Lioté F, Ea HK. Revisiting spatial distribution and biochemical composition of calcium-containing crystals in human osteoarthritic articular cartilage. Arthritis Res Ther. 2013;15(5):R103.
38. Fuerst M, Lammers L, Schäfer F, Niggemeyer O, Steinhagen J, Lohmann CH, Rüther W. Investigation of calcium crystals in OA knees. Rheumatol Int. 2010;30(5):623–31. https://doi.org/10.1007/s00296-009-1032-2. Epub 2009 Jul 29
39. Dessombz A, Nguyen C, Ea HK, Rouzière S, Foy E, Hannouche D, Réguer S, Picca FE, Thiaudière D, Lioté F, Daudon M, Bazin D. Combining µX-ray fluorescence, µXANES and µXRD to shed light on Zn2+ cations in cartilage and meniscus calcifications. J Trace Elem Med Biol. 2013;27(4):326–33.
40. Kiraly AJ, Roberts A, Cox M, Mauerhan D, Hanley E, Sun Y. Comparison of meniscal cell-mediated and chondrocyte-mediated calcification. Open Orthop J. 2017;11:225–33.

6

Beneficial effect of resveratrol on phenotypic features and activity of osteoarthritic osteoblasts

Élie Abed, Aline Delalandre and Daniel Lajeunesse[*] ⓘ

Abstract

Background: Osteoarthritis (OA) is a complex disease, which affects multiple tissues, namely the subchondral bone, articular cartilage and synovial membrane. Alterations of the subchondral bone include an increased, yet under mineralized osteoid matrix, abnormal osteoblast cell phenotype including elevated alkaline phosphatase (ALP) activity, increased release of osteocalcin (OC) and transforming growth factor β-1 (TGF-β1). Previous studies have demonstrated an inhibition of the canonical Wnt signaling (cWnt) pathway in OA osteoblasts (Ob). As resveratrol (RSV) has been shown to upregulate the Wnt signaling pathway in different cell systems, we hypothesized that RSV could be beneficial for OA Ob.

Method: We prepared primary human Ob using the subchondral bone plate of tibial plateaus of OA patients undergoing total knee arthroplasty, or tibial plateaus of normal individuals at autopsy. Sirtuin 1 (Sirt1) expression in normal and OA subchondral bone tissue was evaluated by immunohistochemical analysis. Expression of genes was evaluated by qRT-PCR and protein production by western blot analysis. ALP activity and osteocalcin secretion were evaluated respectively with substrate hydrolysis and enzyme immunoassay. Mineralization levels were evaluated with alizarin red staining. Wnt/β-catenin signaling was evaluated by target gene expression using the TOPflash TCF/lef luciferase reporter assay and intracellular signaling using β-catenin levels in western blot analysis. Extracellular signal-regulated kinase (Erk)1/2 and the Smad1/5/8 pathways were evaluated by western blot analysis.

Results: Sirt1 expression and production were reduced in OA subchondral bone tissue compared to normal tissue. RSV upregulated Sirt1 and its activity, and reduced the expression of leptin. RSV increased Erk1/2 phosphorylation in OA Ob; however, it had no effect on Smad 1/5/8 phosphorylation. RSV had little effect on cell proliferation and only slightly affected the Bax/Bcl2 ratio. The expression of Runx2/Cbfa1 and peroxisome proliferator-activated receptor (PPAR)γ were not affected by increasing doses of RSV. The endogenous increased ALP activity and OC release observed in OA Ob compared to normal Ob were partly corrected only for ALP at high RSV levels but not for OC release. In contrast, RSV increased the mineralization of OA Ob. Moreover, whereas Wnt3a stimulates the Wnt/β-catenin pathway in these cells, RSV further increased the response to Wnt3a.

Conclusion: These data indicate that RSV promotes Sirt1 levels, inhibits the endogenous expression of leptin by OA osteoblasts and can promote the Wnt/β-catenin and Erk1/2 signaling pathways, which are altered in these cells.

Keywords: Osteoarthritis, Subchondral bone, Canonical Wnt signaling, Resveratrol, Mineralization, Sirtuin 1

* Correspondence: daniel.lajeunesse@umontreal.ca
Unité de recherche en Arthrose, Centre de recherche du Centre hospitalier
de l'Université de Montréal (CRCHUM), 900, rue Saint-Denis, Montréal,
Québec H2X 0A9, Canada

Background

The exact mechanism that leads to osteoarthritis (OA) remains unknown; however, recent studies indicate that the subchondral bone tissue is implicated in the progression and/or the initiation of OA [1]. Cartilage damage, loss and failure to repair damage are characteristics of OA. It was believed this was restricted to abnormal chondrocyte function, yet recent studies using both clinical and animal models have underlined the crucial role played by the subchondral bone tissue in this process. Indeed, subchondral bone tissue is abnormal in OA patients and osteoblasts (Ob) from OA subchondral bone have altered functions [2, 3]. The Wnt signaling pathway is crucial for normal skeletal tissue homeostasis and function. In OA patients, the subchondral bone tissue is altered [4–6] and we previously showed that OA subchondral Ob have altered functions [2, 7, 8]. Moreover, we reported that the abnormal expression of phenotypic markers and reduced mineralization of OA Ob are linked with stimulation of the Wnt antagonist dickkopft-2 (DKK2) [9] and sclerostin (SOST) [10], and inhibition of the Wnt agonist, R-spondin 2 (Rspo2) [11].

Resveratrol (3,4′,5-trihydroxystlben (RSV)) is a natural product found in most grape cultivars. Resveratrol is recognized as a major phytoestrogen and has been shown to possess estrogenic activity [12]. Although the effect of RSV was mostly demonstrated in endothelial cells where it alters endothelial activities [13], recent studies have revealed its potential role in Ob. Indeed, RSV was shown to promote Ob proliferation and differentiation of multipotent mesenchymal cells [14] and to enhance the proliferation and differentiation of osteoblastic MC3T3-E1 cells [15] in a mouse cell model of osteoblasts. In contrast, RSV can also suppress the proliferation of osteosarcoma cells via a role in cell apoptosis [16]. Recent studies further demonstrated that RSV plays its role via its modulation of the Wnt/β-catenin signaling pathway by promoting Ob differentiation of multipotent mesenchymal cells [17]. The activation of the Wnt/β-catenin pathway by RSV triggers other signaling pathways such as extracellular signal-regulated kinase (Erk)1/2 in multipotent mesenchymal cells [17], and of note, the activation of the Erk1/2 pathway is responsible for the differentiation of mesenchymal cells into Ob [18].

Osteoarthritic Ob present a number of altered phenotypic features among which increased alkaline phosphatase (ALP) activity, osteocalcin release, and type 1 collagen expression, and reduced in vitro mineralization are but a few examples of these alterations [2, 3, 7, 9, 19]. Recent evidence indicates that alterations in the Wnt/β-catenin signaling pathway are responsible, at least in part, for the alterations of phenotypic features and reduced mineralization observed in OA Ob [7]. Indeed, Wnt/β-catenin activity is reduced in Ob in OA due to elevated levels of the Wnt antagonist DKK2 [9], elevated production of SOST [10], yet another Wnt antagonist, and reduced levels of the Wnt agonist Rspo2 [11].

Osteoarthritic Ob also have altered responses to insulin-like growth factor 1 and leptin treatments in part due to altered Erk1/2 and Smad1/5/8 signaling [20]. Of note, under hypoxic conditions, a situation observed in OA patients [21–24], leptin and DKK2 are further upregulated in these cells compared to cells under normorxic conditions [25]. In vitro mineralization is also altered in osteoblasts in OA [2] in response to alterations in transforming growth factor-β1 (TGF-β1) levels and reduced Wnt/β-catenin signaling activity [9]. In addition, Ob express more hepatocyte growth factor (HGF) than normal Ob in OA, and increased endogenous HGF production stimulates the expression of TGF-β1 and reduces the response to bone morphogenetic protein 2 (BMP-2) and mineralization in osteoblasts in OA [26].

As resveratrol has been shown to regulate the activity of Wnt/β-catenin in mesenchymal stem cells (MSC) cells [17], increase Erk1/2 and Akt, AMPK, Smad 1/5/8, p38, ERK,c-Jun N-terminal kinase, and enhance nuclear factor-κB activity in OM-stimulated cells [27], whereas some of these pathways are altered in Ob in OA, we questioned if RSV could correct these activities and which signaling pathways are involved in the potential response to RSV.

Methods

Patients and clinical parameters

Tibial plateaus were obtained from OA patients undergoing total knee replacement surgery and prepared as previously described [7, 19, 28]. A total of 41 patients (67.9 ± 7.8 years, mean $\pm$ SD; 15 male/26 female patients), who had OA according to the recognized clinical criteria of the American College of Rheumatology, were included [29]. No patients had received medication that would interfere with bone metabolism, including corticosteroids, for 6 months before surgery. A total of 12 subchondral bone specimens from normal individuals (age 64.3 ± 13.1 years, mean $\pm$ SD; 9 male/3 female individuals) were collected at autopsy within 12 h of death. They had not been on any medication that could interfere with bone metabolism or had any bone metabolic disease or abnormal cartilage macroscopic changes. All human samples were acquired following a signed agreement by the patients undergoing knee surgery and, for the specimens collected at autopsy, by the relatives of the deceased, in accordance with the ethics committee guidelines of the Centre de recherche du Centre Hospitalier de l'Université de Montréal (CRCHUM).

Preparation of primary subchondral bone cell culture

Isolation of the subchondral bone plate and cell cultures were prepared as previously described using the medial tibial plateaus where bone sclerosis is observed [19]. At confluence, cells were passaged once at 25,000 cells/cm^2 in 100-mm petri dishes and grown for 5 days in Ham F12/DMEM medium (Sigma-Aldrich, Oakville, Canada) containing 10% FBS. Confluent cells were then incubated in the presence or absence of 1,25(OH)$_2$D$_3$ (50 nM) for 48 h for the determination of biomarkers in the presence of 2% FBS. Supernatants were collected at the end of the incubation and kept at –80 °C prior to assay. Cells were prepared either in ALP buffer for phenotypic determinations or in TRIzol for RT-PCR experiments. Protein determination was by the bicinchoninic acid method [30]. Resveratrol was used at concentrations ranging from 10 nM to 1000 nM following previously published in vitro experiments [14–17], which reflect in vivo doses used in animal studies [13, 31]. Where indicated, phosphorylation of Erk1/2 was inhibited by the selective inhibitor PD98059 at a final concentration of 10 µM.

Phenotypic characterization of human subchondral Ob cell cultures

ALP activity was determined by substrate hydrolysis using p-nitrophenylphosphate of whole cell lysates whereas osteocalcin release in cell supernatants was evaluated using an enzyme immunoassay (EIA) as previously described [7, 19]. Determinations were performed in duplicate for each preparation.

Preparation of Wnt3a-conditioned medium (Wnt3a-CM)

Murine L cell lines transfected with either an empty vector (CRL-2648) or Wnt3a (CRL-2647) were obtained from the American Culture Type Collection (Cedarlane Laboratories Ltd, Burlington, ON, Canada). Control (L-CM) and Wnt3a-conditioned medium (Wnt3a-CM) was prepared using these cells. Briefly, the cells were grown in BGJb medium for 48 h after which conditioned medium (CM) was collected. CM was filtered sterilized, aliquoted and stored at –80 °C prior to use. CM was added to normal and OA Ob at a 10% final concentration.

RT-PCR assays

For RT-PCR assays, total cellular RNA was extracted with the TRIzol^{TM} reagent (Invitrogen, Burlington, ON, Canada) according to the manufacturer's specifications and treated with the DNA-free^{TM} Dnase Treatment and Removal kit (Ambion, Austin, TX, USA) to ensure complete removal of chromosomal DNA. The RNA was quantitated using the RiboGreen RNA quantification kit (Molecular Probes, Eugene, OR, USA). The RT reactions were primed with random hexamers with 1 ug of total RNA in a 100-µl final reaction volume followed by PCR amplification with the Rotor-Gene 6$^®$ RG-3000A (Corbett Research, Mortlake, NSW, Australia) as previously

described [9, 10] using 20 pmol of each specific PCR primer. Gene specific primers were: ALP, F:ACGTGG CTAA GAATGTCATC, R: CTGGTAGGCGATGTCCTTA; osteocalcin (OC), F: ATGAGAGCCCTCACACTC, R: GA AAGCCGATGTGGTCAG; PPARG, F: TCTCTCCGTAAT GGAAGACC, R: GCATTATGAGACATCCCAC; LEP-TIN, F: GGCTTTGGCCCTATCTTTTC, R: GGATAAGG TCAGGATGGGGT; Sirt1, F: GCTGGAACAGGTTGCG GGAA, R: GGGCACCTAGGACATCGAGGA; P300, F: GCAGTGTGCCAAACCAGATG, R: GGGTTTGCCGGG GTACAATA; glyceraldehyde-3-phosphate dehydrogenase (GAPDH), F: CAGAACATCATCCCTGCCTCT, R: GCTT GACAAAGTGGTCGTTGA G; RUNX2, F: AGATGATG ACACTGCCACCTCTG, R: GGGATGAAATGCTTGGG AACTGC; these were added at a final concentration of 200 nM. The data were collected and processed with the GeneAmp 5700 SDS software and given as threshold cycle (Ct). Ct values were converted to number of molecules using standard curves for each target gene and values were expressed as the ratio of the number of molecules of the target gene to GAPDH.

Evaluation of mineralization

Confluent cells were incubated in BGJb medium containing 10% FBS, 50 µg/ml ascorbic acid and 50 µg/ml β-glycerophosphate. This medium was changed every 2 days until day 28. Mineralization of cell cultures was evaluated by quantification of alizarin red staining performed following the extraction procedure of Gregory [32].

Western immunoblotting

Cell extracts were loaded onto polyacrylamide gels and separated by sodium dodecyl sulfate-polyacrylamide gel electrophoresis (SDS-PAGE) under a reducing condition as previously described [2, 3]. Loading of the protein was adjusted according to the cellular protein concentration of each specimen. The proteins were then electrophoretically transferred onto nitrocellulose membranes (Boehringer Mannheim, Penzberg, Germany), and immunoblotting was performed as described in the ECL Plus western blotting detection system manual (Amersham Pharmacia Biotech, UK, England). We used rabbit anti-p300 at a dilution of 1:500 (Santa Cruz Biotechnology), rabbit anti-smad1/5/8 and rabbit anti-p-smad1/5/8 at a dilution of 1:1000 (Cell Signaling Technology, Beverly, MA, USA), rabbit anti-Sirt1 at a dilution of 1:1000 (Cell Signaling), rabbit anti-β-catenin and rabbit anti-phosphorylated β-catenin at dilutions of 1:2000 and 1:1000, respectively (Cell Signaling Technology), rabbit anti-p44/42 and rabbit anti-Phospho-p44/42 mitogen-activated protein kinase (MAPK) (Erk1/2) at dilutions of 1:1000 (Cell Signaling Technology), rabbit anti-Phospho-Smad1/5/8 at dilutions of 1:1000 (Cell Signaling Technology), and rabbit anti-human actin at a dilution of 1:10,000 (Sigma-Aldrich) as primary antibodies; a horseradish peroxidase (HRP)-conjugated goat anti-rabbi t IgG (1:10,000, Upstate Biotechnology, NY, USA) was used as the secondary antibody for the western blot assays. Densitometry analysis of western blot films was performed using the public domain National Institutes of Health (NIH) Image program developed with the Scion Image 1.63 program (Research Services Branch (RSB)). The public domain NIH Image program was developed at the US NIH (http://rsb.info.nih.gov/nih-image/).

TOPflash dual-luciferase reporter assays

Primary normal and OA Ob were plated in 24-well plates at a density of 1.5×10^5 cells/well containing 10% FBS in BGJb medium and left to recover overnight. Plasmid mixtures containing 2 μg TOPflash luciferase construct (Upstate Biotechnology, Lake Placid, NY, USA) and 0.05 μg RENILLA luciferase driven by the SV40 promoter (Promega, Madison, WI, USA) were transfected into cells using FuGENE 6 Transfection Reageant (Roche) according to the manufacturer's protocol. After 24 h transfection, cells were incubated for another 24 h with Wnt3a-CM or L-CM, in the presence of increasing doses of RSV. After the last 24 h of incubation, the cells were lysed and luciferase activity was evaluated using the dual luciferase assay kit (Promega). Values for TOPflash luciferase activity were normalized to those of Renilla activity.

Sirt1 activity assay in OA Ob

Sirt1 activity was determined in whole cell lysates using the Abcam Sirt1 Activity Assay Kit (Fluorometric, ab156065). Cells treated with RSV for 24 h were harvested with cell lysis buffer under non-denaturing conditions. Briefly, medium was removed and cells were rinsed with ice-cold PBS and then 75 ul of 1X ice-cold cell lysis buffer added to each well and incubated on ice for 5 minutes. Cells were scrapped and transferred and sonicated four times for 5 seconds each on ice and centrifuged for 10 minutes at 4 °C. The supernatant is the whole cell lysate. Determinations were performed in triplicate for each preparation.

Detection of Sirt1 in human bone tissue by immunohistochemical analysis

Full-thickness specimens from the tibial plateaus were processed for immunohistochemical analysis using the protocol for immunohistochemical paraffin-embedded staining sections (Abcam, ab64264). Briefly, slides were incubated for 10 minutes in 10 mM sodium citrate buffer pH 6.0 at 80 °C and then slides were cooled on the bench top for 30 minutes. Slides were incubated with PBS, 0.4% Triton 1% BSA for 10 minutes at room temperature. The slides were then incubated with hydrogen peroxide block for 10 minutes followed by protein

block for another 10 minutes at room temperature. The primary antibodies against Sirt1 (1:100, NBP1-49540) were applied overnight at 4 °C in a humidified chamber. Slides were incubated in the presence of a biotin-conjugated goat anti-polyvalent for 10 minutes at room temperature. This was followed by the addition of the streptavidin peroxidase complex for 10 minutes, and slides were counterstained with eosin. Sections were examined under a light microscope (Leitz Orthoplan; Leica) and photographed using a CoolSNAP cf Photometrics camera (Roper Scientific, USA).

Statistical analysis

All quantitative data are expressed as mean ± SEM. The data were analyzed by Student's t test when comparing two groups. In experiments comparing three groups, we performed analysis of variance (ANOVA) and the post-hoc Fisher least significant difference (LSD) protected t test; p values <0.05 were considered statistically significant.

Results

Effect of RSV on altered phenotype in OA Ob

We first evaluated the expression of Sirt1 in normal and OA subchondral bone tissues. As shown in Fig. 1a, Sirt1 was readily observed in normal bone tissue whereas it was much reduced in OA bone tissue. The expression of Sirt1 in ex vivo bone samples also demonstrated robust expression in normal bone explants, whereas it was significantly reduced in OA explants (Fig. 1b). As we previously reported that Sirt1is reduced in OA Ob and leads to alteration of Ob functions [10], we determined that indeed, OA Ob had reduced Sirt1 expression compared to normal Ob (Fig. 1c). Since RSV is known to stimulate Sirt1 activity, we then attempted to determine if RSV treatments could increase Sirt1 expression and production in OA Ob. Indeed, there was almost threefold dose-dependent stimulation by RSV of Sirt1 expression (Fig. 1d), production (Figs. 1e and 2c) and activity (Fig. 1f) in OA Ob. Whereas RSV can stimulate p300 levels in other cell systems [33], the addition of RSV did not significantly affect p300 levels in OA Ob (Fig. 2a-c).

The expression of leptin, which is already elevated in OA Ob, contributes to their abnormal function as we previously reported [28]. RSV is known to regulate leptin expression in other cell systems [31], hence we tested whether this could also be the case for OA Ob. Indeed, RSV dose-dependently decreased the expression of leptin approximately twofold in OA Ob (Fig. 2d). As OA osteoblasts also have altered responses to insulin-like growth factor 1 and leptin treatments [20], in part due to altered Erk1/2, and since in the present study RSV corrected the expression of leptin, we evaluated the effect of RSV treatments on altered Erk1/2 and other signaling

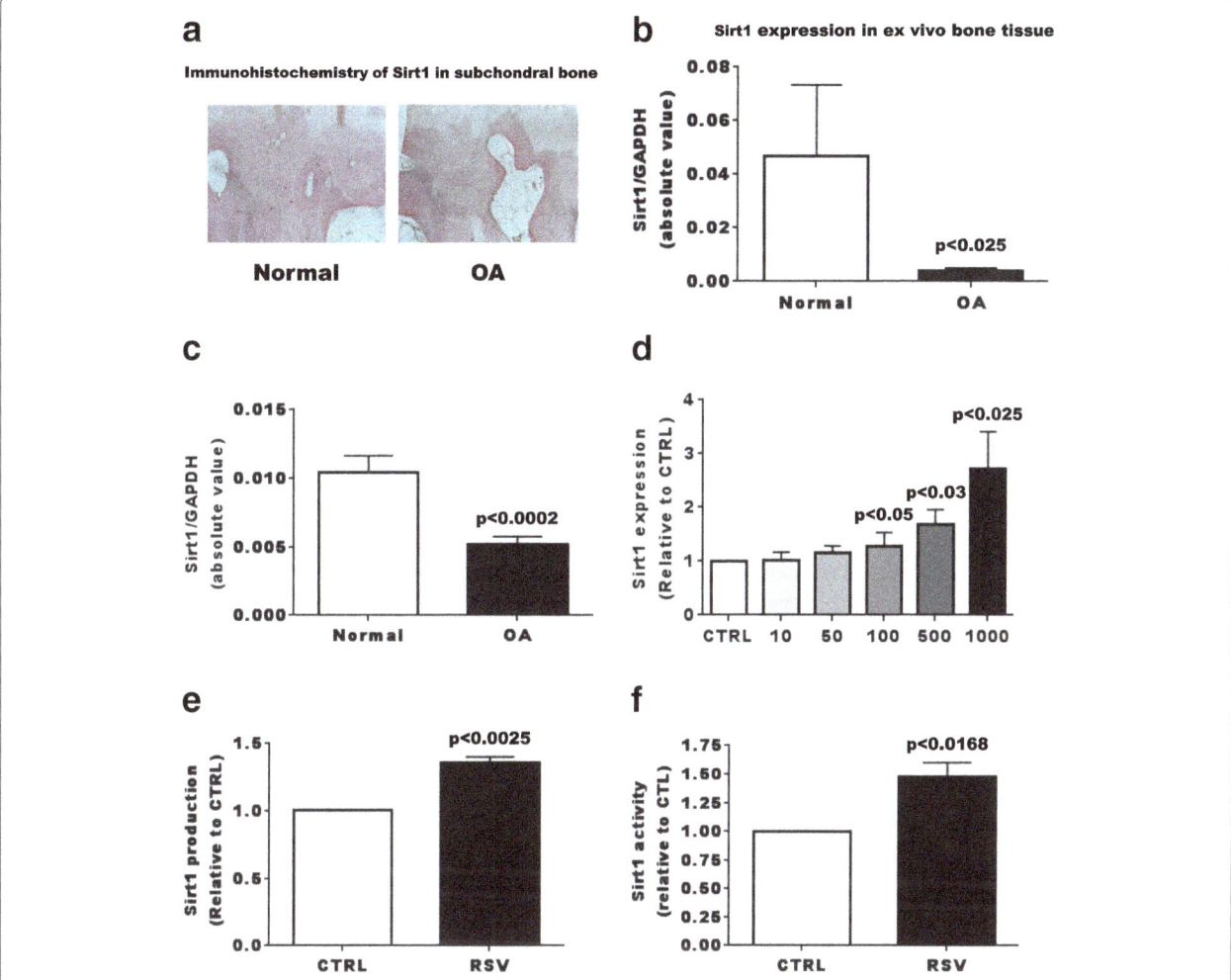

Fig. 1 Effect of resveratol (RSV) on sirtuin 1 (*Sirt1*) and P300 levels. **a** Representative immunohistochemical determination of Sirt1 protein expression in normal subchondral bone tissues and in osteoarthritis (*OA*). **b** Sirt1 expression by normal (*n* = 3) and OA (*n* = 6) ex vivo subchondral bone explants. **c** Sirt1 expression by normal (*n* = 9) and OA osteoblasts (*Ob*) (*n* = 21). **d** Confluent OA Ob were treated with increasing doses of RSV for 24 h and lysed in TRIzol™ for qRT-PCR analysis of Sirt1 messenger RNA expression (*n* = 5). **e** Quantification of Sirt1 levels as detected in Fig. 2c. **f** Sirt1 activity analysis in OA Ob cell lysates in response to RSV (*n* = 3). *GAPDH* glyceraldehyde-3-phosphate dehydrogenase, *CTRL* control

pathways. Our results indicated that RSV increased the phosphorylation of Erk1/2, which is involved in the control of cell proliferation, differentiation and apoptosis (Fig. 2e and f). In contrast, the addition of RSV did not significantly affect the phosphorylation of Smad 1/5/8 levels (Fig. 2e). Using PD 98059 which selectively inhibits the phosphorylation of Erk1/2, we also showed that it prevented the RSV-dependent stimulation of phosphorylated Erk1/2 in OA osteoblasts (Fig. 2g).

As OA Ob grow faster than normal Ob in vitro [20], we determined the importance of RSV in the proliferation and the viability of OA Ob. Our results indicate that RSV had little effect on cell proliferation as assessed by the MTT assay (Fig. 3a) and slightly affected the Bax/Bcl2 ratio, an indicator of cell survival (Fig. 3b). Since the runt-related transcription factor 2 (Runx2/Cbfa1) pathway has been identified as a master regulator of the

Ob-specific expression of osteocalcin [34], which is elevated in OA Ob [2], we therefore analyzed the ability of RSV to control the expression of Runx2/Cbfa1. Our results indicated that RSV had no effect on Runx2/Cbfa1 expression (Fig. 3c). Similarly, increasing doses of RSV did not alter the expression of PPARγ (Fig. 3d).

As alkaline phosphatase activity and osteocalcin release are elevated in OA Ob as compared to normal Ob [2], and since recent studies have shown an association between dietary polyphenols and the prevention of OA [35], we tested the effect of RSV on altered ALP activity and osteocalcin release in human OA Ob. Our results showed that RSV at a high dose only of 500 nM reduced ALP in OA Ob (Fig. 4a), indicating that RSV can partially reverse the abnormal ALP activities observed in OA Ob. However, the addition of RSV did not significantly affect osteocalcin release in OA Ob (Fig. 4b).

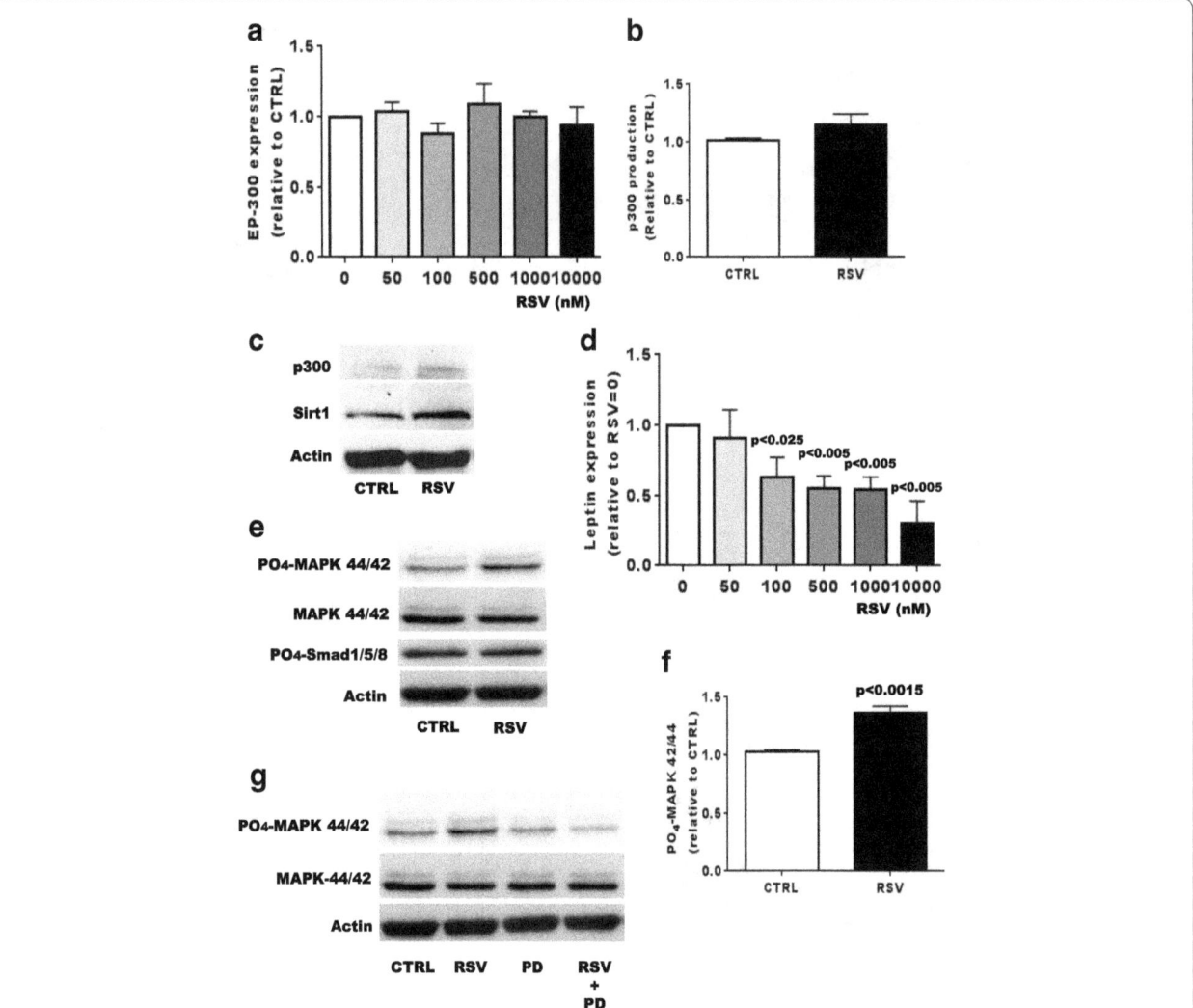

Fig. 2 Effect of resveratol (*RSV*) EP-300 and leptin expression, extracellular signal-regulated kinase (Erk)1/2 and Smad1/5/8 signaling activities in osteoarthritis (*OA*) osteoblasts (*Ob*). Confluent OA Ob were treated with increasing doses of RSV for 24 h and lysed in TRIzol™ for qRT-PCR analysis. **a** EP-300 messenger RNA (mRNA) expression (*n* = 6). **b** EP-300 protein abundance in response to 24 h of RSV treatment at 500 nM. **c** Western blot analysis of EP-300 and sirtuin 1 (*Sirt1*) in response to 24 h of RSV treatment at 500 nM. **d** Leptin mRNA expression (*n* = 6). Results are given as the mean value ± SEM of markers relative to glyceraldehyde-3-phosphate dehydrogenase (*GAPDH*). **e** Representative western blot analysis of OA Ob treated or not with 500 nM of RSV for 1 h. Phosphorylated and non-phosphorylated Erk1/2, phosphorylated Smad1/5/8, and β-actin were detected by western blot analysis (*n* = 6 experiments). **f** Quantification of phosphorylated and non-phosphorylated Erk1/2 levels as detected in **e**. **g** Specific inhibition of RSV-dependent phosphorylated Erk1/2 by PD98059. *CTRL* control, *MAPK* mitogen-activated protein kinase

Under similar conditions, RSV treatments did not affect the gene expression of ALP and OC (data not illustrated).

Effect of RSV on mineralization in OA Ob

The mineralization of OA Ob is reduced compared to normal Ob, as we previously reported [2], and reflects the in vivo situation [5, 36]. The reduction in in vitro mineralization was due to an increase in the endogenous production of TGF-β1 by OA Ob, which could be reduced by stimulating Sirt1 activity in OA Ob with β-nicotinamide mononucleotide (NMN) [10]. Of note,

Sirt1 is expressed in bone cells and promotes bone formation [37] and on the other hand it reduces osteoclastogenesis [38]. Osteoblast deletion of Sirt1 in mice leads to delayed bone mineralization [39]. As RSV stimulates Sirt1 activity [10] and we showed herein that the expression, production and activity of Sirt1 were increased in OA Ob following RSV treatment, we tested whether RSV could play a role on OA Ob mineralization. As shown in Fig. 5a and b, increasing doses of RSV increased the mineralization potential of OA Ob about twofold as assessed by alizarin red staining.

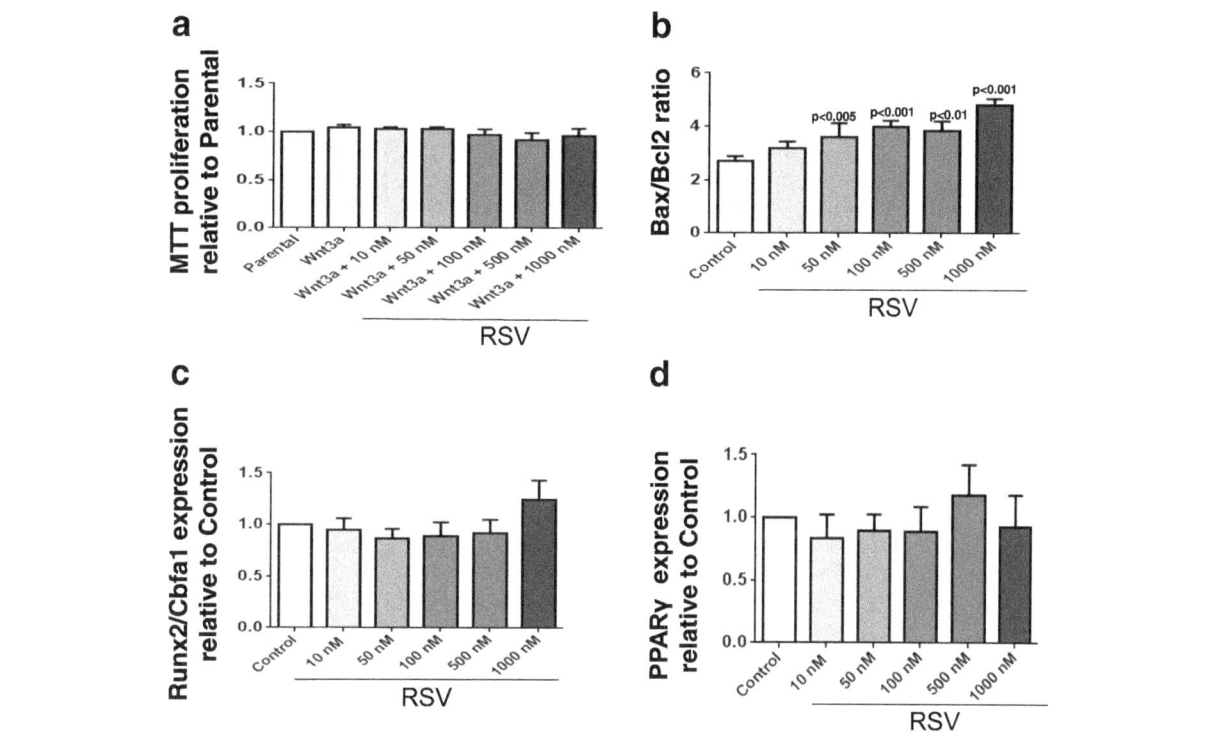

Fig. 3 Effect of resveratol (*RSV*) on proliferation, bax/bcl2, runx2/cbfa1, and peroxisome proliferator-activated receptor γ (*PPARγ*) expression in osteoblasts (Ob) in osteoarthritis (OA). **a** OA Ob were plated at 10,000 cells/cm² and allowed to attach overnight in BGJ medium containing 10% FBS. Cells were then treated with the same medium with 0.5% FBS for 24 h prior to receiving increasing doses of RSV (10 , 50 , 100, 500 or 1000 nM) or the vehicle in the same medium for another incubation of 24 h. Cell proliferation was assessed by the MTT assay (*n* = 5). Confluent OA Ob were treated with increasing doses of RSV for 24 h and lysed in TRIzol™ for qRT-PCR analysis. **b** BAX/BCL2 messenger RNA (mRNA) expression (*n* = 6). **c** Runx2/Cbfa1 mRNA expression (*n* = 7). **d** PPARγ mRNA expression (*n* = 6). Results are given as the mean value ± SEM of markers relative to glyceraldehyde-3-phosphate dehydrogenase

Effect of RSV on DKK2 expression in OA Ob

We previously reported that elevated DKK2 levels are responsible for the elevated ALP in OA Ob and that correcting DKK2 levels by small interfering RNA (siRNA) techniques reduced the level of ALP in OA Ob to that in normal Ob [9]. Since RSV partly corrected the altered elevated ALP, we tested whether RSV could have an effect on the expression of the Wnt antagonist DKK2. Our results indicated that increasing doses of RSV had no effect on DKK2 expression (Fig. 4c), suggesting that RSV acts differently on ALP.

Role of RSV on altered Wnt/β-catenin signaling

We previously reported that OA Ob have an altered Wnt/β-catenin signaling pathway [9], hence we questioned whether RSV treatment could correct this activity. When OA Ob were treated with Wnt3a-CM, the canonical Wnt signaling pathway was increased about fourfold (Fig. 5c). The presence of increasing doses of RSV further stimulated this activity up to sixfold (Fig. 5c). This increase in Wnt/β-catenin signaling activity was accompanied by a significant increase in free β-catenin levels measured by immunoblotting assays (Fig. 5d). We next evaluated what

triggered this increase in β-catenin activity in response to RSV. Using the selective Erk1/2 inhibitor PD98059, which reduced Erk1/2 phosphorylation in OA Ob (Fig. 2g), we observed that it also reduced the RSV-dependent β-catenin activation observed in these cells (Fig. 5e). Indeed, PD98059 reduced RSV-dependent β-catenin levels by 36.1 ± 10.5%.

Discussion

Resveratrol, a natural polyphenol is known for its anti-inflammatory, anti-oxidant, anti-aging, anti-carcinogenic, cardioprotective and neuroprotective properties [40–42]. The protective effect of RSV on articular cartilage degradation was first reported by Elmali et al. in a rabbit model of OA [43]. In human articular chondrocytes, RSV has an anti-apoptotic and anti-inflammatory effects [44, 45]. Similarly, Im et al. demonstrated potent anabolic and anti-catabolic potential of RSV in human adult articular chondrocytes via inhibition of matrix-degrading enzyme [46]. Taken together, these findings suggest that RSV may protect against cartilage degeneration and have protective effects against OA. RSV enhances osteoblast activities in bone tissue, and stimulates Ob proliferation and

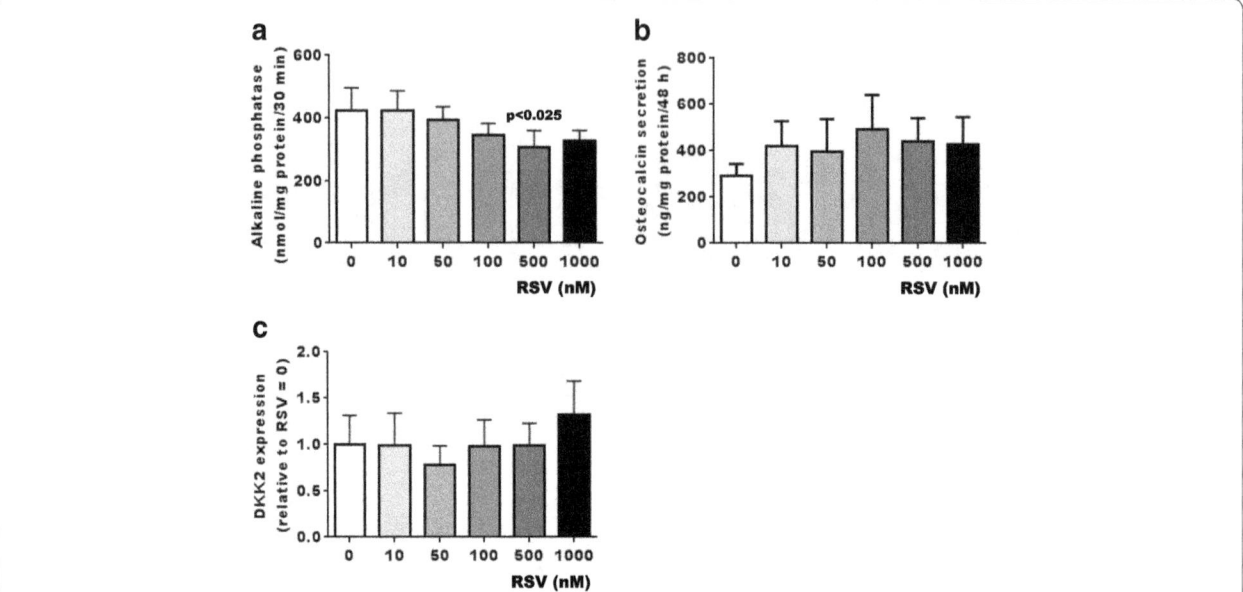

Fig. 4 Effect of resveratol (*RSV*) on alkaline phosphatase (ALP) activity, osteocalcin secretion and dickkopft-2 (*DKK2*) expression in osteoblasts (Ob) in osteoarthritis (OA). Confluent OA Ob were treated with increasing doses of RSV (10, 50, 100, 500 or 1000 nM) or the vehicle for 48 h in presence of 1,25(OH)$_2$D$_3$. Cell culture medium was collected for the determination of osteocalcin secretion and cell lysates were used for the determination of ALP activity. **a** ALP activity in OA ($n = 6$) Ob. **b** Osteocalcin release by OA ($n = 6$) Ob. Confluent OA Ob were treated with increasing doses of RSV for 24 h and lysed in TRIzol™ for qRT-PCR analysis. **c** DKK2 mRNA expression ($n = 4$). Results are given as the mean ± SEM value of markers relative to glyceraldehyde-3-phosphate dehydrogenase

differentiation and therefore promotes bone formation and further suggests a future role for RSV in fracture healing [14]. However, the role of RSV on altered subchondral bone has not yet been elucidated and since the subchondral bone plays a critical role in the process of the initiation and/or the progression of OA, it is necessary to address whether RSV can play a beneficial role in altered subchondral bone in patients with OA.

In the present study, we showed the beneficial effect of RSV on the altered phenotype of human OA Ob and the mechanism by which RSV acts. We previously reported that Sirt1 expression was significantly reduced in OA Ob compared to normal Ob and is responsible, at least in part, for the increased expression of TGF-β1 and SOST, which can both alter the phenotype of human OA Ob [10]. Herein, we demonstrated that Sirt1 expression is reduced in OA subchondral bone tissue, ex vivo explants, and in vitro Ob. Stimulating Sirt1 activity with β-nicotinamide mononucleotide reduced the elevated expression of TGF-β1 and SOST in OA Ob, and corrected the phenotype and altered mineralization of OA Ob [10]. Of note, TGF-β1 is upregulated by leptin, which is elevated in OA Ob and contributes to the abnormal function of these cells as we showed previously [20]. We first demonstrated that RSV increased Sirt1 expression, production and activity in OA Ob. This upregulation of Sirt1 observed in OA Ob following treatment with RSV is consistent with previous studies in which RSV was

identified as an activator of Sirt1 in OA chondrocytes [47]. Second, the expression of leptin, which is elevated in OA Ob and contributes to their abnormal function, was decreased in OA Ob when treated with RSV. Taken together, these results and our previously published data indicate that leptin and TGF-β1 are downstream targets of RSV via its stimulation of Sirt1 activity in OA Ob, a situation that could link reduced Sirt1 levels in OA Ob with a number of abnormal biomarkers in these cells. However, in contrast to previously reported studies [33], we did not establish a link between EP-300 and Sirt1 activation following RSV stimulation in OA Ob.

We previously demonstrated that leptin alters a number of intracellular cell signaling pathways, namely Erk1/2, in OA osteoblasts [20]. Since stimulating SIRT1 activity with RSV reduced the elevated expression of leptin in OA Ob, we therefore questioned whether this could correct the abnormal phenotype and altered mineralization observed in OA Ob. Our study revealed that RSV has an effect on the altered intracellular Erk1/2 signaling pathway, while it was without effect on the Smad1/5/8 signaling pathway in OA Ob. Indeed, RSV treatments increased the phosphorylation of Erk1/2, which is involved in the control of cell proliferation, differentiation and apoptosis.

It has been demonstrated by Li et al. that RSV inhibits proliferation and promotes apoptosis of osteosarcoma cells [16]. As OA Ob proliferate faster than normal Ob,

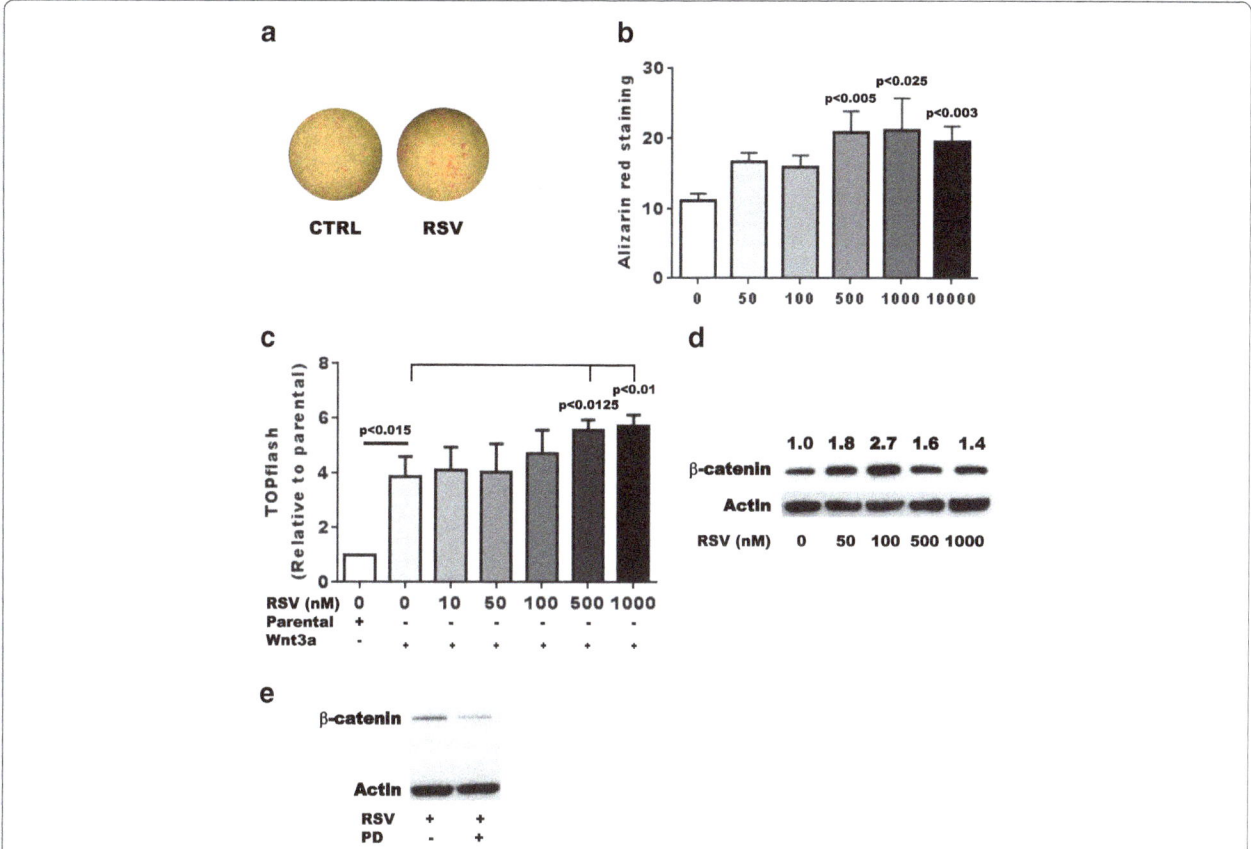

Fig. 5 Effect of resveratrol (*RSV*) on Wnt/β-catenin signaling activity and mineralization in osteoblasts (Ob) in osteoarthritis (OA). OA osteoblasts were stimulated with increasing doses of RSV (10, 50, 100, 500 or 1000 nM) for up to 28 days. **a** Representative alizarin red staining of normal Ob. **b** Quantification of alizarin red staining as a function of time and chronic effect of RSV exposure in OA Ob (*n* = 6). Cells were treated for 4 h with vehicle or increasing doses of RSV. **c** TOPflash activity in OA Ob in response to parental and Wnt3a conditioned medium either in the presence or absence of RSV for 24 h. Values are reported relative to values in parental samples (*n* = 5 experiments). **d** Western blot analysis of β-catenin expression in OA Ob in response to Wnt3a in the presence of RSV. Representative of four experiments. **e** Western blot analysis of the effect of PD98059 on RSV-dependent β-catenin activation in OA Ob. Representative of three experiments. *CTRL* control

we determined the importance of RSV in the proliferation and the viability of OA Ob cells. Our results indicated that RSV had little effect on cell proliferation and slightly affected the Bax/Bcl2 ratio, an indicator of cell survival. These results indicate that RSV could not correct the abnormal proliferation of human OA Ob. However it has been shown that RSV induced the proliferation and differentiation of human bone marrow-derived mesenchymal stem cells (MSC) [48] and of the Ob precursor cell line derived from mouse calvaria, MC-3 T3 cells [15]. As OA Ob proliferate faster and are more differentiated than human bone marrow-derived MSC and the Ob precursor MC-3 T3 cells, this would explain again that RSV has a different role to play in well-differentiated cells vs pre-osteoblasts, hence that its effect depends on the state of differentiation and the type of cells.

The Runx2 pathway has been identified as a master regulator of Ob-specific expression of OC, which is elevated in OA Ob [37]. We therefore analyzed the ability of RSV to control the Runx2 and PPARγ in OA Ob. Our results indicate that RSV had no effect on Runx2 expression and on PPARγ. These results confirmed that RSV could not regulate Runx2 and therefore it was expected that it would not correct the abnormal OC release in OA Ob. However, RSV partially corrected the abnormal ALP activities in OA Ob, whereas the addition of RSV did not significantly affect elevated OC release in OA Ob. In contrast, RSV promotes the activity of ALP in rat bone marrow-derived MSC [47], indicating again that RSV has a different role depending on the context and the type of cells.

Previous reports from our laboratory [2, 10, 26] and other investigators [4, 5] have shown a reduction in mineralization in OA Ob and in OA bone tissue, respectively, and reflects the in vivo situation. The reduction in in vitro mineralization was due to an increase in TGF-β1, which was slightly reduced by stimulating Sirt1 activity in OA Ob with NMN. As RSV stimulate Sirt1 activity, we tested whether RSV could play a role on OA

Ob mineralization. We showed that increasing doses of RSV in OA Ob increased their mineralization potential about twofold as assessed by alizarin red staining.

Zhou et al. demonstrated that RSV elevates the expression of β-catenin in the early stages of MSC differentiation and that knockdown of *SIRT1* inhibits Wnt/β-catenin signaling, while RSV treatment or overexpression of *SIRT1* activates Wnt/β-catenin signaling [49]. Indeed, in the present study, we observed that RSV increased the Wnt3a-dependent Wnt/β-catenin activity in OA Ob using the dual TOPflash/Renilla reporter assay. This increase in Wnt/β-catenin signaling was accompanied by an increase in free β-catenin levels measured by immunoblotting assays in OA Ob. We previously reported that the abnormal expression of phenotypic markers and reduced mineralization of OA Ob are linked with the stimulation of the Wnt antagonist DKK2 [9] and SOST [10] and the inhibition of the Wnt agonist, R-spondin 2 [11]. Since RSV partly corrected the altered elevated ALP, yet increased abnormal Wnt signaling and altered mineralization in human OA Ob, we tested whether RSV could have an effect on the elevated expression of the Wnt antagonist DKK2 in OA Ob, which is responsible in part for the altered ALP in these cells. Our results indicated that increased dose response to RSV had no effect on DKK2, suggesting that RSV acts differently on ALP activity bypassing DKK2. Mak et al. showed that the antagonist DKK1 inhibits Wnt3a-induced β-catenin in MSC cells and that RSV abolishes this inhibitory effect [50]. Moreover, they showed that RSV increases Wnt signaling by reducing the level of glycogen synthase kinase 3β (GSK-3β), which phosphorylates and destabilizes β-catenin, and that phosphorylation of GSK-3β requires Erk1/2. Indeed our result indicated that RSV increases the phosphorylation of ERK1/2 and increases Wnt signaling in OA Ob.

Conclusion

These data indicate that RSV inhibits the endogenous expression of leptin by OA osteoblasts and promotes the Wnt/β-catenin and Erk1/2 signaling pathways, which are altered in these cells. This last situation could explain the role of RSV in the in vitro mineralization, which is altered in these cells. These data suggest the potential role of RSV in OA.

Abbreviations

1,25(OH)$_2$D$_3$: Active form of vitamin D$_3$; ALP: Alkaline phosphatase; BSA: Bovine serum albumin; cWnt: Canonical Wnt/β-catenin signalling; DKK2: Dickkopft-2; DMEM: Dulbecco's modified Eagle's medium; EP300: E1A binding protein p300; Erk: Extracellular signal-regulated kinase; FBS: Fetal bovine serum; GAPDH: Glyceraldehyde-3-phosphate dehydrogenase; MAPK: Mitogen-activated protein kinase; MSC: Mesenchymal stem cells; NMN: β-Nicotinamide mononucleotide; OA: Osteoarthritis; Ob: Osteoblasts; OC: Osteocalcin; OM: Osteogenic induction medium; PPARγ: Peroxisome proliferator-activated receptor γ; qRT-PCR: Quantitative reverse transcriptase-polymerase chain reaction; RSV: Resveratol; Runx2: Since runt-related transcription factor 2; SIRT1: Sirtuin 1; SOST: Sclerostin; TFG-β1: Transforming growth factor β-1; TOPflash: TCF/Lef luciferase assay; WB: Western blot

Acknowledgements

The authors wish to thank all participants in this study.

Funding

This study was supported by grant MOP-49501 from the Canadian Institutes for Health Research (CIHR) to Daniel Lajeunesse. Élie Abed received a post-doctoral fellowship from Fonds de la Recherche du Québec-Santé (FRQ-S).

Authors' contributions

EA performed the experiments, participated in the statistical analysis and the interpretation of data and drafted the manuscript. JMP and JPP participated in the interpretation of data and reviewed the manuscript. ND provided the human OA knee samples, participated in the interpretation of data and reviewed the manuscript. DL participated in the design of the study, performed the statistical analysis and the interpretation of data and drafted the manuscript. All authors read and approved the final manuscript.

Authors' information

Élie Abed, Ph.D., Research Associate. Aline Delalandre, B.Sc., Research Associate. Daniel Lajeunesse, Ph.D., Laboratory Director.

Competing interests

The authors declare that they have no competing interests.

Consent for publication

Not applicable.

References

1. Goldring MB, Goldring SR. Osteoarthritis. J Cell Physiol. 2007;213(3):626–34.
2. Couchourel D, Aubry I, Delalandre A, Lavigne M, Martel-Pelletier J, Pelletier JP, Lajeunesse D. Altered mineralization of human osteoarthritic osteoblasts is due to abnormal collagen type 1 production. Arthritis Rheum. 2009;60(5):1438–50.
3. Massicotte F, Aubry I, Martel-Pelletier J, Pelletier JP, Fernandes J, Lajeunesse D. Abnormal insulin-like growth factor 1 signaling in human osteoarthritic subchondral bone osteoblasts. Arthritis Res Ther. 2006;8(6):R177.
4. Li B, Aspden RM. Mechanical and material properties of the subchondral bone plate from the femoral head of patients with osteoarthritis or osteoporosis. Ann Rheum Dis. 1997;56:247–54.
5. Mansell JP, Bailey AJ. Abnormal cancellous bone collagen metabolism in osteoarthritis. J Clin Invest. 1998;101:1596–603.
6. Mansell JP, Tarlton JF, Bailey AJ. Biochemical evidence for altered subchondral bone collagen metabolism in osteoarthritis of the hip. Br J Rheumatol. 1997;36:16–9.
7. Hilal G, Martel-Pelletier J, Pelletier JP, Ranger P, Lajeunesse D. Osteoblast-like cells from human subchondral osteoarthritic bone demonstrate an altered phenotype in vitro: possible role in subchondral bone sclerosis. Arthritis Rheum. 1998;41:891–9.
8. Loots GG, Keller H, Leupin O, Murugesh D, Collette NM, Genetos DC. TGF-beta regulates sclerostin expression via the ECR5 enhancer. Bone. 2012;50(3):663–9.
9. Chan TF, Couchourel D, Abed E, Delalandre A, Duval N, Lajeunesse D. Elevated Dickkopf-2 levels contribute to the abnormal phenotype of human osteoarthritic osteoblasts. J Bone Miner Res. 2011;26(7):1399–410.
10. Abed E, Couchourel D, Delalandre A, Duval N, Pelletier JP, Martel-Pelletier J, Lajeunesse D. Low sirtuin 1 levels in human osteoarthritis subchondral osteoblasts lead to abnormal sclerostin expression which decreases Wnt/beta-catenin activity. Bone. 2014;59:28–36.

11. Abed E, Chan TF, Delalandre A, Martel-Pelletier J, Pelletier JP, Lajeunesse D. R-spondins are newly recognized players in osteoarthritis that regulate Wnt signaling in osteoblasts. Arthritis Rheum. 2011;63(12):3865–75.

12. Hwang KA, Choi KC. Anticarcinogenic effects of dietary phytoestrogens and their chemopreventive mechanisms. Nutr Cancer. 2015;67(5):796–803.

13. Pendurthi UR, Williams JT, Rao LV. Resveratrol, a polyphenolic compound found in wine, inhibits tissue factor expression in vascular cells: a possible mechanism for the cardiovascular benefits associated with moderate consumption of wine. Arterioscler Thromb Vasc Biol. 1999;19(2):419–26.

14. Dai Z, Li Y, Quarles LD, Song T, Pan W, Zhou H, Xiao Z. Resveratrol enhances proliferation and osteoblastic differentiation in human mesenchymal stem cells via ER-dependent ERK1/2 activation. Phytomedicine. 2007;14(12):806–14.

15. Mizutani K, Ikeda K, Kawai Y, Yamori Y. Resveratrol stimulates the proliferation and differentiation of osteoblastic MC3T3-E1 cells. Biochem Biophys Res Commun. 1998;253(3):859–63.

16. Li Y, Backesjo CM, Haldosen LA, Lindgren U. Resveratrol inhibits proliferation and promotes apoptosis of osteosarcoma cells. Eur J Pharmacol. 2009;609(1-3):13–8.

17. Zhou H, Shang L, Li X, Zhang X, Gao G, Guo C, Chen B, Liu Q, Gong Y, Shao C. Resveratrol augments the canonical Wnt signaling pathway in promoting osteoblastic differentiation of multipotent mesenchymal cells. Exp Cell Res. 2009;315(17):2953–62.

18. Hipskind RA, Bilbe G. MAP kinase signaling cascades and gene expression in osteoblasts. Front Biosci. 1998;3:d804–16.

19. Massicotte F, Lajeunesse D, Benderdour M, Pelletier JP, Hilal G, Duval N, Martel-Pelletier J. Can altered production of interleukin 1ß, interleukin-6, transforming growth factor-ß and prostaglandin E2 by isolated human subchondral osteoblasts identify two subgroups of osteoarthritic patients. Osteoarthritis Cartilage. 2002;10:491–500.

20. Mutabaruka MS, Aoulad Aissa M, Delalandre A, Lavigne M, Lajeunesse D. Local leptin production in osteoarthritis subchondral osteoblasts may be responsible for their abnormal phenotypic expression. Arthritis Res Ther. 2010;12:R20.

21. Imhof H, Breitenseher M, Kainberger F, Trattnig S. Degenerative joint disease: cartilage or vascular disease? Skeletal Radiol. 1997;26:398–403.

22. Arnoldi CC, Linderholm H, Mussbichler H. Venous engorgement and intraosseous hypertension in osteoarthritis of the hip. J Bone Joint Surg (Br). 1972;54(3):409–21.

23. Aaron RK, Dyke JP, Ciombor DM, Ballon D, Lee J, Jung E, Tung GA. Perfusion abnormalities in subchondral bone associated with marrow edema, osteoarthritis, and avascular necrosis. Ann NY Acad Sci. 2007;1117:124–37.

24. Lee JH, Dyke JP, Ballon D, Ciombor DM, Rosenwasser MP, Aaron RK. Subchondral fluid dynamics in a model of osteoarthritis: use of dynamic contrast-enhanced magnetic resonance imaging. Osteoarthritis Cartilage. 2009;17(10):1350–5.

25. Bouvard B, Abed E, Yelehe-Okouma M, Bianchi A, Mainard D, Netter P, Jouzeau JY, Lajeunesse D, Reboul P. Hypoxia and vitamin D differently contribute to leptin and dickkopf-related protein 2 production in human osteoarthritic subchondral bone osteoblasts. Arthritis Res Ther. 2014;16(5):459.

26. Abed E, Bouvard B, Martineau X, Jouzeau JY, Reboul P, Lajeunesse D. Elevated hepatocyte growth factor levels in osteoarthritis osteoblasts contribute to their altered response to bone morphogenetic protein-2 and reduced mineralization capacity. Bone. 2015;75:111–9.

27. Lee YM, Shin SI, Shin KS, Lee YR, Park BH, Kim EC. The role of sirtuin 1 in osteoblastic differentiation in human periodontal ligament cells. J Periodontal Res. 2011;46(6):712–21.

28. Hilal G, Massicotte F, Martel-Pelletier J, Fernandes JC, Pelletier JP, Lajeunesse D. Endogenous prostaglandin E2 and insulin-like growth factor 1 can modulate the levels of parathyroid hormone receptor in human osteoarthritic osteoblasts. J Bone Miner Res. 2001;16:713–21.

29. Altman RD, Asch E, Bloch DA, Bole G, Borenstein D, Brandt KD, Christy W, Cooke TD, Greenwald R, Hochberg M, et al. Development of criteria for the classification and reporting of osteoarthritis. Classification of osteoarthritis of the knee. Arthritis Rheum. 1986;29:1039–49.

30. Smith PK, Krohn RI, Hermanson GT, Mallia AK, Gartner FH, Provenzano MD, Fujimoto EK, Goeke NM, Olson BJ, Klenk DC. Measurement of protein using bicinchoninic acid. Anal Biochem. 1985;150:76–85.

31. Yaylali A, Ergin K, Cecen S. Effect of resveratrol on leptin and Sirtuin 2 expression in the kidneys in streptozotocin-induced diabetic rats. Anal Quant Cytopathol Histopathol. 2015;37(4):243–51.

32. Gregory CA, Gunn WG, Peister A, Prockop DJ. An alizarin red-based assay of mineralization by adherent cells in culture: comparison with cetylpyridinium chloride extraction. Anal Biochem. 2004;329(1):77–84.

33. Zhang E, Guo Q, Gao H, Xu R, Teng S, Wu Y. Metformin and resveratrol inhibited high glucose-induced metabolic memory of endothelial senescence through SIRT1/p300/p53/p21 Pathway. PLoS One. 2015;10(12), e0143814.

34. Liu DD, Zhang JC, Zhang Q, Wang SX, Yang MS. TGF-beta/BMP signaling pathway is involved in cerium-promoted osteogenic differentiation of mesenchymal stem cells. J Cell Biochem. 2013;114(5):1105–14.

35. Shen CL, Smith BJ, Lo DF, Chyu MC, Dunn DM, Chen CH, Kwun IS. Dietary polyphenols and mechanisms of osteoarthritis. J Nutr Biochem. 2012;23(11):1367–77.

36. Li B, Aspden RM. Composition and mechanical properties of cancellous bone from the femoral head of patients with osteoporosis or osteoarthritis. J Bone Miner Res. 1997;12:641–51.

37. Tseng PC, Hou SM, Chen RJ, Peng HW, Hsieh CF, Kuo ML, Yen ML. Resveratrol promotes osteogenesis of human mesenchymal stem cells by upregulating RUNX2 gene expression via the SIRT1/FOXO3A axis. J Bone Miner Res. 2011;26(10):2552–63.

38. Shakibaei M, Buhrmann C, Mobasheri A. Resveratrol-mediated SIRT-1 interactions with p300 modulate receptor activator of NF-kappaB ligand (RANKL) activation of NF-kappaB signaling and inhibit osteoclastogenesis in bone-derived cells. J Biol Chem. 2011;286(13):11492–505.

39. Cohen-Kfir E, Artsi H, Levin A, Abramowitz E, Bajayo A, Gurt I, Zhong L, D'Urso A, Toiber D, Mostoslavsky R, et al. Sirt1 is a regulator of bone mass and a repressor of Sost encoding for sclerostin, a bone formation inhibitor. Endocrinology. 2011;152(12):4514–24.

40. Lancon A, Frazzi R, Latruffe N. Anti-oxidant, anti-inflammatory and anti-angiogenic properties of resveratrol in ocular diseases. Molecules. 2016;21(3):304.

41. Liu FC, Tsai YF, Tsai HI, Yu HP. Anti-inflammatory and organ-protective effects of resveratrol in trauma-hemorrhagic injury. Mediators Inflamm. 2015;2015:643763.

42. Venigalla M, Sonego S, Gyengesi E, Sharman MJ, Munch G. Novel promising therapeutics against chronic neuroinflammation and neurodegeneration in Alzheimer's disease. Neurochem Int. 2016;95:63–74.

43. Elmali N, Esenkaya I, Harma A, Ertem K, Turkoz Y, Mizrak B. Effect of resveratrol in experimental osteoarthritis in rabbits. Inflamm Res. 2005;54(4):158–62.

44. Shakibaei M, Csaki C, Nebrich S, Mobasheri A. Resveratrol suppresses interleukin-1beta-induced inflammatory signaling and apoptosis in human articular chondrocytes: potential for use as a novel nutraceutical for the treatment of osteoarthritis. Biochem Pharmacol. 2008;76(11):1426–39.

45. Csaki C, Keshishzadeh N, Fischer K, Shakibaei M. Regulation of inflammation signalling by resveratrol in human chondrocytes in vitro. Biochem Pharmacol. 2008;75(3):677–87.

46. Im HJ, Li X, Chen D, Yan D, Kim J, Ellman MB, Stein GS, Cole B, Kc R, Cs-Szabo G, et al. Biological effects of the plant-derived polyphenol resveratrol in human articular cartilage and chondrosarcoma cells. J Cell Physiol. 2012; 227(10):3488–97.

47. Kim HJ, Braun HJ, Dragoo JL. The effect of resveratrol on normal and osteoarthritic chondrocyte metabolism. Bone Joint Res. 2014;3(3):51–9.

48. Ornstrup MJ, Harslof T, Sorensen L, Stenkjaer L, Langdahl BL, Pedersen SB. Resveratrol increases osteoblast differentiation in vitro independently of inflammation. Calcif Tissue Int. 2016;99(2):155–63.

49. Zhou Y, Zhou Z, Zhang W, Hu X, Wei H, Peng J, Jiang S. SIRT1 inhibits adipogenesis and promotes myogenic differentiation in C3H10T1/2 pluripotent cells by regulating Wnt signaling. Cell Biosci. 2015;5:61.

50. Mak W, Shao X, Dunstan CR, Seibel MJ, Zhou H. Biphasic glucocorticoid-dependent regulation of Wnt expression and its inhibitors in mature osteoblastic cells. Calcif Tissue Int. 2009;85(6):538–45.

7

Glycation marker glucosepane increases with the progression of osteoarthritis and correlates with morphological and functional changes of cartilage in vivo

Catherine Legrand[1†], Usman Ahmed[2,3†], Attia Anwar[2], Kashif Rajpoot[4], Sabah Pasha[2], Cécile Lambert[1], Rose K. Davidson[5], Ian M. Clark[5], Paul J. Thornalley[2,3], Yves Henrotin[1,6] and Naila Rabbani[2,3*] (iD)

Abstract

Background: Changes of serum concentrations of glycated, oxidized, and nitrated amino acids and hydroxyproline and anticyclic citrullinated peptide antibody status combined by machine learning techniques in algorithms have recently been found to provide improved diagnosis and typing of early-stage arthritis of the knee, including osteoarthritis (OA), in patients. The association of glycated, oxidized, and nitrated amino acids released from the joint with development and progression of knee OA is unknown. We studied this in an OA animal model as well as interleukin-1β-activated human chondrocytes in vitro and translated key findings to patients with OA.

Methods: Sixty male 3-week-old Dunkin-Hartley guinea pigs were studied. Separate groups of 12 animals were killed at age 4, 12, 20, 28 and 36 weeks, and histological severity of knee OA was evaluated, and cartilage rheological properties were assessed. Human chondrocytes cultured in multilayers were treated for 10 days with interleukin-1β. Human patients with early and advanced OA and healthy controls were recruited, blood samples were collected, and serum or plasma was prepared. Serum, plasma, and culture medium were analyzed for glycated, oxidized, and nitrated amino acids.

Results: Severity of OA increased progressively in guinea pigs with age. Glycated, oxidized, and nitrated amino acids were increased markedly at week 36, with glucosepane and dityrosine increasing progressively from weeks 20 and 28, respectively. Glucosepane correlated positively with OA histological severity ($r = 0.58$, $p < 0.0001$) and instantaneous modulus ($r = 0.52–0.56$; $p < 0.0001$), oxidation free adducts correlated positively with OA severity ($p < 0.0009–0.0062$), and hydroxyproline correlated positively with cartilage thickness ($p < 0.0003–0.003$). Interleukin-1β increased the release of glycated and nitrated amino acids from chondrocytes in vitro. In clinical translation, plasma glucosepane was increased 38% in early-stage OA ($p < 0.05$) and sixfold in patients with advanced OA ($p < 0.001$) compared with healthy controls.

Conclusions: These studies further advance the prospective role of glycated, oxidized, and nitrated amino acids as serum biomarkers in diagnostic algorithms for early-stage detection of OA and other arthritic disease. Plasma glucosepane, reported here for the first time to our knowledge, may improve early-stage diagnosis and progression of clinical OA.

Keywords: Glycation, Oxidative stress, Citrullination, Inflammation, Machine learning

* Correspondence: n.rabbani@warwick.ac.uk
†Catherine Legrand and Usman Ahmed contributed equally to this work.
[2]Warwick Systems Biology, University of Warwick, Clinical Sciences Research Laboratories, University Hospital, Coventry CV2 2DX, UK
[3]Warwick Medical School, Clinical Sciences Research Laboratories, University of Warwick, University Hospital, Coventry CV2 2DX, UK
Full list of author information is available at the end of the article

Background

Osteoarthritis (OA) is a pathogenesis in movable joints characterized by cell stress and extracellular matrix degradation initiated by micro- and macroinjury. Pathogenesis involves low-grade inflammation mediated by innate and adaptive immunity and maladaptive repair responses. It initially manifests in molecular changes related to drivers of pathogenesis and culminates in anatomic and/or physiologic derangements of increasing severity [1].

Current diagnosis of OA is based on radiographic criteria and clinical symptoms, such as joint space width, pain, and loss of function. The related established cartilage lesions are irreversible with current treatments. Magnetic resonance imaging has been applied to early-stage OA diagnosis, but its use is limited by cost, availability, and absence of a validated scoring system. Measurement of soluble biomarkers in plasma or serum

offers an alternative approach for early-stage diagnosis, assessment of progression, and therapeutic monitoring [2]. Development of early-stage diagnosis and effective earlier conservative interventions would likely decrease morbidity and cost of care.

Optimum candidate biomarkers in OA are molecules or molecular fragments present in cartilage, bone, or synovium [3]. Damaging posttranslational modifications of proteins in the joint—glycation, oxidation, and nitration—are considered part of the pathogenic process in OA, impairing biomechanical properties of cartilage [4]. A source of blood-based biomarkers relevant to damaging modifications of cartilage and other proteins are trace-level glycated, oxidized, and nitrated amino acids (Fig. 1), part of which originates from the arthritic joint. We recently reported patterns of changes of these metabolites in synovial fluid and plasma of patients with early and advanced stages of OA and other arthritic disease of

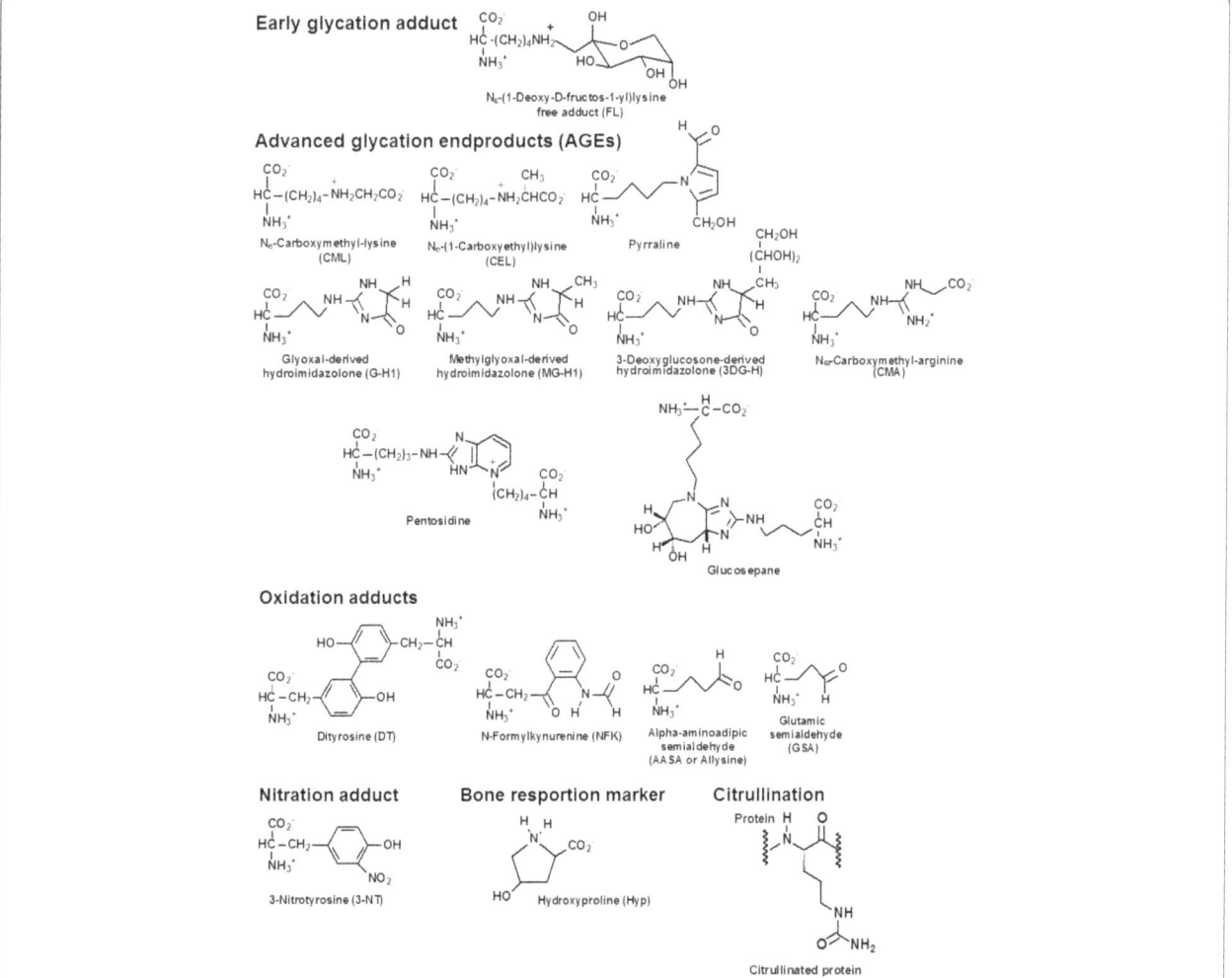

Fig. 1 Protein glycation, oxidation, and nitration free adducts, bone resorption marker hydroxyproline, and citrullinated protein. For glycation, oxidation, and nitration adduct residues of proteins, the NH_3^+- and $-CO_2^-$ termini are part of the peptide backbone of the protein as -NH- and –CO- residues, respectively

the knee compared with subjects with good skeletal health. Patterns of analyte change were distinctive for type of arthritis. Data-driven combination of plasma or serum levels of glycated, oxidized, and nitrated amino acids with anticyclic citrullinated peptide (anti-CCP) antibody status and hydroxyproline (Hyp) by machine learning techniques with two different diagnostic algorithms applied sequentially provided high sensitivity and specificity for diagnosis and typing of early-stage arthritic disease [5]. The application of this diagnostic approach may be further substantiated by gaining insight into the temporal relationship of changes in glycated, oxidized, and nitrated amino acids in serum during development of experimental OA, where correlation with changes in joint histology and thickness and biomechanical properties of cartilage may be made. It is currently unknown how levels of serum glycated, oxidized, and nitrated proteins and amino acids change longitudinally in experimental models of OA and how the changes relate to morphological and functional changes of cartilage in the developing arthritic joint. Glucosepane (GSP) is a further major glycation-derived crosslink of joint proteins [6, 7] that we did not study in our previous work but was considered in the present study [5].

In this work, we studied the progression of histological and biomechanical properties in the Dunkin-Hartley guinea pig model of spontaneous OA. This animal model is the gold standard for studying aging-related OA, is recommended by the Osteoarthritis Research Society International (OARSI), and is defined as a spontaneous model of OA [8, 9]. It has advantages over other animal models in that the guinea pig knee joint structure is similar to that of the human knee and develops OA with many histopathological similarities to human pathology, related to both age and body weight [10]. The development of OA during a younger life period than in human subjects involves a shorter period for protein damage adduct accumulation than in human subjects, and hence changes in serum concentrations of glycated, oxidized, and nitrated amino acids may be smaller than those found in human subjects [5]. Nevertheless, serum GSP emerged in this animal model and in an in vitro model of chondrocyte inflammation as a key new glycated amino acid biomarker. This translated well to clinical early and advanced OA. This further advances the potential role of glycated, oxidized, and nitrated amino acids as biomarker features in diagnostic algorithms for early-stage detection and typing of OA and other arthritic disease.

Methods
Spontaneous OA in Dunkin-Hartley guinea pig
Sixty male 3-week-old Dunkin-Hartley guinea pigs, purchased from Charles River Laboratories (Paris, France) with identification by microchip, were used in the study.

They were bred under pathogen-free conditions with free access to water. In experimental studies, they were housed three per solid-bottom cage and fed with a standard guinea pig chow (Special Diets Service, Essex, England) containing vitamin C (394 mg/kg) and vitamin D_3 (1973 IU/kg), allowing 2 weeks for acclimatization. Polyvinyl chloride pipes were added to the cages to improve housing conditions and minimize stress. Separate groups of 12 animals were sacrificed and analyzed at age 4, 12, 20, 28 and 36 weeks. There was no repeated analysis of animals in the study. The number of animals per group was chosen according to the OARSI recommendation [11]. Animal body weight and food consumption were recorded weekly. Blood samples were collected by intracardiac puncture under general anesthesia (sodium pentobarbital 200 mg/kg intraperitoneally) immediately before animals were killed. Blood samples were centrifuged ($2000 \times g$, 5 minutes), and serum was stored at $-80\ °C$ until analysis. Samples were centrifuged within 1 hour of collection. All experimental procedures and protocols were reviewed and approved by the Institutional Animal Care and Use Ethics Committee of the University of Liège (Belgium) (reference 1648).

Histology
At the time animals were killed, cartilage samples were processed for histological evaluation. The right knee joint (femoral condyles and tibial plateaus) from each animal was fixed for 24 hours in 4% paraformaldehyde, followed by decalcification in hydrochloric acid (DC2 medium; Labonord, Templemars, France) for 4 hours at 4 °C before embedding in paraffin. The right kidney and a piece of the liver were fixed in 4% paraformaldehyde and embedded in paraffin.

Sections (6 μm) of the femoral condyles and tibial plateaus were cut with a microtome in the central area not covered by meniscus following the Cushin plane, as recommended by OARSI [11]. Three sections at 200-μm intervals were stained with hematoxylin, Fast Green, and Safranin-O, and one supplementary central section was stained with toluidine blue. Each compartment of the section (tibial median, tibial lateral, femoral median, and femoral lateral) was scored by two trained experts blinded from sample identity following OARSI recommendations for the guinea pig model. Briefly, the evaluation considered the cartilage surface integrity (0–8), the proteoglycan content (0–6), the cellularity (0–3), the tidemark integrity (0–1), and the osteophyte (0–3), with a maximum of 21 per compartment. The mean score of three sections was calculated for each knee compartment. To assess the global OA score, scores of each compartment were added, giving a maximal score of 84. Lateral and medial synovial membranes were also scored (synovial lining cells hyperplasia 0–2, villous hyperplasia

0–3, degree of cellular infiltration by perivascular lymphocytes and mononuclear cells 0–5), and the mean of lateral and median membrane was calculated to assess the global synovial score (maximum score of 10) [11].

Biomechanical testing by Mach-1® micromechanical tester

The left knee joint (femoral condyles and tibial plateaus) of each animal was used for testing the biomechanical properties of articular cartilage assessed using a Mach-1® micromechanical tester (Mach-1; Biomomentum Inc., Laval, QC, Canada) [12]. Prior to testing, samples were thawed at room temperature in PBS for 30 minutes to equilibrate before starting experiments. Subsequently, the femoral condyle or tibial plateau was fixed with LOC-TITE® 4013 glue (Henkel, Stamford, CT, USA) in a small plastic container (Additional file 1: Figure S2). Throughout the testing, each sample was kept moist with PBS. Using top-view pictures of each sample, at least 50 positions per articular surface were tested using the automated indentation and thickness-mapping protocol. The instantaneous modulus—a measure of cartilage stiffness and cartilage thickness—was calculated using the Mach-1 analysis software (see Additional file 1).

Primary culture of human chondrocytes

Human chondrocytes were cultured in multilayers in six-well plates and treated with interleukin-1β (IL-1β) [13]. Chondrocytes were isolated from human articular cartilage taken during the installation of total knee prosthesis. Cartilage samples were obtained from four adults (two men and two women) whose mean age was 70 years (range, 51–81 years). All specimens used were obtained with informed consent. This procedure was approved by the Ethics Committee of the Catholic University of Louvain (project no. B403201214793). Full-depth articular cartilage was excised and immersed in DMEM (with phenol red and 4.5 g/L glucose) supplemented with 4-(2-hydroxyethyl)-1--piperazineethanesulfonic acid (HEPES) 10 mM, penicillin 100 U/ml, and streptomycin 0.1 mg/ml (all from Lonza, Verviers, Belgium). After three washings, chondrocytes were released from cartilage by sequential enzymatic digestions with 0.5 mg/ml hyaluronidase type IV S (Sigma-Aldrich, Bornem, Belgium) for 30 minutes at 37 °C, 1 mg/ml pronase E (Merck, Leuven, Belgium) for 1 hour at 37 °C, and 0.5 mg/ml collagenase from *Clostridium histolyticum* type IA (Sigma-Aldrich) for 16 to 20 hours at 37 °C. The enzymatically isolated cells were then filtered through a nylon mesh (70 μm), washed three times, counted, and filled to the density of 0.25×10^6 cells/ml of DMEM (with phenol red and 4.5 g/L glucose) supplemented with 10% FBS, 10 mM HEPES, 100 U/ml penicillin, 0.1 mg/ml streptomycin, 2 mM glutamine (all from Lonza), and 20 μg/ml proline (Sigma-Aldrich). After 21 days of culture, chondrocytes were treated in triplicate with recombinant

human IL-1β (1.7 ng/ml; Roche Pharmaceuticals, Brussels, Belgium). The seeding density of the chondrocytes in the six-well plates was 50,000 cells/cm². There was no passage of the cells; the cells overlap and form an extracellular matrix. Culture medium and IL-1β treatment were replaced at 3 and 6 days, and conditioned medium was removed at 3, 6, and 10 days and stored at – 20 °C until analysis.

Patients, healthy subjects, and sampling

Patient recruitment, characteristics, and sampling were similar to those previously described [14]. Briefly, patients with early-stage OA (eOA) ($n = 28$), early-stage rheumatoid arthritis (eRA) ($n = 35$), and inflammatory joint disease other than rheumatoid arthritis (often self-resolving) (non-RA) ($n = 32$) were recruited. Criteria for eOA were subjects presenting with new-onset knee pain, normal radiographs of the symptomatic knee, and routine exploratory arthroscopy with macroscopic findings classified as grade I/II on the Outerbridge scale, and recruited at the Orthopaedic Clinics, University Hospital Coventry & Warwickshire (UHCW), Coventry, UK. Patients with eRA and non-RA were recruited within 5 months of the onset of symptoms of inflammatory arthritis at the Rapid Access Rheumatology Clinic, City Hospital, Birmingham, UK. Synovial fluid and peripheral venous blood samples were collected at initial presentation, and diagnostic outcomes were determined at follow-up. Diagnosis of eRA was made according to the 1987 American Rheumatism Association criteria [15]. Diagnosis of non-RA was made when alternative rheumatological diagnoses explained the inflammatory arthritis [16]. Criteria for these clinical classifications are similar to those suggested in consensus position statements and best practice statements [16, 17]. Healthy controls were recruited at participating clinical centers ($n = 29$) at UHCW. For healthy control subjects, inclusion criteria were no history of joint symptoms, arthritic disease, or other morbidity, and exclusion criteria were a history of injury or pain in either knee, taking medication (excepting oral contraceptives and vitamins), and any abnormality at physical examination of the knee.

Recruitment of patients with advanced OA ($n = 38$) immediately prior to total knee replacement (TKR) surgery (advanced osteoarthritis [aOA], pre-TKR) was done with written informed consent from patients referred for TKR to the Norfolk and Norwich University Hospitals NHS Trust (NNUH), Norwich, UK. Patients were screened for study eligibility criteria as described previously [14]. Eligible patients were males or postmenopausal females scheduled for TKR. This study was approved by the National Research Ethics Service Committee East of England, Cambridge South, UK (approval no. 2012ORTH06L [104-07-12]). All study procedures were performed in accordance with relevant laboratory guidelines and institutional regulations.

Peripheral venous blood samples were collected with ethylenediaminetetraacetic acid (EDTA) anticoagulant from healthy subjects and patients with eOA after overnight fasting. Venous blood samples for the eRA, non-RA, and aOA study groups were collected in the nonfasted state. For analytes studied, diurnal variation in plasma and serum was 13–25%, depending on the analyte, as described previously. Blood samples were centrifuged ($2000 \times g$, 10 minutes), and the plasma and synovial fluid supernatant was removed and stored at $-80\ °C$ until analysis. Samples were centrifuged within 1 hour of collection. Serum was available for eRA and non-RA study groups, and plasma was used for all others. Serum was comparable to plasma because nonprotein analytes were assessed. To confirm this, venous blood samples were collected with informed consent from human volunteers ($n = 6$; 4 female, 2 male; age 47.8 ± 15.8 years; BMI $25.9 \pm 4.0\ kg/m^2$). Ethical approval was given by East Midlands Regional Ethics Committee (reference 16/EM/0095). Serum and plasma (with EDTA anticoagulant) was prepared and assayed for the concentrations of glycated, oxidized, and nitrated amino acids as described below. There was no significant difference between analyte levels in serum and plasma by Wilcoxon signed-rank test.

Analysis of glycated, oxidized, and nitrated protein and amino acids in serum/plasma

Glycation, oxidation, and nitration adduct residues and related precursor unmodified amino acid residues in plasma/serum protein were quantified in exhaustive enzymatic digests, with correction for autohydrolysis of hydrolytic enzymes [18, 19]. The concentrations of glycated, oxidized, and nitrated amino acids (free adducts) and hydroxyproline in plasma/serum were determined similarly in 10 kDa ultrafiltrate of plasma/serum and cell culture medium. Ultrafiltrate of plasma/serum (50 µl) was collected by microspin ultrafiltration (10 kDa cutoff) at 4 °C. Retained protein was diluted with water to 500 µl and washed in four cycles of concentration to 50 µl and dilution to 500 µl with water over the microspin ultrafilter at 4 °C. The final washed protein (100 µl) was delipidated and hydrolyzed enzymatically as described previously [19, 20]. Protein hydrolysate (25 µl, 32 µg equivalent) or ultrafiltrate (5 µl) was mixed with stable isotopic standard analytes (amounts as given previously) and analyzed by LC-MS/MS. Samples were analyzed using an ACQUITY™ ultra-high-performance liquid chromatography system with a Xevo-TQS LC-MS/MS mass spectrometer (Waters, Manchester, UK). Samples are maintained at 4 °C in the autosampler during batch analysis. The columns were 2.1×50-mm and 2.1×250-mm, 5-µm particle size Hypercarb™

(Thermo Fisher Scientific, Waltham, MA, USA) in series with programmed switching at 30 °C. Chromatographic retention was necessary to resolve oxidized analytes from their amino acid precursors to avoid interference from partial oxidation of the latter in the electrospray ionization source of the mass spectrometric detector. Analytes were detected by electrospray positive ionization and mass spectrometry multiple reaction monitoring (MRM) mode, where analyte detection response was specific for mass/charge ratio of the analyte molecular ion and major fragment ion generated by collision-induced dissociation in the mass spectrometer collision cell. The ionization source and desolvation gas temperatures were 120 °C and 350 °C, respectively; cone gas and desolvation gas flow rates were 99 and 900 L/h; and the capillary voltage was 0.60 kV. Argon gas (0.5 Pa) was in the collision cell. For MRM detection, molecular ion and fragment ion masses and collision energies optimized to $\pm$ 0.1 Da and ± 1 eV, respectively, were programmed [19]. In all sample analyses, the investigator was blinded from the sample identity. Analytes determined were as follows: glycation adducts N^ε-fructosyl-lysine (FL), N^ε-carboxymethyl-lysine (CML), N^ε-carboxyethyl-lysine (CEL), N^ω-carboxymethylarginine (CMA), glyoxal-derived hydroimidazolone (G-H1), methylglyoxal-derived hydroimidazolone (MG-H1), 3-deoxyglucosone-derived hydroimidazolone isomers (3DG-H), GSP, and pentosidine; oxidation adducts dityrosine (DT), N-formylkynurenine (NFK), α-aminoadipic semialdehyde (AASA), and glutamic semialdehyde (GSA); nitration adduct 3-nitrotyrosine (3-NT); and related amino acids [19] (see Fig. 1 for structures and expansion of acronyms). The biochemical and clinical significance is described elsewhere [6]. Protein adduct residues (normalized to their amino acid residue precursors; mmol/mol amino acid modified) and serum or plasma free adduct concentrations (µM or nM) are given. In culture medium, free adduct concentrations were corrected for cell number by normalizing to cellular DNA content.

Citrullinated protein and hydroxyproline

Serum citrullinated protein (CP) and Hyp were analyzed by stable isotopic dilution analysis LC-MS/MS, as previously described [20].

Machine learning

We developed algorithms using the clinical analyte data to distinguish the following four groups of subjects and patients: healthy control, eOA, eRA, and non-RA. The diagnostic algorithms were trained on the dataset using support vector machines [21]. The algorithm was validated by twofold cross-validation using five randomized repeat trials for improved robustness. A two-stage approach was taken: (1) to distinguish between disease and healthy control and (2) to distinguish between eOA, eRA, and non-RA. We used accuracy of case and control classification to optimize algorithm features. Diagnostic characteristics, including area under the ROC (AUROC), are given with 95% CI determined via bootstrap analysis. The contribution of each feature in the algorithms to classification accuracy was assessed by determining the change in AUROC when a feature was omitted from the algorithm and retrained; a negative change represents a valuable feature, and a positive change an adverse feature, for classification accuracy. Data were analyzed using MATLAB version R2017A software (MathWorks, Natick, MA, USA).

Statistical analysis

Results are expressed as mean ± SEM unless otherwise stated. Following a normality test, one-way analysis of variance (ANOVA) with Tukey's posttest was performed for histology, MACH-1, and amino acid analytes. Pearson's correlations were performed between global OA score, parameters of MACH-1, and amino acid biomarkers. Given the asymmetric distribution of biomarkers, a logarithmic transformation was considered to satisfy the hypothesis of normality. ANOVA was applied to compare each biomarker between age groups. The same analysis was used to compare the different parameters between age groups. The association between the log-transformed biomarkers and the parameters was assessed by Pearson's correlation. A multiple regression model (including as independent variables age, the parameter of interest, and an interaction term between these two factors) was constructed in order to investigate the influence of this parameter in the biomarker-age relationship (potential confounding factor). The results were considered to be significant at the 5% critical level ($p < 0.05$). There was no repeated analysis of the guinea pigs or human subjects, so repeated measures analysis is not applicable. For longitudinal analysis of multilayer cultures, to investigate a possible difference between the two groups, a mixed model with an undefined covariance matrix was applied to the data. The independent variables considered in this model were time, IL-1β treatment, and interaction between them. This statistical approach allowed us to compare biomarker production curves between the two groups while taking into account the presence of correlated data. For significance tests and correlation analysis of 14 glycated, oxidized, and nitrated amino acids and hydroxyproline analyzed in serum filtrate and 14 glycation, oxidation, and nitration adduct residues and CP in serum protein (15 analytes in each sample type), analyzed without preconceived hypothesis, a Bonferroni correction of 15 was applied. The predictive ability of these analytes for development of OA was studied by developing a partial least squares (PLS) regression model.

The model was trained to learn to predict OA histological score from concentrations of serum glycated, oxidized, and nitrated amino acids (FL, CML, CEL, MG-H1, G-H1, 3DG-H, CMA, AASA, GSP, GSA, NFK, DT, 3-NT, pyrraline, Hyp, and CP) with the 4–36 weeks guinea pig study groups. Subsequent to training, the model was used to predict OA histological score for each guinea pig. The residual error between model predictions and the actual OA histological score was estimated as root mean squares error. Error at each individual stage and the overall error at all stages were estimated. Data analysis was performed with SAS version 9.4 for Windows statistical software (SAS Institute, Cary, NC, USA).

Results

Spontaneous OA in Dunkin-Hartley guinea pig

All 60 guinea pigs were examined daily during the study. Two guinea pigs died at study weeks 30 and 31. Guinea pig body weights at the time the animals were killed were (in grams, mean ± SD): week 4, 282 ± 9; week 12, 723 ± 54; week 20, 887 ± 61; weak 28, 978 ± 78; and week 36, 1016 ± 80. During the study, the five groups showed similar gains in body weight, with no difference observed between study groups of the same age. Food consumption declined progressively with guinea pig age (*see* Additional file 1). The liver and kidney were examined after animals were killed. No abnormalities were observed; the liver and adrenal gland weights were similar between guinea pigs of the same study group.

Histological assessment of cartilage lesions as recommended by OARSI showed that guinea pigs spontaneously developed severe knee OA (Fig. 2). In all animals, the global histological score increased significantly with age until week 28 and then stabilized between weeks 28 and 36 (Fig. 3a). A significant and progressive increase of synovial score between weeks 4 and 36 was observed (Fig. 3b). The global histological score correlated positively with the global synovial histological score ($r = 0.55$, $p < 0.001$).

Cartilage thickness and biomechanical properties were assessed by the Mach-1® micromechanical tester. Cartilage thickness of the knee joint was decreased at the condyle and tibial plateau regions from 12 to 20 weeks and remained at a stable low level thereafter (Fig. 3c and d). Instantaneous modulus of the articular cartilage increased progressively in the condyle at weeks 12 and 20 and remained at a stable high level thereafter, and it increased progressively from weeks 20 to 36 in the tibial plateau region (Fig. 3e and f). There were negative correlations of condyle and tibial plateau cartilage thickness with increased OA histological score and positive correlations with instantaneous modulus (Fig. 3g–j). Detailed histological analysis showed that the structure of the

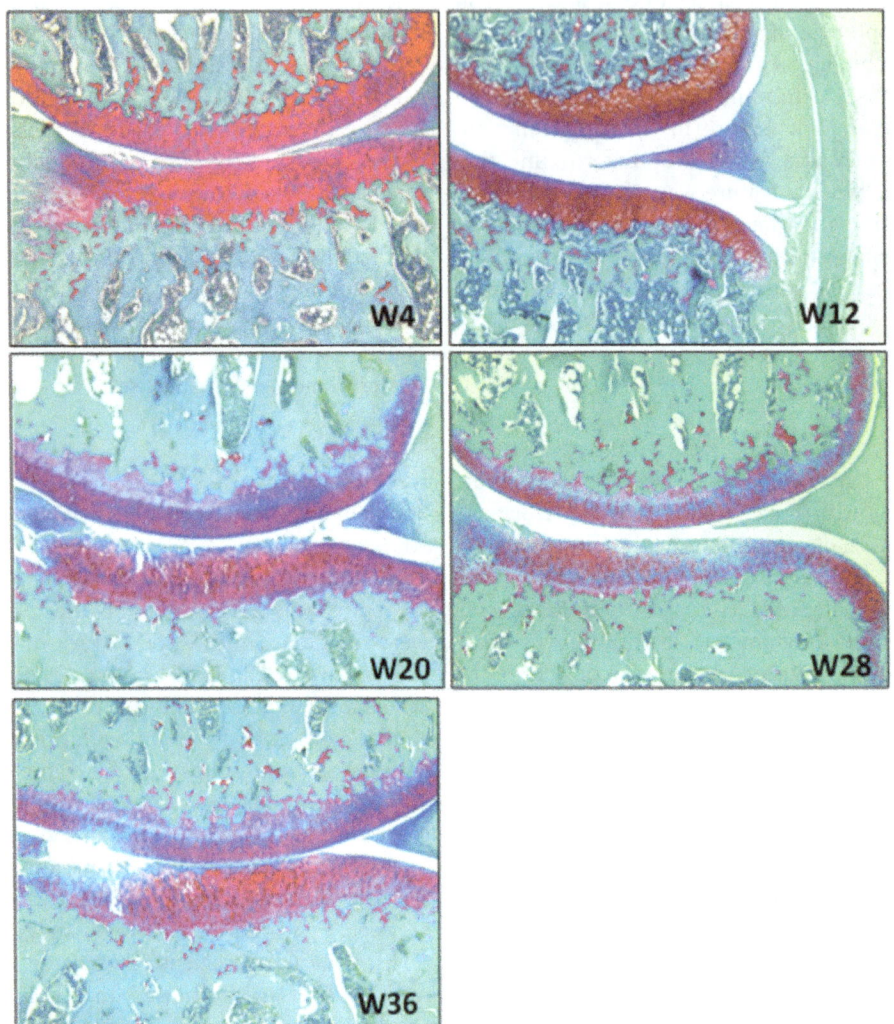

Fig. 2 Representative pictures of medial compartment of right guinea pig knees of each group over time. Safranin-O/Fast Green/hematoxylin staining, 4 × magnification. W4–W36 (week 4 – week 6) inset indicates the age of the guinea pig donor analyzed

cartilage and the proteoglycan content correlated with the instantaneous modulus of the femoral condyle ($r = 0.58$, $p < 0.001$; $r = 0.52$, $p < 0.001$). At the tibial plateaus, the strongest associations were found between the cartilage structure and integrity of tidemark and the instantaneous modulus ($r = 0.44$, $p < 0.002$; $r = 0.43$, $p < 0.002$, respectively).

Analysis of glycated, oxidized, and nitrated amino acids and protein in serum

For glycated amino acids, serum concentrations of FL, CEL, and G-H1 were unchanged from 4 to 28 weeks and then increased two- to threefold at week 36 when OA was severe (Fig. 4a–c). Pyrraline free adduct was decreased at weeks 20 and 28 compared with 4, 12, and 36 weeks (Fig. 4d). Pyrraline is an advanced glycation endproduct (AGE) sourced exclusively from food, which may explain this disparate time-course profile [22].

CMA free adduct showed a similar trend (Fig. 4e). CML, MG-H1, and 3DG-H free adducts initially decreased at 12 and 20 weeks compared with the 4-week baseline levels, returned to baseline levels at 28 weeks, and then increased two- to threefold at 36 weeks (Fig. 4f–h). In contrast, GSP free adduct was unchanged at 12 weeks and then increased progressively from 20 to 36 weeks to threefold higher than baseline levels (Fig. 4i).

For oxidized amino acids, serum DT, NFK, and GSA free adducts increased progressively from 28 to 36 weeks to two- to threefold higher than baseline levels, increasing slightly later in OA development than GSP (Fig. 4j–l). AASA free adduct was decreased at 12 weeks and increased at 36 weeks (Fig. 4m). Serum 3-NT concentration was decreased by 29–32% at 12–36 weeks compared with baseline (Fig. 4n).

For OA-linked markers, bone resorption marker serum Hyp was decreased at weeks 12–28 with

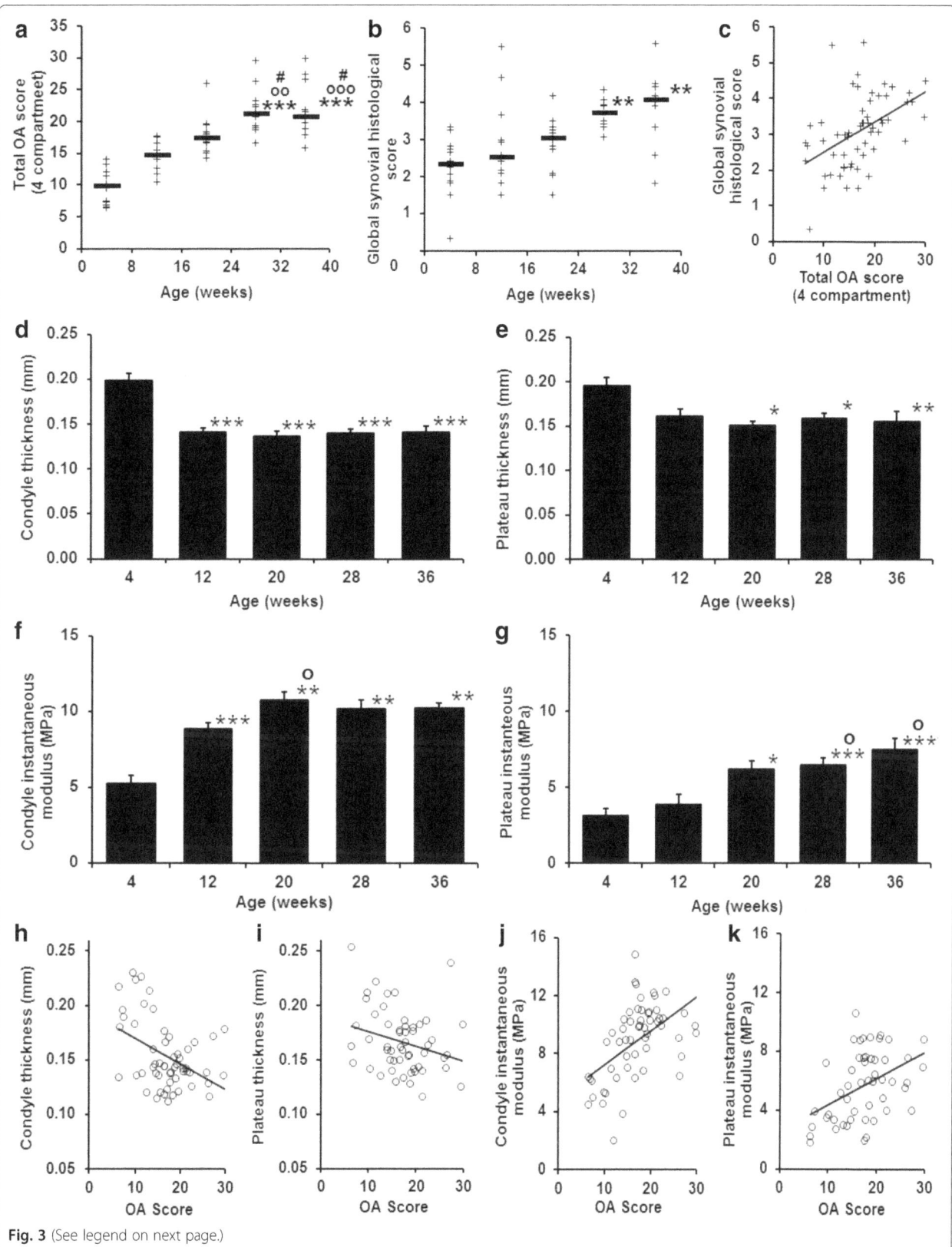

Fig. 3 (See legend on next page.)

(See figure on previous page.)

Fig. 3 Development of osteoarthritis in Dunkin-Hartley guinea pigs. **a** Total OA score at four sites in each group. **b** Global synovial histological score in each group. Horizontal bars indicate median values. **c** Correlation of global synovial histological score with total OA score ($r = 0.55$, $p = 7 \times 10^{-6}$; Spearman). Thickness (in millimeters) (**d** and **e**) and instantaneous modulus (MPa) (**f** and **g**) in femoral condyles and tibial plateau, respectively. Data are mean ± SEM ($n = 12$ in each group, except $n = 10$ at week 36). **h–k** Correlations of cartilage thickness and instantaneous modulus on global OA histological score in condyle and tibial plateau. Correlation coefficients are (**h**) $r = -0.35$, $p < 0.01$; (**i**) $r = -0.27$, $p < 0.05$; (**j**) $r = 0.58$, $p < 0.001$; and (**k**) $r = 0.44$, $p < 0.002$. Significance (**a–f**): * $p < 0.05$; ** $p < 0.01$; and *** $p < 0.001$ with respect to 4-week study group; o, oo, and ooo, $p < 0.05$, $p < 0.01$, and $p < 0.001$ with respect to 12-week study group; and # $p < 0.05$ with respect to 20-week study group; one-way analysis of variance with Tukey posttest

respect to baseline level, and serum CP was decreased by 50–71% from weeks 20 to 36 (Fig. 4o and p).

For glycation, oxidation, and nitration of serum protein, most adduct residue contents decreased from 12 to 20 weeks and remained decreased thereafter, exceptions being glycation adducts FL and pentosidine and oxidation adduct DT, which increased (*see*

Additional file 1). Changes of serum free adducts and serum protein adducts are summarized in heat maps (Fig. 4q and r).

In correlation analysis, most serum glycation and oxidation free adducts were correlated with each other, the correlations being driven mainly by the marked increase of most analytes at 36 weeks. Exceptions were positive

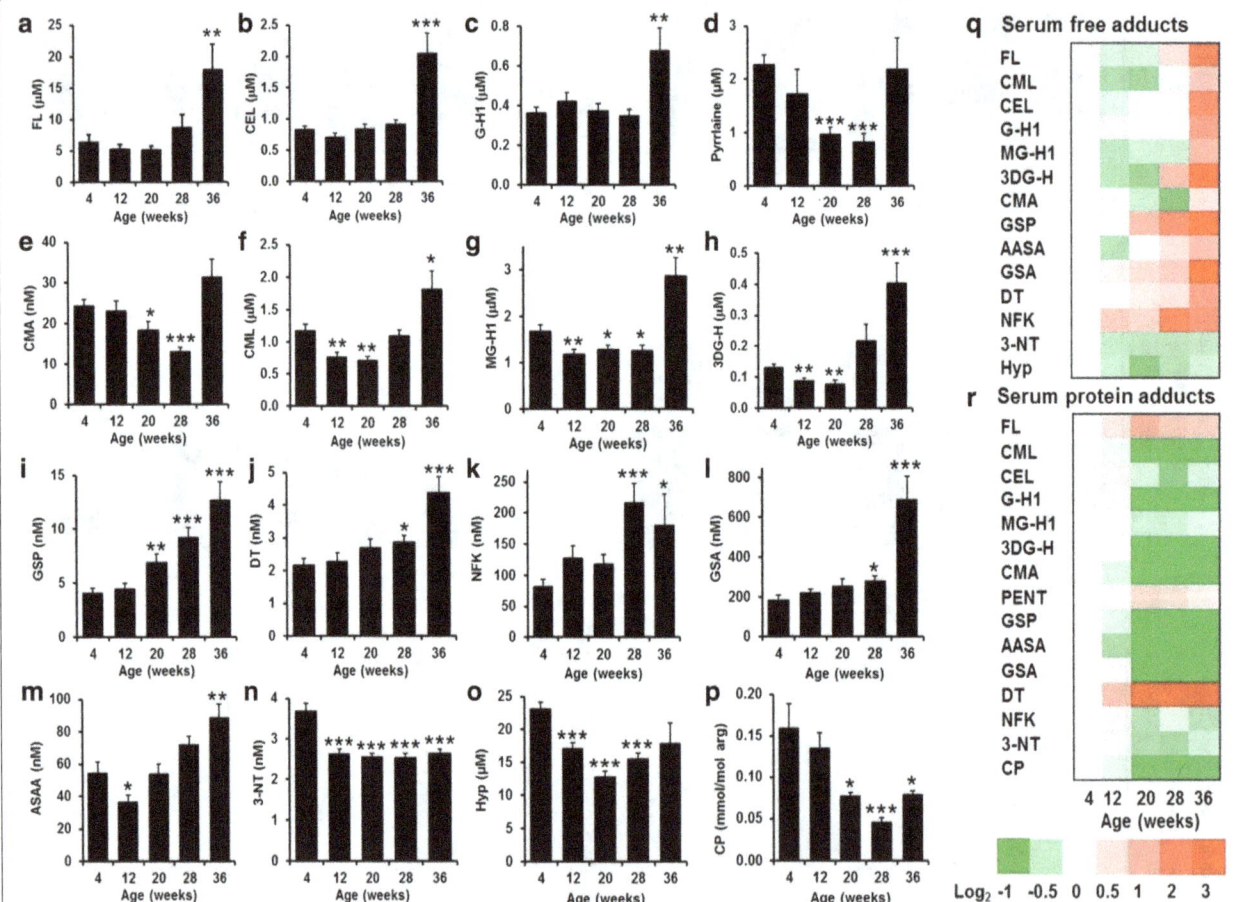

Fig. 4 Serum protein glycation, oxidation, and nitration adducts and hydroxyproline and citrullinated protein during development of osteoarthritis in Dunkin-Hartley guinea pigs. Left side, center panels: Time course changes of serum glycation, oxidation, and nitration free adducts. **a** N^ε-Fructosyl-lysine (FL). **b** N^ε(1-carboxyethyl)lysine (CEL). **c** glyoxal-derived hydroimidazolone (G-H1). **d** Pyrraline. **e** N^ω-carboxymethylarginine (CMA). **f** N^ε(1-carboxymethyl)lysine (CML). **g** Methylglyoxal-derived hydroimidazolone (MG-H1). **h** 3-Deoxyglucosone-derived hydroimidazolone (3DG-H). **i** Glucosepane (GSP). **j** Dityrosine (DT). **k** N-formylkynurenine (NFK). **l** Glutamic semialdehyde (GSA). **m** α-Aminoadipic semialdehyde (AASA). (**n**) 3-Nitrotyrosine (3-NT). Other serum markers were Hydroxyproline (Hyp) (**o**) and citrullinated protein (CP) (**p**). Data are mean ± SEM. Significance: * $p < 0.05$, ** $p < 0.01$ and *** $p < 0.001$ by one-way analysis of variance with Tukey posttest. Right side panels: Heat map representation of changes: **q** serum glycation, oxidation, and nitration free adducts and Hyp. **r** Serum protein glycation, oxidation, and nitration adduct residues and CP

correlations of pyrraline with CMA and 3-NT free adducts and a negative correlation with NFK, and positive correlation of serum Hyp with CML. There were no correlations of glycation, oxidation, and nitration free adducts with serum CP. In contrast, serum CP correlated positively with levels of most glycation, oxidation, and nitration adduct residues of serum protein, except for FL and DT, where the correlations were negative (*see* Additional file 1).

For associations of protein glycation, oxidation, and nitration free adducts with the global histological score, GSP, AASA, GSA, DT, and NFK correlated positively with global histological score after correction for multiple analyte measurements. GSP had the highest correlation coefficient and significance ($r = 0.58$, $p < 0.0001$). In contrast, 3-NT free adduct correlated negatively with the global histological score. For cartilage thickness, 3-NT and Hyp correlated positively, and GSA negatively, at condyle and tibial plateau sites. Hyp had the highest correlation coefficient and significance (condyle $r = 0.47$, $p = 0.0003$; plateau $r = 0.39$, $p = 0.003$). Six free adducts correlated positively with instantaneous modulus; GSP had the highest correlation coefficient and significance (condyle $r = 0.52$ and plateau $r = 0.56$; $p < 0.0001$). CMA and 3-NT free adducts and CP correlated negatively with instantaneous modulus; 3-NT free adduct (condyle $r = - 0.46$, $p = 0.0004$; plateau $r = - 0.41$, $p = 0.003$) and CP (femoral condyle $r = - 0.53$, $p < 0.0001$), remaining significant after Bonferroni correction (Table 1).

A PLS regression model of serum glycated, oxidized, and nitrated amino acids, Hyp, and CP on total OA histological

score was computed. After training, the model was used to predict total OA histological score for each guinea pig. The outcome indicated that the model predicted histological score well in the early development of OA (4, 12, and 20 weeks) with declining predictive performance in more advanced stages (28 and 36 weeks) (*see* Additional file 1).

Multilayer primary human chondrocytes culture
From days 6 through 10, the production of CEL, G-H1, CMA, GSP, NFK, and 3-NT was increased with IL-1β treatment compared with control. In mixed model statistical study, all amino acid analytes increased over time, and increases of G-H1, CEL, and 3-NT were higher with IL-1β treatment compared with the control (Fig. 5).

Plasma/serum glucosepane free adduct in clinical OA and application for clinical diagnosis and typing of early-stage arthritis of the knee
With the emergence of serum GSP free adduct as a potential marker of OA from the guinea pig study and chondrocyte studies, we analyzed serum GSP in patients and healthy controls, including a study group with aOA, pre-TKR surgery. Clinical characteristics were presented previously [14, 20]. Plasma GSP free adduct was increased 38% in eOA, sixfold in aOA, pre-TKR, twofold in non-RA, and threefold in eRA (Table 2). Developing diagnostic algorithms for early-stage arthritic disease, we found that optimum performance to discriminate between healthy controls and early-stage arthritis of any type was achieved with features in the algorithm: serum Hyp, glycation free adducts (CEL, GSP, MG-H1, 3DG-H, G-H1, and

Table 1 Correlation of glycation, oxidation, and nitration free adducts and citrullinated protein with global histological score and joint biomechanical properties measured by Mach-1 parameters

| | | Global histological score | | Thickness | | | | Instantaneous modulus | | | |
| | | | | Condyle | | Plateau | | Condyle | | Plateau | |
		r	p Value	r	p Value	r	p Value	r	p Value	r	p Value
Glycation	FL	0.33	0.012							0.30	0.031
	G-H1	0.26	0.046								
	CMA							− 0.32	0.017		
	3DG-H	0.27	0.044								
	GSP	0.58	< 0.0001[a]					0.52	< 0.0001[a]	0.56	< 0.0001[a]
Oxidation	AASA	0.38	0.0029[a]					0.27	0.043	0.40	0.004
	GSA	0.36	0.0062[a]	− 0.29	0.033	− 0.33	0.015			0.35	0.013
	Dityrosine	0.42	0.0009[a]					0.34	0.010	0.36	0.010
	NFK	0.42	0.0011[a]					0.37	0.006	0.33	0.018
Nitration	3-NT	− 0.46	0.0003[a]	0.33	0.013	0.29	0.034	− 0.46	0.0004[a]	− 0.41	0.003[a]
Hyp				0.47	0.0003[a]	0.39	0.003[a]	− 0.38	0.0037		
CP		− 0.52	< 0.0001[a]					− 0.53	< 0.0001[a]	− 0.33	0.018

Abbreviations: FL N^ε^-fructosyl-lysine, G-H1 Glyoxal-derived hydroimidazolone, CMA N^ω^-carboxymethylarginine, 3DG-H 3-Deoxyglucosone-derived hydroimidazolone isomers, GSP Glucosepane, AASA α-Aminoadipic semialdehyde, GSA Glutamic semialdehyde, NFK N-formylkynurenine, 3-NT 3-Nitrotyrosine, Hyp Hydroxyproline, CP Citrullinated protein
[a]Correlation coefficient significant after Bonferroni correction of 15 was applied

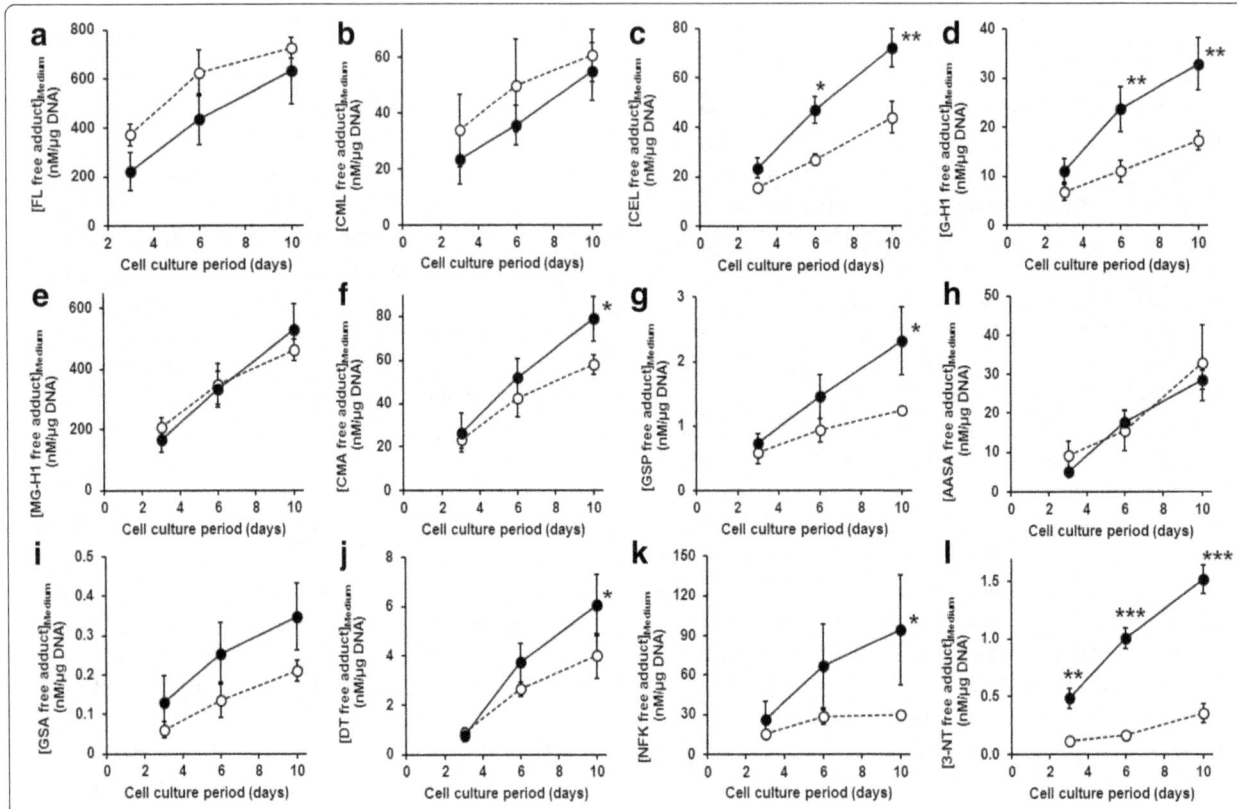

Fig. 5 Concentrations of glycation, oxidation, and nitration free adducts in multilayer culture supernatant. Analyte concentrations in the culture medium, normalized to cell DNA content. Key: dashed lines = control; solid lines = + IL-1β. Free adduct: **a** FL. **b** CML. **c** CEL. **d** G-H1. **e** MG-H1. **f** CMA. **g** GSP. **h** AASA. **i** GSA. **j** DT. **k** NFK. **l** 3-NT. Data are mean ± SEM ($n = 4$). * $p < 0.05$, ** $p < 0.01$, and *** $p < 0.001$. Through longitudinal statistical study, we found that all biomarkers increased significantly over time ($p < 0.0001$). Comparison of the time-course curves showed that levels of G-H1, CEL, and 3-NT were increased with IL-1β treatment compared with control ($p = 0.0023$, $p = 0.0071$, and $p < 0.0001$, respectively)

CMA), oxidation free adducts (NFK, methionine sulfoxide [MetSO], and DT), and nitration free adduct 3-NT (Algorithm 1). This had sensitivity 90.4%, specificity 83.2%, and AUROC 0.93; random selection is 0.50. In assessing the relative importance of each feature in classification accuracy, ΔAUROC on feature omission was (largest to smallest): CEL, − 0.067; GSP, − 0.063; Hyp, − 0.026; NFK, − 0.024; MetSO, − 0.014; MG-H1, − 0.011; 3DG-H, − 0.009; G-H1, − 0.008; 3-NT, − 0.004; DT, − 0.0005; and CMA, − 0.00008.

In a subsequent step for patients with early-stage arthritis, optimum performance to discriminate between types of arthritis included features in the algorithm: anti-CCP-Ab positivity assessment with glycation free adducts (3DG-H, CML, FL, GSP, and CEL) and oxidation and nitration free adducts (MetSO and 3-NT, respectively). This distinguished eOA from eRA and non-RA with sensitivity 94.0%, specificity 96.1%, and AUROC 0.98; random selection is 0.33 (Table 3 and Additional file 1). In assessing relative importance of each feature in classification accuracy, mean

Table 2 Plasma or serum glucosepane free adduct in patients with early and advanced osteoarthritis and other early-stage arthritic disease

Study group	No.	Age (yr)	Gender (M/F)	Glucosepane (nM)
Control	29	34.4 ± 8.2	14/15	13.6 (10.1–18.1)
eOA	28	43.3 ± 13.3*	12/16	18.7 (13.3–35.5)*,ooo
aOA, pre-TKR	38	70.7 ± 8.9***	15/23	76.3 (61.2–97.5)***
Non-RA	32	51.7 ± 18.1**	14/16	31.2 (20.3–45.2)**,ooo
eRA	35	60.4 ± 15.7***	13/22	46.1 (31.1–77.8)***,ooo

Abbreviations: eOA Early-stage osteoarthritis, *aOA* Advanced osteoarthritis, *TKR* Total knee replacement, *RA* Rheumatoid arthritis, *eRA* Early-stage rheumatoid arthritis

Data are median (lower – upper quartile). Significance: 5-group comparison – $p < 0.001$ (*Kruskal-Wallis*). For binary comparisons: *, ** and ***, $p < 0.05$, $p < 0.01$ and $p < 0.001$ with respect to plasma levels of healthy controls; ooo, $p < 0.001$ with respect to plasma levels of aOA, pre-TKR (*Mann-Whitney U*)

ΔAUROC on feature omission for the three classifications was as follows: anti-CCP antibody status, – 0.116; 3DG-H, – 0.089; CML, – 0.082; FL, – 0.073; GSP, – 0.066; MetSO, – 0.034; CEL, – 0.027; and 3-NT, – 0.023.

Discussion

In this study, we showed that serum concentrations of trace-level glycated, oxidized, and nitrated amino acids increase with development of OA in an experimental spontaneous model of knee joint OA. Multiple regression models, adjusted for body weight, suggested that these changes were not due to changes in body weight. GSP free adduct emerged as a biomarker that strongly and positively correlated with global OA histological score and instantaneous modulus measure of stiffness of articular cartilage, increasing with OA severity. Plasma GSP free adduct was modestly and markedly increased in early-stage and severe, advanced clinical OA, respectively. Inclusion of plasma GSP free adduct in a diagnostic algorithm with other trace-level glycated, oxidized, and nitrated amino acids improved detection and arthritis type classification of early-stage clinical OA. We also found that IL-1β, a key cytokine involved in OA pathogenesis, increased the release of GSP and other glycation, oxidation, and nitration free adduct release from chondrocytes, suggesting that inflammation-driven proteolysis may increase free adduct release in vivo. This provides further evidence that, taken together with our previous reports [5, 10, 20], suggests that measurement of trace-level damaged amino acids in serum or plasma are potential biomarkers for diagnosis, progression of severity and therapeutic monitoring in OA and other arthritic disease.

In advanced OA in guinea pigs at 36 weeks, serum concentrations of glycated and oxidized amino acids were increased compared with week 4 control, except for pyrraline, CMA, and 3-NT. From previous studies of Dunkin Hartley guinea pigs, the development of knee joint cartilage, proteoglycan, and bone structure is mature at 12 weeks [23]. Beyond this time, there is increased cartilage density associated with change in cartilage crosslink structure, and from 28 weeks, increased degradation of cartilage [24, 25]. Previous studies found increased markers of cartilage degradation, keratan sulfate, cartilage oligomeric matrix protein, and collagenase-generated fragments of collagen II [26] as well as markers of bone metabolism (urinary hydroxylysyl-pyridinoline and lysyl-pyridinoline, and serum osteocalcin), consistent with this [27]. We suggest that increases in glycated and oxidized amino acids are due to enhanced proteolysis of articular cartilage and bone remodeling, leading to increased flux of release of glycation and oxidation free adducts into the vasculature for urinary excretion. There is also an expected contribution from increased uptake of some glycated amino acids from food for some analytes (see below). Increased glycated and oxidized amino acid release from cartilage may occur without further change in its thickness through increased cartilage turnover and/or swelling [28]. The earlier increase in serum GSP from week 20 may relate to restructuring and decrease of cartilage crosslinks found during this period.

Pyrraline is an AGE derived only from food [22] and hence provides an objective biomarker of food consumption [29]. Serum CMA free adduct correlated positively with pyrraline

Table 3 Characteristics of diagnostic algorithms for diagnosis and typing of early-stage arthritis: predictive algorithm outcomes for twofold cross-validation

Algorithm features	Algorithm 1: plasma Hyp and GSP, G-H1, MG-H1, 3DG-H, CEL, CMA, MetSO, 3-NT, NFK, and DT free adducts	Algorithm 2: anti-CCP-Ab positivity assessment and plasma GSP, FL, 3DG-H, CML, CEL, MetSO, and 3-NT free adducts		
Classification	Disease vs control	eOA vs non-RA and eRA	eRA vs non-RA and eOA	Non-RA vs eRA and eOA
Accuracy (%)	88.4 (86.9–90.0)	95.5 (93.7–97.3)	78.1 (74.3–82.0)	78.9 (74.7–83.2)
Sensitivity (%)	90.4 (88.7–92.1)	94.0 (88.8–99.3)	69.1 (54.4–83.7)	67.5 (46.2–88.8)
Specificity (%)	83.2 (77.4–89.0)	96.1 (92.6–99.6)	83.2 (71.8–94.6)	84.6 (77.1–92.1)
AUROC	0.93 (0.92–0.94)	0.98 (0.97–0.99)	0.86 (0.81–0.90)	0.88 (0.86–0.90)
Positive likelihood ratio	8.26 (5.77–10.75)	16.11 (9.56–22.66)	7.66 (2.94–12.37)	4.96 (3.31–6.60)
Negative likelihood ratio	0.11 (0.10–0.13)	0.06 (0.01–0.11)	0.34 (0.20–0.48)	0.36 (0.14–0.57)
Positive predictive value (%)	93.6 (91.7–95.6)	92.8 (86.5–99.0)	76.3 (65.1–87.4)	71.8 (62.7–80.8)
Negative predictive value (%)	77.3 (74.4–80.2)	97.5 (95.3–99.6)	84.4 (79.0–89.8)	86.2 (78.9–93.4)
F-score	0.92 (0.91–0.93)	0.93 (0.90–0.96)	0.69 (0.62–0.75)	0.64 (0.49–0.79)

Abbreviations: MetSO Methionine sulfoxide, *FL* N^ϵ-fructosyl-lysine, *G-H1* Glyoxal-derived hydroimidazolone, *MG-H1* Methylglyoxal-derived hydroimidazolone, *CMA* N^ω-carboxymethylarginine, *3DG-H* 3-Deoxyglucosone-derived hydroimidazolone isomers, *GSP* Glucosepane, *NFK* N-formylkynurenine, *3-NT* 3-Nitrotyrosine, *Hyp* Hydroxyproline, *eOA* Early-stage osteoarthritis, *TKR* Total knee replacement, *RA* Rheumatoid arthritis, *eRA* Early-stage rheumatoid arthritis, *DT* Dityrosine, *CCP* Cyclic citrullinated peptide, *CML* N^ϵ-carboxymethyl-lysine, *CEL* N^ϵ-carboxyethyl-lysine

Data are mean (95% CI). Analyte data other than GSP (Table 2) employed in algorithm development were reported previously [5]

and may be sourced mainly from the diet in this study. There was a progressive decline in food consumption by the guinea pigs from week 4 to week 36. Gait and mobility are impaired in advanced OA in this model [30], but in the present study decreased food consumption may have been linked to pain with loss of appetite and decreased voluntary activity. The guinea pigs typically show a progressive increase in body weight [31], as found in the present study (see Additional file 1). Serum pyrraline free adduct concentration showed a trend similar to that of food consumption with decreases at weeks 20 and 28, diverging from this with an anomalous increase at week 36. CML, MG-H1, and 3DG-H usually have significant contributions from the diet [29, 32, 33]. The decreases of serum CML, MG-H1, and 3DG-H free adduct concentrations at 12 weeks may be related to the initial decline in food consumption. Progressive decreased food consumption may explain decreases in serum CMA, CML, MG-H1, and 3DG-H free adduct concentrations at 20 weeks, as well as decreases in serum CMA and MG-H1 at 28 weeks. The lack of decrease in serum CML and 3DG-H free adduct concentrations at 28 weeks may relate to increasing release of these analytes from the joints with increasing OA progression. Reversal of the decrease in serum pyrraline concentration at 36 weeks is not linked to food consumption, but rather to increased efficiency of uptake of pyrraline from ingested food, likely mediated by increased intestinal amino acid transporter activity. Similar increased dietary uptake of CMA, CML, MG-H1, and 3DG-H is expected and may contribute to the increases of these serum analytes at 36 weeks. The mechanism by which this occurs merits further investigation.

The negative correlations of serum 3-NT free adduct with global histological score and condyle and plateau instantaneous modulus may be due to changes in 3-NT free adduct from digestion of nitrated proteins in the ingested chow and decreased food intake as OA developed because serum 3-NT free adduct correlated positively with serum pyrraline free adduct. A similar but more limited effect was found for serum CMA free adduct.

The amino acid analytes with strongest correlation to histological and biomechanical features of developing OA were GSP and DT free adducts. GSP is formed by degradation of FL residues and subsequent proteolysis of GSP-modified protein. Although GSP is present in food proteins, it is not usually absorbed from the diet. The strong link of serum GSP free adduct concentration to global OA histological score and cartilage stiffness is likely due to GSP being of an exclusive endogenous source, a major protein crosslink and formation by joint proteolysis. This also translated to increase plasma or serum levels of GSP in clinical OA. Serum DT free adduct may have emerged as a biomarker of global OA histological score for similar reasons and also its likely increased formation associated with inflammation.

We also measured protein glycation, oxidation, and nitration adduct residues and citrullination in serum protein during OA development. These showed markedly different changes with age (cf. Fig. 4q and r). This demonstrates the importance of analyzing protein glycation residues and free adduct separately. Most protein modifications were decreased as OA developed. Exceptions were FL, pentosidine, and DT. The concurrent decrease of many different modifications suggests the underlying cause may be increased capillary permeability with increased residence time of albumin in the interstitial fluid, where protein concentration and rates of protein modification are usually lower than in the vascular compartment [34]. Increased capillary permeability may be driven by increased inflammatory reaction from 3 to 12 weeks of age in this guinea pig model [35] and also by increased prostaglandin E_2, a dilatator of blood vessels [10]. Levels of FL and pentosidine may be increased by decline in glucose tolerance related to insulin resistance driven by increased IL-1β [35], producing increased early-stage protein glycation and increased pentose-derived metabolite precursors of pentosidine [36]. The anomalous increase in DT while other oxidative markers are decreasing suggests a specific effect. Formation of DT occurs enzymatically by dual oxidase (DUOX) [37]. DUOX expression is increased through activation of activating transcription factor 2in inflammatory signaling [38]. Similar effects were found previously in plasma and synovial fluid protein in clinical early- and advanced-stage OA [5, 20]. This is a likely consequence of systemic low-grade inflammation in OA and indicates relevance of the Dunkin-Hartley guinea pig model of OA for clinical translation.

Serum CP decreased as OA developed in Dunkin-Hartley guinea pigs. The mechanism of this remains unclear, but it corroborates with our earlier clinical studies where there was higher plasma CP in patients with eOA than in patients with aOA [20]. The increased inflammatory mediators in OA are thought to reach their zenith in early-stage disease and then decrease in advanced disease [39]. Inflammatory mechanisms linked to CP formation through expression of protein arginine deiminases may be a component of this and may explain the decline of serum CP in advanced OA.

We studied the effect of IL-1β on flux of protein glycation, oxidation, and nitration, as judged by increased concentration of protein glycation, oxidation, and nitration free adducts in culture medium. IL-1β increased flux of formation of CEL, G-H1, CMA, GSP, DT, NFK, and 3-NT. This model was not confounded by change in uptake of protein glycation, oxidation, and nitration free adducts (cf. effects in Dunkin-Hartley guinea pigs). The upper limit of the concentration of IL-1β in human synovial fluid is about 20 pg/ml in patients with severe knee OA [40]. We used a higher concentration, as previously [41–43], to model the effects of continuous exposure to IL-1β in vivo at the steady-state concentration, with additions at 3-day intervals and half-life of 2.5 hours of IL-1β [44].

We applied plasma or serum glycated, oxidized, and nitrated amino acid with Hyp and anti-CCP antibody status for diagnosis and type of early-stage arthritic disease. For classification of good vs early-stage arthritic disease (any), the relative importance of algorithm features was as follows: CEL > GSP > Hyp > NFK > MetSO > MG-H1 > 3DG-H > G-H1 > 3-NT > DT > CMA. The high importance of GSP corroborates with the early changes in serum GSP free adduct found in experimental spontaneous OA in the present study, and the importance of Hyp corroborates results of our earlier studies [20]. The importance of methylglyoxal-derived AGEs, CEL, and MG-H1 is a new development and supports the emergence of the role of dicarbonyl stress in aging and chronic disease [45]. For classification of early-stage arthritic disease, the relative importance of algorithm features was as follows: anti-CCP antibody positivity > 3DG-H > CML > FL > GSP > MetSO > CEL > 3-NT. This reflects the high prevalence of anti-CCP antibody positivity in eRA. The three next most important features are glycation adducts, which may also suggest there are distinct contributions of glycation to eOA, eRA, and non-RA. Combination of estimates of serum trace-level glycated, oxidized, and nitrated amino acids and Hyp may therefore improve diagnosis of early-stage arthritic disease, including progression of experimental spontaneous OA, as supported by predictions with the PLS regression model.

Conclusions
We conclude that trace-level damaged amino acids in serum may be valuable biomarkers in OA, particularly GSP.

Additional file

Additional file 1: Supplementary text: description of measurement and outcome of guinea pig food consumption. **Figure S1.** (a) MACH-1 mechanical testing system. (b) View of a guinea pig femoral condyle with a position grid superimposed; **Figure S2.** Body weight of guinea pigs during the study. **Figure S3.** Partial least squares (PLS) regression model of serum glycated, oxidized, and nitrated amino acids Hyp and CP on total OA histological score. **Table S1.** Serum glycated, oxidized, nitrated, and citrullinated protein in the guinea pig model of osteoarthritis; **Table S2.** Correlation between glycation, oxidation, and nitration free adducts and hydroxyproline. **Table S3.** Correlations between glycated, oxidized, nitrated, and citrullinated serum protein. **Table S4.** Confusion matrix and nCorrect. (DOCX 735 kb)

Abbreviations
3DG-H: 3-Deoxyglucosone-derived hydroimidazolone isomers; 3-NT: 3-Nitrotyrosine; AASA: α-Aminoadipic semialdehyde; AGE: Advanced glycation endproduct; aOA: Advanced osteoarthritis; AUROC: Area under the receiver operating characteristic curve; CCP: Cyclic citrullinated peptide; CEL: N^ϵ-carboxyethyl-lysine; CMA: N^ω-carboxymethylarginine; CML: N^ϵ-carboxymethyl-lysine; CP: Citrullinated protein; DT: Dityrosine; DUOX: Dual oxidase; EDTA: Ethylenediaminetetraacetic acid; eOA: Early-stage osteoarthritis; eRA: Early-stage rheumatoid arthritis; FL: N^ϵ-fructosyl-lysine; G-H1: Glyoxal-derived hydroimidazolone; GSA: Glutamic semialdehyde; GSP: Glucosepane; HEPES: 4-(2-Hydroxyethyl)-1-piperazineethanesulfonic acid; Hyp: Hydroxyproline; IL-1β: Interleukin-1β; MetSO: Methionine sulfoxide; MG-H1: Methylglyoxal-derived hydroimidazolone; MRM: Multiple reaction monitoring; NFK: N-formylkynurenine; Non-RA: Inflammatory joint disease other than rheumatoid arthritis (often self-resolving); OA: Osteoarthritis; OARSI: Osteoarthritis Research Society International; PLS: Partial least squares; TKR: Total knee replacement

Acknowledgements
We thank Matthew L. Costa (Warwick Medical School, Clinical Sciences Research Laboratories, University of Warwick, University Hospital, Coventry, UK), Andrew Filer and Karim Raza (Sandwell and West Birmingham Hospital NHS Trust, Birmingham, West Midlands, UK) for assistance with eOA, eRA and non-RA patient and healthy subject recruitment as well as with clinical sample collection.

Funding
This study was supported by grants from the University of Warwick (Warwick Impact Fund award) and Val Smith's Legacy gift (to NR). Research work of YH and CLe was funded by the Walloon government programme CWALITY Multicart (number 1318276).

Authors' contributions
CLe and CLa performed cell culture and animal experiments supervised by YH. UA, AA, and SP performed protein damage marker, citrullinated protein, and hydroxyproline analysis. RKD and IMC performed the clinical study on TKR patients. UA, AA, SP, PJT, and NR collected and assembled the data. CLe, UA, KR, CLa, PJT, YH, and NR analyzed and interpreted the data. PJT, NR, and YH contributed to study conception and design. CLe, PJT, and NR drafted the report. PJT provided statistical expertise. YH and NR obtained funding. All authors reviewed and revised the manuscript critically, and all authors read and approved the final version to be published.

Competing interests
The authors declare that they have no competing interests.

Author details
[1]Bone and Cartilage Research Unit, Arthropôle Liège, Institute of Pathology, Level 5, CHU Sart-Tilman, 4000 Liège, Belgium. [2]Warwick Systems Biology, University of Warwick, Clinical Sciences Research Laboratories, University Hospital, Coventry CV2 2DX, UK. [3]Warwick Medical School, Clinical Sciences Research Laboratories, University of Warwick, University Hospital, Coventry CV2 2DX, UK. [4]School of Computer Science, University of Birmingham, Birmingham, UK. [5]School of Biological Sciences, University of East Anglia, Norwich, UK. [6]Department of Physical Therapy and Rehabilitation, Princess Paola Hospital, Vivalia, Marche-en-Famenne, Belgium.

References
1. Kraus VB, Blanco FJ, Englund M, Karsdal MA, Lohmander LS. Call for standardized definitions of osteoarthritis and risk stratification for clinical trials and clinical use. Osteoarthritis Cartilage. 2015;23(8):1233–41.
2. Kraus VB, Burnett B, Coindreau J, Cottrell S, Eyre D, Gendreau M, Gardiner J, Garnero P, Hardin J, Henrotin Y, et al. Application of biomarkers in the development of drugs intended for the treatment of osteoarthritis. Osteoarthritis Cartilage. 2011;19(5):515–42.

3. Lotz M, Martel-Pelletier J, Christiansen C, Brandi M-L, Bruyère O, Chapurlat R, Collette J, Cooper C, Giacovelli G, Kanis JA, et al. Value of biomarkers in osteoarthritis: current status and perspectives. Ann Rheum Dis. 2013;72(11):1756–63.

4. Hardin JA, Cobelli N, Santambrogio L. Consequences of metabolic and oxidative modifications of cartilage tissue. Nat Rev Rheumatol. 2015; 11(9):521–9.

5. Ahmed U, Anwar A, Savage RS, Thornalley PJ, Rabbani N. Protein oxidation, nitration and glycation biomarkers for early-stage diagnosis of osteoarthritis of the knee and typing and progression of arthritic disease. Arthritis Res Ther. 2016;18(1):250.

6. Thornalley PJ, Rabbani N. Detection of oxidized and glycated proteins in clinical samples using mass spectrometry - a user's perspective. Biochim Biophys Acta. 2014;1840(2):818–29.

7. Sell DR, Biemel KM, Reihl O, Lederer MO, Strauch CM, Monnier VM. Glucosepane is a major protein cross-link of the senescent human extracellular matrix: relationship with diabetes. J Biol Chem. 2005; 280(13):12310–5.

8. Kuyinu EL, Narayanan G, Nair LS, Laurencin CT. Animal models of osteoarthritis: classification, update, and measurement of outcomes. J Orthop Surg Res. 2016;11:19.

9. Jimenez PA, Glasson SS, Trubetskoy OV, Haimes HB. Spontaneous osteoarthritis in Dunkin Hartley Guinea pigs: histologic, radiologic, and biochemical changes. Lab Anim Sci. 1997;47(6):598–601.

10. Horcajada MN, Sanchez C, Membrez Scalfo F, Drion P, Comblain F, Taralla S, Donneau AF, Offord EA, Henrotin Y. Oleuropein or rutin consumption decreases the spontaneous development of osteoarthritis in the Hartley Guinea pig. Osteoarthritis Cartilage. 2015;23(1):94–102.

11. Kraus VB, Huebner JL, DeGroot J, Bendele A. The OARSI histopathology initiative - recommendations for histological assessments of osteoarthritis in the Guinea pig. Osteoarthritis Cartilage. 2010;18(Suppl 3):S35–52.

12. Sim S, Chevrier A, Garon M, Quenneville E, Lavigne P, Yaroshinsky A, Hoemann CD, Buschmann MD. Electromechanical probe and automated indentation maps are sensitive techniques in assessing early degenerated human articular cartilage. J Orthop Res. 2017;35(4):858–67.

13. Harmand MF, Duphil R, Blanquet P. Proteoglycan synthesis in chondrocyte cultures from osteoarthrotic and normal human articular-cartilage. Biochim Biophys Acta. 1982;717(2):190–202.

14. Davidson R, Gardner S, Jupp O, Bullough A, Butters S, Watts L, Donell S, Traka M, Saha S, Mithen R, et al. Isothiocyanates are detected in human synovial fluid following broccoli consumption and can affect the tissues of the knee joint. Sci Rep. 2017;7(1):3398.

15. Arnett FC, Edworthy SM, Bloch DA, McShane DJ, Fries JF, Cooper NS, Healey LA, Kaplan SR, Liang MH, Luthra HS, et al. The American rheumatism association 1987 revised criteria for the classification of rheumatoid arthritis. Arthritis Rheum. 1988;31(3):315–24.

16. Raza K, Falciani F, Curnow SJ, Ross EJ, Lee CY, Akbar AN, Lord JM, Gordon C, Buckley CD, Salmon M. Early rheumatoid arthritis is characterized by a distinct and transient synovial fluid cytokine profile of T cell and stromal cell origin. Arthritis Res Ther. 2005;7(4):R784–95.

17. Ryd L, Brittberg M, Eriksson K, Jurvelin JS, Lindahl A, Marlovits S, Moller P, Richardson JB, Steinwachs M, Zenobi-Wong M. Pre-osteoarthritis: definition and diagnosis of an elusive clinical entity. Cartilage. 2015;6(3):156–65.

18. Ahmed N, Thornalley PJ. Chromatographic assay of glycation adducts in human serum albumin glycated in vitro by derivatisation with aminoquinolyl-N-hydroxysuccimidyl-carbamate and intrinsic fluorescence. Biochem J. 2002;364:15–24.

19. Rabbani N, Shaheen F, Anwar A, Masania J, Thornalley PJ. Assay of methylglyoxal-derived protein and nucleotide AGEs. Biochem Soc Trans. 2014;42(2):511–7.

20. Ahmed U, Anwar A, Savage RS, Costa ML, Mackay N, Filer A, Raza K, Watts RA, Winyard PG, Tarr J, et al. Biomarkers of early stage osteoarthritis, rheumatoid arthritis and musculoskeletal health. Sci Rep. 2015;5:9259.

21. Sajda P. Machine learning for detection and diagnosis of disease. Annu Rev Biomed Eng. 2006;8:537–65.

22. Foerster A, Henle T. Glycation in food and metabolic transit of dietary AGEs (advanced glycation end-products): studies on the urinary excretion of pyrraline. Biochem Soc Trans. 2003;31:1383–5.

23. Teeple E, Fleming BC, Mechrefe AP, Crisco JJ, Brady MF, Jay GD. Frictional properties of Hartley Guinea pig knees with and without proteolytic disruption of the articular surfaces. Osteoarthritis Cartilage. 2007;15(3):309–15.

24. de Bri E, Reinholt FP, Svensson O. Primary osteoarthrosis in Guinea pigs: a stereological study. J Orthop Res. 1995;13(5):769–76.

25. Zamli Z, Robson Brown K, Tarlton JF, Adams MA, Torlot GE, Cartwright C, Cook WA, Vassilevskaja K, Sharif M. Subchondral bone plate thickening precedes chondrocyte apoptosis and cartilage degradation in spontaneous animal models of osteoarthritis. Biomed Res Int. 2014;2014:10.

26. Huebner JL, Kraus VB. Assessment of the utility of biomarkers of osteoarthritis in the Guinea pig. Osteoarthritis Cartilage. 2006;14(9):923–30.

27. Huebner JL, Hanes MA, Beekman B, TeKoppele JM, Kraus VB. A comparative analysis of bone and cartilage metabolism in two strains of Guinea-pig with varying degrees of naturally occurring osteoarthritis. Osteoarthritis Cartilage. 2002;10(10):758–67.

28. Quasnichka HL, Anderson-MacKenzie JM, Bailey AJ. Subchondral bone and ligament changes precede cartilage degradation in Guinea pig osteoarthritis. Biorheology. 2006;43(3–4):389–97.

29. Xue M, Weickert MO, Qureshi S, Ngianga-Bakwin K, Anwar A, Waldron M, Shafie A, Messenger D, Fowler M, Jenkins G, et al. Improved glycemic control and vascular function in overweight and obese subjects by glyoxalase 1 inducer formulation. Diabetes. 2016;65(8):2282–94.

30. Brismar BH, Lei W, Hjerpe A, Svensson O. The effect of body mass and physical activity on the development of Guinea pig osteoarthrosis. Acta Orthop Scand. 2003;74(4):442–8.

31. Bendele AM, Hulman JF. Effects of body weight restriction on the development and progression of spontaneous osteoarthritis in Guinea pigs. Arthritis Rheum. 1991;34(9):1180–4.

32. Ahmed N, Mirshekar-Syahkal B, Kennish L, Karachalias N, Babaei-Jadidi R, Thornalley PJ. Assay of advanced glycation endproducts in selected beverages and food by liquid chromatography with tandem mass spectrometric detection. Mol Nutr Food Res. 2005;49(7):691–9.

33. Liardon R, de Weck-Gaudard D, Philipossian G, Finot PA. Identification of N^ε-carboxymethyllysine: a new Maillard reaction product, in rat urine. J Agric Food Chem. 1987;35:427–31.

34. Masania J, Malczewska-Malec M, Razny U, Goralska J, Zdzienicka A, Kiec-Wilk B, Gruca A, Stancel-Mozwillo J, Dembinska-Kiec A, Rabbani N, et al. Dicarbonyl stress in clinical obesity. Glycoconj J. 2016;33:581–9.

35. Huebner JL, Seifer DR, Kraus VB. A longitudinal analysis of serum cytokines in the Hartley Guinea pig model of osteoarthritis. Osteoarthritis Cartilage. 2007;15(3):354–6.

36. Wang F, Zhao Y, Niu Y, Wang C, Wang M, Li Y, Sun C. Activated glucose-6-phosphate dehydrogenase is associated with insulin resistance by upregulating pentose and pentosidine in diet-induced obesity of rats. Horm Metab Res. 2012;44(13):938–42.

37. Edens WA, Sharling L, Cheng GJ, Shapira R, Kinkade JM, Lee T, Edens HA, Tang XX, Sullards C, Flaherty DB, et al. Tyrosine cross-linking of extracellular matrix is catalyzed by Duox, a multidomain oxidase/peroxidase with homology to the phagocyte oxidase subunit gp91 phox. J Cell Biol. 2001;154(4):879–91.

38. Ha EM, Lee KA, Seo YY, Kim SH, Lim JH, Oh BH, Kim J, Lee WJ. Coordination of multiple dual oxidase-regulatory pathways in responses to commensal and infectious microbes in Drosophila gut. Nat Immunol. 2009;10(9):949–57.

39. Abramson SB, Attur M. Developments in the scientific understanding of osteoarthritis. Arthritis Res Ther. 2009;11(3):227–36.

40. Ye G, Peng CA, Gao ZG, Xiao J, Mei L. Effects of arthroscopic knee surgery on IL-1β, CXCL13 and TNF-α in the knee joint fluid of knee osteoarthritis patients and their correlation with clinical outcomes. Int J Clin Exp Pathol. 2017;10(2):1690–6.

41. Henrotin YE, Sanchez C, Deberg MA, Piccardi N, Guillou GB, Msika P, Reginster JYL. Avocado/soybean unsaponifiables increase aggrecan synthesis and reduce catabolic and proinflammatory mediator production by human osteoarthritic chondrocytes. J Rheumatol. 2003;30(8):1825–34.

42. Sanchez C, Mathy-Hartert M, Deberg MA, Ficheux H, Reginster JYL, Henrotin YE. Effects of rhein on human articular chondrocytes in alginate beads. Biochem Pharmacol. 2003;65(3):377–88.

43. Sanchez C, Deberg MA, Burton S, Devel P, Reginster JYL, Henrotin YE. Differential regulation of chondrocyte metabolism by oncostatin M and interleukin-6. Osteoarthritis Cartilage. 2004;12(10):801–10.

44. Moors MA, Mizel SB. Proteasome-mediated regulation of interleukin-1β turnover and export in human monocytes. J Leukoc Biol. 2000;68(1):131–6.

45. Rabbani N, Xue M, Thornalley PJ. Methylglyoxal-induced dicarbonyl stress in aging and disease: first steps towards glyoxalase 1-based treatments. Clin Sci. 2016;130:1677–96.

8

Could low birth weight and preterm birth be associated with significant burden of hip osteoarthritis?

Sultana Monira Hussain*[iD], Ilana N. Ackerman, Yuanyuan Wang, Ella Zomer and Flavia M. Cicuttini

Abstract

Background: Approaches for the prevention and treatment of hip osteoarthritis (OA) remain limited. There are recent data suggesting that low birth weight (LBW) and preterm birth may be risk factors for hip osteoarthritis. This has the potential to change the current paradigm of hip osteoarthritis prevention by targeting early life factors. The aim of this review was to examine the available evidence for an association of LBW and preterm birth with hip OA. The potential cost implications associated with total hip arthroplasty were also evaluated.

Methods: Ovid Medline, EMBASE, and Cinahl were searched up until August 2017 using MeSH terms and key words. Methodological quality was evaluated using the National Heart Lung and Blood Institute (NHLBI) quality assessment tool. Qualitative evidence synthesis was performed to summarise the results. Bradford Hill's criteria for causation including the temporal relationship, consistency, strength of the association, specificity, dose-response relationship, and analogy were used to assess the evidence for causation. Economic modelling was used to calculate the potential economic burden associated with LBW or preterm birth related total hip arthroplasty using Australian data from 2012 to 2015.

Results: Five studies, ranging from high to low quality, were included. Hip bone shape abnormalities examined included developmental hip dysplasia and immature hip, and hip osteoarthritis included osteophytes and total hip arthroplasty. A causal link between low birth weight or preterm birth and hip osteoarthritis was found. Of the 30,477 total hip arthroplasties performed for hip osteoarthritis in Australia in 2015, 5791 were estimated to be born preterm and 5273 with low birth weight. This equated to a potential total hip arthroplasty cost of AU$145,136,082 and AU$132,150,222 for these subgroups, respectively.

Conclusion: Available data suggest that low birth weight and preterm birth are associated with hip bone shape abnormalities and hip osteoarthritis requiring total hip arthroplasty, with a substantial associated financial burden. Given the current lack of effective treatment and prevention strategies for hip osteoarthritis, this offers a new avenue for reducing the future burden of hip osteoarthritis.

Keywords: Low birth weight, Preterm birth, Hip osteoarthritis, Total hip arthroplasty, Economic evaluation

* Correspondence: monira.hussain@monash.edu
School of Public Health and Preventive Medicine, Monash University,
Melbourne, VIC 3004, Australia

Background

Hip osteoarthritis (OA) is a common joint disease with one in four people developing symptomatic hip OA in their lifetime [1]. There are limited treatment and preventive strategies for hip OA; as a result, end-stage disease is treated by total hip arthroplasty (THA), imposing a burden on health systems internationally [2, 3]. In Australia, almost one in eight people have a lifetime risk of undergoing THA [3]. The number of THAs per annum in Australia has risen steadily over time, with an increase of 65% from 2003 to 2015 [4]. To reduce the burden of this disease, new approaches to prevention are needed.

There is increasing evidence for the importance of hip bone shape in the pathogenesis of hip OA [5, 6]. For example, recent studies have shown that mild acetabular dysplasia [7] and alterations in hip bone shape and geometry [6] predate the onset of hip OA. Events in early life may be risk factors for hip OA and these may be mediated by changes in hip bones. Potential mechanisms affecting the bone include differences in bone accretion for a fetus in an intrauterine environment versus a preterm infant in an extrauterine environment [8], and greater bone mineral content in a full-term-born baby compared with a preterm infant [9, 10]. Both low birth weight (LBW) and preterm born babies frequently suffer from metabolic bone disease which is often asymptomatic and self-limiting [11] and has been linked to thickening of the chondrocostal junctions of the long bones [12]. Preterm birth has also been linked to reduced bone mass [13] and underdeveloped acetabula [14]. Post-delivery, these infants demonstrate an altered hip position (with hip extension) compared with the position of intrauterine life (flexed and abducted hip) and this may contribute to an increased incidence or greater severity of acetabular dysplasia [15, 16]. It is perhaps unsurprising, therefore, that LBW and preterm birth have been associated with the pathology of hip OA. If this association exists between LBW, preterm birth, and hip structure, it could facilitate a paradigm shift for the monitoring and prevention of hip OA. Hip joint abnormalities exist as a continuum, and subtle morphological abnormalities of hip bone, i.e. mild acetabular dysplasia or a shallow acetabulum, are associated with late-onset of primary hip OA [17, 18]. As hip OA is a chronic long-term condition, to understand the risk factors and pathogenesis of hip OA we need to consider the stages of hip OA across the life-course from early changes in hip bone shape to established hip OA and end-stage joint disease requiring joint replacement surgery. Without considering these earlier stages, simply trying to identify hip OA will not be helpful as the prevalence of hip OA in those aged < 40 years is very low.

A substantial number of babies are born with LBW in developed countries. Based on data from 2015 and 2016,

6.2% of infants are born LBW (< 2500 g) and 8% are born preterm (at < 37 completed weeks gestation) in Australia [19], which is lower than the prevalence of LBW and preterm births in the United States (8.0% LBW and < 12.0% preterm) [20, 21], the United Kingdom (7.6% LBW) [22], and the Organisation for Economic Co-operation and Development average (6.6% LBW) [23]. A steady increase in the number of LBW and preterm born infants is expected since the average age of mothers in developed countries is increasing [24]; older mothers (≥ 35 years) [25] are at higher risk of delivering LBW and preterm born babies than mothers aged 20 to 34 years. Additionally, the survival rate of LBW and preterm birth infants has increased almost 80% in the past 30 years [9]. Thus, determining whether LBW or preterm birth increases the risk of abnormal hip bone shape and hip OA, and subsequent THA in later life and the potential economic burden, will be important to inform future resource allocation and hip OA prevention initiatives.

In this study, we aimed to examine the available evidence for an association of LBW and preterm birth with hip OA, and to examine the evidence for potential causation based on the Bradford Hill criteria. Considering the range of definitions used to describe OA-related changes and outcomes, we have collectively termed 'hip pathologies', hip joint abnormalities, hip OA, and hip arthroplasty for hip OA as 'Hip OA'. Given the huge burden associated with both hip OA and LBW and preterm birth, we also considered the potential cost implications associated with THA.

Methods

Systematic review

This systematic review was conducted and reported in accordance with the Preferred Reporting Items for Systematic Review and Meta-Analysis (PRISMA) guidelines [26].

Search strategy

Ovid Medline, CINAHL, and EMBASE databases were searched between January 1947 and August 2017 using MeSH terms (after exploding) and key words to identify studies examining the association between LBW or preterm birth and hip bone abnormality and hip OA. The MeSH and key terms used to define hip bone abnormality and hip OA included "hip" and "osteoarthritis" or "degenerative arthritis" or "coxarthritis" or "dysplasia" or "joint space narrowing" or "osteophytes" or "bone shape" or "bone geometry" or "neck shaft angle" or "hip deformity" or "femora acetabular impingement" or "pincer deformity" or "cam deformity". For LBW and preterm birth, the MeSH and key terms used were "birth weight" or "low birth weight" or "preterm birth" or "prematurity" or "preterm". Searches were limited to human studies and those published in English.

Study selection

Two authors (SMH and YW) independently assessed study eligibility using a three-stage determination method, reviewing the title, abstract, and then full text. Any disagreement between the two authors was resolved by consensus reviewing the criteria. Studies were only included if they assessed hip bone abnormality and hip OA including developmental dysplasia of the hip (DDH), hip instability at childhood, hip deformity, hip osteophytes, joint space narrowing, symptomatic hip OA, radiological hip OA, magnetic resonance imaging (MRI) changes of the hip, hip bone shape, hip bone geometry, hip neck-shaft angle, hip deformity, THA for hip OA, and either LBW or preterm birth or both LBW and preterm birth. Case reports, conference abstracts, and review articles were excluded, as were studies without a comparison group. The reference lists of the included articles and review articles identified were searched to identify any additional relevant studies.

Data extraction and synthesis

Two authors (SMH and YW) extracted data independently on study design, participant characteristics (number, gender, and age), definition and prevalence of hip bone abnormality and hip OA, duration of follow-up, measures of LBW or preterm birth, adjustment for confounding factors, and associations between LBW or preterm birth and hip bone abnormality and hip OA. A third author (FMC) assessed the consistency of extracted data. Although a meta-analysis was planned, significant heterogeneity across the studies (predominantly different ages of the study populations, different methods for defining and assessing hip bone abnormality and hip OA, and different sources of birth weight data) precluded the pooling of data for analysis.

Risk of bias assessment

Two authors (INA and YW) independently assessed the risk of bias of included studies using the National Heart Lung and Blood Institute (NHLBI) quality assessment tool for observational studies [27]. This tool includes 14 criteria for cohort and cross-sectional studies and 12 criteria for case-control studies to assess the internal validity and risk of bias, and scores the quality of a study as 'high' (low risk of bias), 'fair' (moderate risk of bias), or 'low' (high risk of bias).

Bradford Hill criteria for causation

The Bradford Hill criteria [28] were used to examine the evidence for a causal relationship between LBW and hip OA, and between preterm birth and hip OA. These criteria are commonly used to assess the adequacy of evidence for a causal relationship between an exposure and a consequence. These criteria include temporal relationship, consistency, strength of the association, specificity, dose-response relationship, and analogy.

Economic evaluation

An economic evaluation was undertaken to estimate the costs associated with THA likely attributable to LBW or preterm birth at a national level. Trends in the national prevalence of LBW and preterm birth were examined using annual birth data published by the Australian Institute of Health and Welfare [29, 30]. Data from Australian Orthopaedic Association National Joint Replacement Registry annual reports were used to establish the incidence of THA performed for OA in 2015 [31]. Data on the likelihood of having THA due to LBW or preterm birth were obtained from a recent Australian data linkage study [32], with additional summary data provided by the authors. These proportions were applied in separate calculations to annual THA incidence data to estimate the number of THA procedures performed for the LBW and preterm birth populations in 2015. The costs associated with THA were estimated from a health system perspective [33]. Published episode of care costs for THA were inflated to 2016 prices (AUD $22,817 per THA) [33] and multiplied by the number of estimated THA procedures in 2015 to calculate the total cost of THA.

Results

Systematic review

Search results

Database searches identified 231 records (CINAHL, n = 49; Ovid Medline, n = 46; and EMBASE, n = 136), of which 69 articles were duplicates. Of the remaining 162 articles, 154 were excluded after title and abstract screening as these studies did not assess hip OA in relation to LBW or preterm birth. Full-text screening was performed for eight articles. Three were excluded as they did not include an appropriate comparison, leaving five included studies (Fig. 1). No additional articles were identified from reference lists.

Summary of included studies

Table 1 provides an overview of the included studies. The included studies comprised two cohort [32, 34], one case-control [35], and two cross-sectional studies [36, 37] published between 1993 and 2015. Two studies originated from Australia [32, 35], two from the UK [34, 36], and one from Turkey [37]. All the studies included men and women.

Assessment of hip pathology and hip OA

Hip bone abnormality included self-reported DDH [35], α-angle of the hip joint (suggestive of immature or pathologic hip) by ultrasound examination [37], and hip deformity by footprint angle and hip rotation [36]. Hip

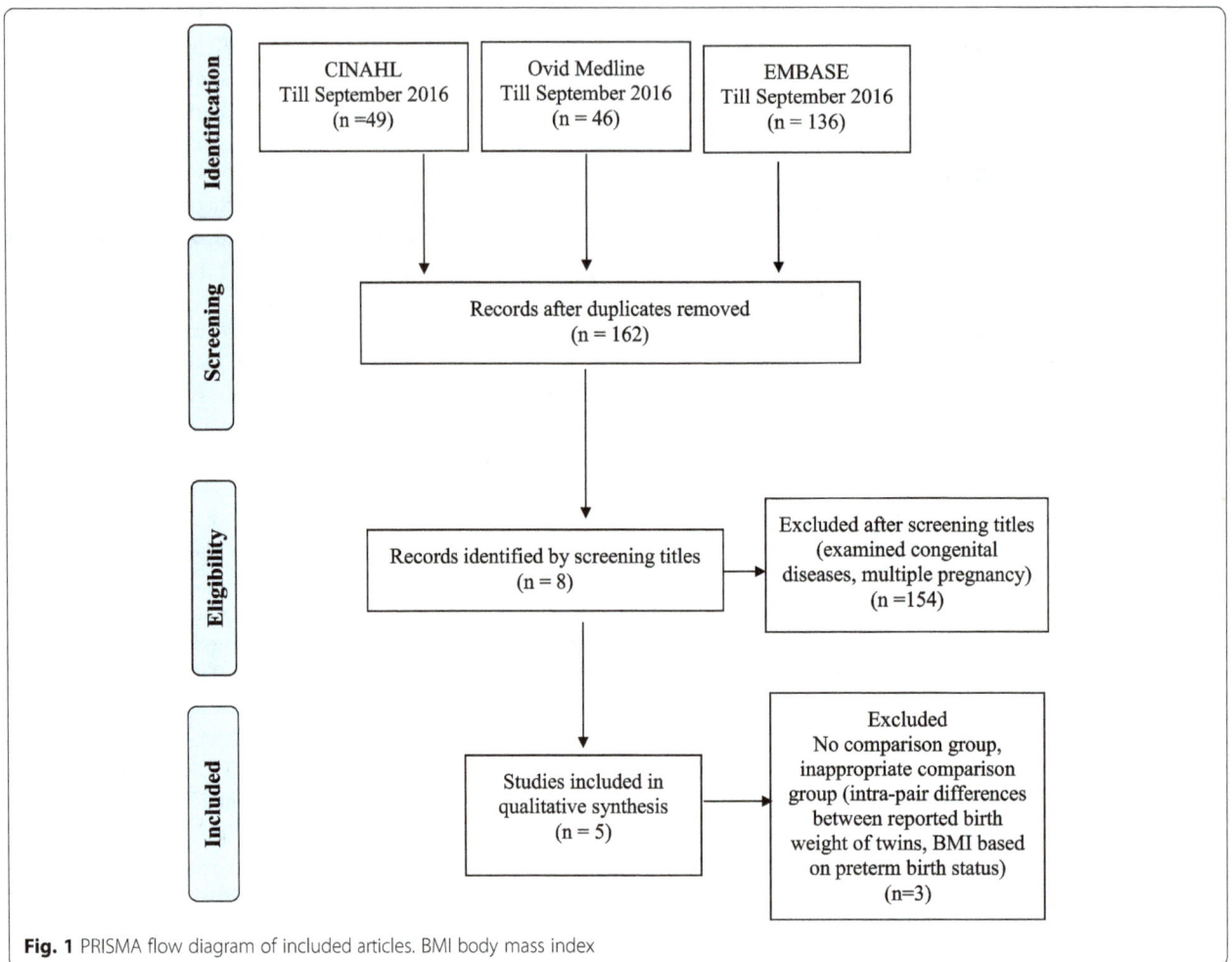

Fig. 1 PRISMA flow diagram of included articles. BMI body mass index

OA was defined by American College of Rheumatology (ACR) algorithms based on the presence of osteophytes and overall Kellgren and Lawrence (K-L) score assessed from hip radiographs [34], and hip arthroplasty for OA [32].

Assessment of low birth weight or preterm birth

Two studies reported both LBW and preterm birth data [32, 36], while the remainder collected data only on LBW [34, 35] or preterm birth [37]. Birth weight information was collected from hospital records [36, 37] and birth registries [34, 35] for four of the included studies. One study collected self-reported birth weight data and whether the participant was born ≥ 2 weeks preterm [32]. In this study, 10% of the participants had birth weight data from hospital records compared against their self-reported data for validation [32].

Prevalence of hip bone abnormality and hip OA

One study reported that self-reported DDH was present among 0.75% of the population [35]. Two studies [32, 34] reporting hip OA prevalence showed a 2.1% prevalence

when hip OA was defined by THA [32], and 3.2% for men and 6.0% for women when the disease was defined as clinical hip OA [34].

Risk of bias

A risk of bias assessment was undertaken for each of the included studies. The overall quality assessment is shown in Table 1, with details of quality assessment presented in Additional file 1: Table S1 for cohort and cross-sectional studies and Additional file 1: Table S2 for case-control studies. Of the two cohort studies, one was classified as high quality [32] and the other was classified as fair quality [34]. The other studies, one case-control [35] and two cross-sectional [36, 37] studies, were considered of low quality. Limitations associated with the cohort studies included the categorisation of birth weight data (i.e. birth weight data was not treated as a continuous variable) [32] and the lack of sample size justification and loss to follow-up [34]. The two cross-sectional studies did not provide information on temporality and also failed to adjust for potential confounders [36, 37]. In the case-control study, the

Table 1 Characteristics of studies included in the systematic review

Author, country, and year	Study population and % women	Age of study population (mean ± SD)	Hip OA or hip pathologies related to hip OA	Prevalence % outcome (OA, DDH, α-angle, hip deformity) (men, women)	Follow-up time (mean ± SD)	Quality of study[a]
Hip bone shape abnormality						
Case-control study						
Chan et al., Australia, 1997 [35]	All live births during 1986–93 n = 151,257 47%	28 days to 5 years	Self-reported DDH, birth registry	0.75% DDH	N/A	Low
Cross-sectional studies						
Orak et al., Turkey, 2015 [37]	Infants born in one hospital n = 467 44%	Preterm 31.11 ± 2.51 weeks Term 40.22 ± 0.36 weeks	α-angle < 60 ° of the hip joint suggestive of immature or pathologic hip	NR	N/A	Low
Davis et al., UK, 1993 [36]	Infants born in one hospital n = 33 55%	3–4.5 years	Hip deformity by footprint angle and hip rotation	NR	N/A	Low
Hip OA						
Cohort studies						
Hussain et al., Australia 2015 [32]	n = 3604 participants 60%	No arthroplasty 51.8 ± 10.0 Hip arthroplasty 59.0 ± 9.5	Hip arthroplasty for hip OA	2.1%	9.3 ± 2.1	High
Clynes et al., UK 2014 [34]	n = 444 50%	Median 75 years (IQR 73–77)	American College of Rheumatology algorithm to define hip OA Radiographic Kellgren and Lawrence (KL) score of hip to count osteophytes	Men 3.2% Women 6.0%	13 years	Fair

DDH developmental dysplasia of the hip, *IQR* interquartile range, *N/A* not applicable, *NR* not reported, *OA* osteoarthritis, *SD* standard deviation
[a] Evaluated using the National Heart Lung and Blood Institute (NHLBI) quality assessment tool for observational studies [27]

processes used to identify or select cases and controls was problematic, and the process for measuring exposure was not clearly defined [35]. The study population and research question were defined clearly in all the studies.

Association between LBW or preterm birth and hip bone abnormality

One low-quality case-control study found that participants born with LBW were less likely to develop DDH [35]. The two low-quality cross-sectional studies reported conflicting results regarding birth weight and hip bone abnormality. One study showed that LBW and preterm birth were associated with deformation of the lower limb including the hip [36], while the other study found that preterm babies had less prevalence of abnormal α-angle of the hip joint (< 60 °, suggestive of immature hip development) compared with full-term babies [37]. Neither study adjusted for potential confounders (Table 2).

Association between LBW or preterm birth and hip OA

Two cohort studies examined the relationship between LBW or preterm birth and hip OA [32, 34] (Table 2). In

a high-quality cohort study, LBW and preterm birth were independently associated with increased incidence of THA for OA [32]. A stronger association was evident for preterm birth than for LBW [32]. The other fair-quality cohort study showed that lower birth weight (as a continuous variable) was associated with hip osteophytes but not clinical hip OA (defined using algorithms developed by the ACR) [34].

Evidence for causation using the Bradford Hill criteria for causation

Table 3 presents the Bradford Hill criteria, an explanation of each criterion, and evidence for a causal relationship between LBW, preterm birth, and hip OA in relation to each criterion. While there was evidence for causation with respect to six items of the Bradford Hill criteria (consistency, strength of the association, dose-response relationship, specificity, analogy, and temporal relationship), there was no or limited evidence for the remaining three criteria (plausibility, reversibility, and coherence). Overall, this approach suggests that there is modest evidence for a cause-effect relationship, with most of the criteria being

Table 2 Association between low birth weight or preterm birth and hip pathology/osteoarthritis

Author and year	Low birth weight/ preterm measurement	Confounder adjusted for	Results	Conclusion
Hip bone shape abnormality				
Case-control study				
Chan et al., 1997 [35]	Birth weight from the birth registry	Maternal age, region of residence, parity, oligohydramnios, presentation and method of delivery, baby's sex, birth weight, gestation	Low birth weight and DDH, where birth weight 3000–3500 g is referent Birth weight < 2000 g OR 0.30 (95% CI 0.12–0.77) Birth weight 2000–2500 g OR 0.52 (95% CI 0.31–0.88)	Those who were born with low birth weight (< 2500 g) were less likely to develop DDH
Cross-sectional studies				
Orak et al., 2015 [37]	Hospital-recorded birth weight	Unadjusted	Preterm born and α-angle of the hip joint suggestive of immature or pathologic hip Preterm born babies with α-angle < 60 ° = 2.7% Full-term born babies with α-angle < 60 ° = 28.5% ($p < 0.001$, Fisher's exact test)	These results suggest that prematurity is not a predisposing factor for immature hip predictive of DDH
Davis et al., 1993 [36]	Hospital-recorded birth weight	Unadjusted	Low birth weight and preterm birth with hip deformity Out-toeing 62% in low birth weight vs 35% in the term babies Total rotation of hip preterm group 119.20 (19.6) vs term group 99.20 (9.6) ($p < 0.003$)	Deformation of the lower limb including hip frequently seen in preterm babies during early infancy
Hip OA				
Cohort studies				
Hussain et al., 2015 [32]	Self-reported birth weight and whether born ≥ 2 weeks preterm	Age, sex, BMI, hypertension, diabetes mellitus, smoking, and physical activity	Low birth weight and hip arthroplasty HR 2.02 (95% CI 1.10–3.73) Preterm birth HR 2.53 (95% CI 1.30–4.92)	Individuals born with LBW or at preterm are at increased risk of hip arthroplasty for OA in adult life
Clynes et al., 2014 [34]	Birth weight from the birth registry	Age, sex, BMI, smoking and alcohol	Lower birth weight and radiographic hip OA OR 0.78 (95% CI 0.48–1.27) Lower birth weight and osteophytes in hip OR 1.51 (95% CI 1.13–2.01)	Individuals with lower birth weights were more likely to have hip osteophytes but not hip arthritis

BMI body mass index, *CI* confidence interval, *DDH* developmental dysplasia of the hip, *HR* hazard ratio, *LBW* low birth weight, *OA* osteoarthritis, *OR* odds ratio

present between LBW, preterm birth, and hip pathology/hip OA.

Modelling the economic burden
Table 4 presents national trends in LBW and preterm births in Australia from 2009 to 2014. The proportion of LBW births and preterm births has remained steady over this period (representing 6.4% and 8.0% of all live births in 2014, respectively), although absolute numbers have increased over time in line with an increasing number of births nationwide. A total of 34,321 primary THA procedures were performed in Australia in 2015 and, of these, 30,477 (88.8%) were performed for hip OA [31]. The proportion of study participants undergoing THA who were born with LBW or preterm was 17.3% and 19.0%, respectively [32]. Based on these data [32], 5273

THA procedures performed for OA were estimated as attributable to LBW, while 5791 THA procedures for OA were estimated as attributable to preterm birth. This equates to a total annual cost for THA of AUD $132,150,222 and AUD $145,136,082 for the LBW and preterm populations, respectively.

Discussion
In this study, we examined the available evidence for an association between LBW and preterm birth, and the evidence for potential causation based on the Bradford Hill criteria [28]. Considering available data from two high- to fair-quality cohort studies and plausible causation evidence [28], there is a strong indication to support the hypothesis that both LBW and preterm birth are risk factors for hip OA. This has the potential for

Table 3 Evidence for a causal relationship between low birth weight and preterm birth and hip osteoarthritis according to the Bradford Hill criteria

Bradford Hill criterion and description	Hip osteoarthritis
Temporal relationship This is an essential criterion. For a possible risk factor to be the cause of a disease, it must come before the disease. This is generally easier to establish from cohort studies than from cross-sectional or case-control studies, when measurements of the possible cause and the effect are made at the same time	Criterion met: Yes Hussain et al. [32] In a cohort study people born with low birth weight (LBW) or preterm underwent hip arthroplasty for hip osteoarthritis (OA) at an average age of 59.0 (standard deviation (SD) 9.5) years Clynes et al. [34] Participants of the Hertfordshire Cohort Study who were born LBW had more osteophytes in the hip joint detected by x-ray at the age median of 75 (interquartile range (IQR) 73–77) years
Plausibility A risk factor associated with a disease is more likely to be the cause of the disease if the association found is consistent with knowledge obtained from other sources, such as animal experiments and experiments on biological mechanisms. However, this criterion must be used with care as a lack of plausibility may simply reflect a lack of scientific knowledge	Criterion met: No
Consistency If similar results have been found in different populations using different study designs, the association is more likely to be causal as it is unlikely that all studies were subject to the same types of errors (chance, bias or confounding). However, a lack of consistency does not exclude a causal association, as different exposure levels and other conditions may reduce the impact of the causal factor in certain studies	Criterion met: Yes Different stages of hip OA including hip arthroplasty for OA [32], osteophytes in hip joint [34], and hip shape deformity [36] were found in different populations using different study designs, including two cohort studies [32, 34] and a cross-sectional study [57]
Strength of an association The strength of an association is measured by the size of the relative risk. A strong association is more likely than a weak association to be causal, as a weak association could more easily be the result of confounding or bias	Criterion met: Yes A strong association was observed in one study [32]
Dose-response relationship Further evidence of a causal relationship is provided if increasing levels of exposure lead to an increasing risk of disease	Criterion met: Yes A dose-response relationship was observed in one study [34]
Specificity If a particular exposure increases the risk of a certain disease but not the risk of other diseases, this is strong evidence in favour of a cause-effect relationship. However, one-to-one relationships between exposure and disease are rare, and lack of specificity should not be used to say that a relationship is causal	Criterion met: Yes Low birth weight and preterm birth is associated with hip arthroplasty for OA [32] and hip osteophytes [34] but not knee arthroplasty for OA [32] or knee osteophytes [34]
Reversibility When the removal of a possible risk factor results in a reduced risk of disease, the likelihood that this association is causal is increased. Ideally, this should be assessed by conducting a randomized intervention trial. For many exposures or diseases, such randomised trials are not possible in practice	Criterion met: Not applicable for this condition
Coherence The suggested cause-effect relationship should essentially be consistent with the natural history and biology of the disease	Criterion met: No
Analogy The causal relationship will be further supported if there are similarities with other (well-established) cause-effect relationships	Criterion met: Yes Reduced bone mineral density [45] and bone mineral content [10] are found in preterm infants, even when age is corrected for term. Radiological changes, including characteristics of rickets, are identifiable in 23% of infants weighing < 1500 g [58]

high healthcare burden since the estimated cost to the Australian health system for THA attributable to LBW and preterm birth would exceed AUD$132 million and AUD$145 million, respectively, based on current estimates. However, the full healthcare costs are likely to be significantly higher, given the additional costs of non-surgical management for less severe hip OA including pain medications and physiotherapy.

Two cohort studies with high to moderate quality and one low-quality cross-sectional study showed that LBW and preterm birth are associated with either hip deformation [36], hip OA [34], or THA for hip OA [32]. Data from the Australian Diabetes, Obesity and Lifestyle Study showed that people with LBW and preterm birth were at higher risk of THA compared with those with normal weight and full-term births, respectively [32].

Table 4 Trends in preterm births and low birth weight in Australia

Year	Number of births	Low birth weight births[a] (%[b])	Pre-term births[c] (%[b])
2009	296,791	18,347 (6.2)	22,645 (7.6)
2010	297,357	18,522 (6.2)	22,952 (7.7)
2011	299,588	18,829 (6.3)	23,282 (7.8)
2012	309,861	19,243 (6.2)	24,671 (8.0)
2013	307,277	19,597 (6.4)	24,582 (8.0)
2014	310,330	19,833 (6.4)	24,826 (8.0)

Data obtained from the Australian Institute of Health and Welfare [19, 29, 30, 59]
[a] Babies with a weight at birth < 2500 g
[b] Proportion of all live births for the specified year
[c] Babies born at 20–36 weeks gestation

Similarly, data from the Hertfordshire Cohort Study showed that individuals with lower birth weight were more likely to have hip osteophytes in adulthood; however, there was no relationship between LBW and clinical hip OA as defined by ACR criteria [34]. The ACR criteria specify that hip pain must be present together with radiographic changes to support a diagnosis of hip OA [38]. This diagnostic approach accounts for the known discordance between radiographic findings and symptoms [39]. For example, approximately 85% of people with structural changes indicative of hip OA do not experience frequent hip pain [40]. In another study, 20.1% of individuals with self-reported hip pain had features of clinical hip OA [41]. Thus, making a comparison between radiographic and clinical definitions of hip OA is problematic.

The association between LBW or preterm birth and hip bone abnormality has not always been clear. There was conflicting evidence regarding LBW or preterm birth and hip bone abnormality in three low-quality studies. One cross-sectional study reported that LBW and preterm birth were associated with hip deformity [36]. In contrast, the other cross-sectional study and the only case-control study reported that there was no relationship between LBW or preterm birth, and immature hip and DDH, respectively [35, 37]. There might be several reasons for these discordant findings. For instance, the study that showed LBW and preterm birth were associated with hip deformity measured hip deformity when the children were 3–4 years old [36], while the other study performed ultrasonography to measure hip angle predictive of immature hip predictive of DDH at the gestational age of 40 weeks, regardless of the participant's actual birth week [37]. It has been shown that a number of infants who progress to hip dysplasia have unstable hips at infancy [42], and hence in most cases dysplasia is diagnosed during late childhood [43]. Furthermore, there is no agreement as to what constitutes an 'abnormal' hip [44]. In the case-control study, DDH was self-reported and therefore may have captured only severe cases [35] and failed to show an association.

Examination of Bradford Hill criteria provided further supportive evidence for a causal relationship between LBW and preterm birth and hip OA. Results from the cohort studies supported a temporal relationship between LBW or preterm birth and hip arthroplasty due to hip OA [32], and between LBW and hip osteophytes [34]. There is also some evidence for a "dose-response relationship" between LBW and severity of hip OA, described in one recent cohort study as the lower the birth weight, the higher the likelihood of having osteophytes [34]. Consistent findings were observed using a different spectrum of hip pathology/hip OA including dysplasia [36], osteophytes [34], and arthroplasty [32] of the hip. There was some evidence of specificity as lower birth weight was associated with hip osteophytes but not osteophytes in other joints [34]. In addition, there is evidence of analogy. For example, reduced bone mineral density [45] and bone mineral content [10] are found in preterm infants, even when age is corrected for term. Further work is needed to clarify the role of LBW and preterm birth in the development of hip OA.

The aetiology of hip OA is multifactorial. Both congenital and developmental diseases of the hip, such as mild acetabular dysplasia, may increase the risk of developing of hip OA in adulthood [5, 46]. Preterm babies are born with an incomplete acetabulum at birth [14]. These infants often develop a postural deformation of the legs which persists until early childhood [36] which may be due to an underdeveloped or shallow, upwardly sloping acetabulum [7], decreased joint surface area [47], or lax ligaments holding the ball in place [36]. These factors may influence the structural development of the hip joint, resulting in an abnormal hip joint shape. The important role of hip bone shape and geometry in the aetiology of hip OA has been established [5]. Premature and LBW babies represent a uniquely vulnerable population in which bone growth and mineral acquisition are critical with regards to bone turnover [48]. A case-control study found reduced peak bone mass at the femoral neck in very low birth weight babies [13]. There is emerging evidence that preterm birth and very low birth weight results in a decrease in bone formation and an increase in bone resorption [9, 48] that reduces osteoclast apoptosis [49] and increases cartilage degeneration [50], which may be another potential pathway for the development of hip OA. Furthermore, there might be other mediating factors, i.e. catch-up growth during infancy, high levels of physical activity during puberty, and childhood obesity which, in conjunction with low birth weight and preterm birth, might contribute to hip OA. However, these speculations should be interpreted with caution and more studies are needed to support this hypothesis. If proven to contribute to the development of hip OA, modifying hip position through postural support [15, 16] and perhaps the use of double nappies [51] may be beneficial for these babies. Similarly, it may be that swaddling that forces the hips into extension and adduction, which is a common practice in some Middle East countries and in the US [52], and is having a resurgence in English-speaking countries [53], may predispose to dysplasia and should be discouraged in these babies. Furthermore, these babies should be targeted for hip dysplasia screening even in the absence of overt hip changes; they could also be identified as being at increased risk of hip OA and be considered for preventive strategies as evidence for this emerges. Given the lack of modifiable risk factors for hip OA and with the increasing number of LBW and preterm births, this has the potential to have a major impact on reducing the future burden of hip OA.

Data from the landmark Global Burden of Disease study have shown that the prevalence of hip OA is highest among high-income countries [54] and prevalence is expected to increase with gains in life expectancy. No conventional factors, such as age, body mass index (BMI), or physical activity, fully explain the pathogenesis of the disease [5]. The burden of LBW and preterm birth is also substantial and is increasing internationally [20] with increases in maternal age [30]. In the year 2000 in the US, 55% of all LBW infants were born to women aged 45 years or over [21]. The average age of mothers in Australia has risen from 29.7 years in 2004 to 30.2 years in 2014, and the proportion of mothers aged 35 years and over has increased from 20% in 2004 to 22% in 2014 [30]. This has key health system implications as the age of mothers continues to rise. This study highlights the need to identify babies at risk of developing hip OA, with early assessment of hip joint development among preterm babies and those of LBW and ongoing monitoring of at-risk individuals in childhood and adolescence.

In this study, we performed a systematic literature search with a comprehensive risk of bias assessment. A major limitation of this review is the lack of available studies. However, it is important to note that research into the development and epidemiology of hip OA is generally limited, despite the high burden of disease. One of the

included studies used THA for hip OA as a surrogate marker of hip OA and probably has underestimated the association between LBW/preterm birth and hip OA (given that not all individuals with moderate or severe hip OA will undergo hip arthroplasty). However, the study was performed in Australia where there is a publicly funded universal health system (Medicare) and people without private health insurance have access to arthroplasty surgery under this system. The evidence of LBW and preterm birth being risk factors for abnormal hip bone shape, and hip OA was established by applying the Bradford Hill criteria of causation in two high- to fair-quality cohort studies and a few poor-quality case-control and cross-sectional studies. Thus, it is clear that further research is required to determine the influence of LBW and preterm birth in the pathological process of hip OA development. LBW could be due to prematurity (59% to 70% of low birth weight babies) [55, 56], intrauterine growth restriction, or both. In this review, we included either separate or combined preterm birth or LBW data based on how they were examined in the primary study. It is therefore not possible to draw conclusions as to how low birth weight alone, low birth weight along with preterm birth, or preterm birth alone contributes to the pathophysiology of hip OA.

The LBW and preterm populations were treated separately for the economic evaluation, although there will undoubtedly be some overlap between these groups. The THA costs are based on average costs for an episode of care and cannot account for individual differences in arthroplasty costs. Finally, our analysis does not include the indirect or out-of-pocket costs of THA.

Conclusion

Despite the lack of high-quality studies in this area, our findings suggest that LBW and preterm birth are potential risk factors for hip bone shape abnormalities and hip OA requiring THA in adulthood. Based on our calculations, this could have substantial financial implications for healthcare systems. Given the current lack of effective treatment and preventive strategies for hip OA, this is an area where further research is needed to reduce the burden of hip OA. For example, the individuals born preterm or with LBW may be identified as an "at-risk group" for future end-stage hip OA; this will enable targeted monitoring and early interventions that could potentially reduce the population burden of THA in later life.

Abbreviations

ACR: American College of Rheumatology; DDH: Developmental dysplasia of the hip; K-L: Kellgren and Lawrence; LBW: Low birth weight; MRI: Magnetic resonance imaging; NHLBI: National Heart Lung and Blood Institute; OA: Osteoarthritis; PRISMA: Preferred Reporting Items for Systematic Review and Meta-Analysis; THA: Total hip arthroplasty

Funding

The systematic review and economic evaluation was not funded by any funding body. YW is the recipient of a National Health and Medical Research Council (NHMRC) Career Development Fellowship (Clinical Level 1, APP1065464).

Authors' contributions

SMH, FMC, INA, and YW were involved in the conception of the systematic review. SMH and INA assessed the eligibility of studies to be included and extracted data. INA and YW were involved in the quality assessment of the included studies. EZ performed the economic modelling. SMH drafted the initial manuscript. SMH, INA, YW, EZ, and FMC were involved in interpretation of the data. All the authors revised the manuscript and gave final approval. FMC is the guarantor.

Consent for publication

All authors have completed the Unified Competing Interest form at www.icmje.org/coi_disclosure.pdf (available on request from the corresponding author) and declare that: 1) SMH, INA, YW, EZ, and FMC have no support from any company for the submitted work; 2) SMH, INA, YW, EZ, and FMC have no relationships with any companies that might have an interest in the submitted work in the previous 3 years; 3) their spouses, partners, or children have no financial relationships that may be relevant to the submitted work; and 4) SMH, INA, YW, EZ, and FMC have no financial interests that may be relevant to the submitted work. All the authors have consented for publication and have checked the reliability of the published data.

Competing interests

The authors declare that they have no competing interests.

References

1. Murphy LB, Helmick CG, Schwartz TA, Renner JB, Tudor G, Koch GG, Dragomir AD, Kalsbeek WD, Luta G, Jordan JM. One in four people may develop symptomatic hip osteoarthritis in his or her lifetime. Osteoarthr Cartil. 2010;18(11):1372–9.
2. Kurtz S, Ong K, Lau E, Mowat F, Halpern M. Projections of primary and revision hip and knee arthroplasty in the United States from 2005 to 2030. J Bone Joint Surg Am. 2007;89(4):780–5.
3. Ackerman IN, Bohensky MA, de Steiger R, Brand CA, Eskelinen A, Fenstad AM, Furnes O, Graves SE, Haapakoski J, Makela K, et al. Lifetime risk of primary total hip replacement surgery for osteoarthritis from 2003–2013: a multi-national analysis using national registry data. Arthritis Care Res (Hoboken). 2017;69(11):1659-67.
4. Australian Orthopaedic Association. National Joint Replacement Registry. Annual Report. Adelaide: AOA; 2016.
5. Ganz R, Leunig M, Leunig-Ganz K, Harris WH. The etiology of osteoarthritis of the hip: an integrated mechanical concept. Clin Orthop Relat Res. 2008; 466:264–72.
6. Agricola R, Heijboer MP, Bierma-Zeinstra SM, Verhaar JA, Weinans H, Waarsing JH. Cam impingement causes osteoarthritis of the hip: a nationwide prospective cohort study (CHECK). Ann Rheum Dis. 2013;72(6): 918–23.
7. Birrell F, Silman A, Croft P, Cooper C, Hosie G, Macfarlane G. Syndrome of symptomatic adult acetabular dysplasia (SAAD syndrome). Ann Rheum Dis. 2003;62(4):356–8.
8. Cooper C, Westlake S, Harvey N, Javaid K, Dennison E, Hanson M. Review: developmental origins of osteoporotic fracture. Osteoporos Int. 2006;17(3): 337–47.
9. Miller ME. The bone disease of preterm birth: a biomechanical perspective. Pediatr Res. 2003;53(1):10–5.
10. Beltrand J, Alison M, Nicolescu R, Verkauskiene R, Deghmoun S, Sibony O, Sebag G, Levy-Marchal C. Bone mineral content at birth is determined both by birth weight and fetal growth pattern. Pediatr Res. 2008;64(1):86–90.
11. Wood CL, Wood AM, Harker C, Embleton ND. Bone mineral density and osteoporosis after preterm birth: the role of early life factors and nutrition. Int J Endocrinol. 2013;2013:902513.
12. Bozzetti V, Tagliabue P. Metabolic bone disease in preterm newborn: an update on nutritional issues. Ital J Pediatr. 2009;35:20.
13. Smith CM, Wright NP, Wales JK, Mackenzie C, Primhak RA, Eastell R, Walsh JS. Very low birth weight survivors have reduced peak bone mass and reduced insulin sensitivity. Clin Endocrinol. 2011;75(4):443–9.
14. Timmler T, Wierusz-Kozlowska M, Wozniak W, Markuszewski J, Lempicki A. Development and remodeling of the hip joint of preterm neonates in sonographic evaluation. Ortop Traumatol Rehabil. 2003;5(6):703–11.
15. Downs JA, Edwards AD, McCormick DC, Roth SC, Stewart AL: Effect of intervention on development of hip posture in very preterm babies. Arch Dis Child 1991, 66(7 Spec No):797–801.
16. Coughlin M, Lohman MB, Gibbins S. Reliability and effectiveness of an infant positioning assessment tool to standardize developmentally supportive positioning practices in the neonatal intensive care unit. Newborn Infant Nurs Rev. 2010;10(2):104–6.
17. Sandell LJ. Etiology of osteoarthritis: genetics and synovial joint development. Nat Rev Rheumatol. 2012;8(2):77–89.
18. Murphy NJ, Eyles JP, Hunter DJ. Hip osteoarthritis: etiopathogenesis and implications for management. Adv Ther. 2016;33(11):1921–46.
19. Hilder L, Zhichao Z, Parker M, Jahan S, Chambers GM. Australia's mothers and babies 2012. Perinatal statistics series no. 30. Cat. no. PER 69. Canberra: AIHW; 2014.
20. Blencowe H, Cousens S, Oestergaard MZ, Chou D, Moller AB, Narwal R, Adler A, Vera Garcia C, Rohde S, Say L, et al. National, regional, and worldwide estimates of preterm birth rates in the year 2010 with time trends since 1990 for selected countries: a systematic analysis and implications. Lancet. 2012;379(9832):2162–72.
21. Martin JA, Hamilton BE, Ventura SJ, Menacker F, Park MM. Births: final data for 2000. Natl Vital Stat Rep. 2002;50(5):1–101.
22. Glinianaia SV, Ghosh R, Rankin J, Pearce MS, Parker L, Pless-Mulloli T. No improvement in socioeconomic inequalities in birthweight and preterm birth over four decades: a population-based cohort study. BMC Public Health. 2013;13(1):345.
23. OECD. Health at a Glance 2015: OECD Indicators. Paris: OECD Publishing; 2015. http://dx.doi.org/10.1787/health_glance-2015-en.
24. Bongaarts J, Blanc AK. Estimating the current mean age of mothers at the birth of their first child from household surveys. Popul Health Metrics. 2015;13:25.
25. Goisis A, Remes H, Barclay K, Martikainen P, Myrskyla M. Advanced maternal age and the risk of low birth weight and preterm delivery: a within-family analysis using Finnish population registers. Am J Epidemiol. 2017;186(11):1219–26.
26. Moher D, Liberati A, Tetzlaff J, Altman DG, Group P. Preferred reporting items for systematic reviews and meta-analyses: the PRISMA statement. Ann Intern Med. 2009;151(4):264–9. W264
27. National Heart Lung and Blood Institute website. Development and use of quality assessment tools. Available online at; http://www.nhlbi.nih.gov/health-pro/guidelines/in-develop/cardiovascular-risk-reduction/tools/cohort#. Accessed 17 May 2016.
28. Hill AB. The environment and disease: association or causation? Proc R Soc Med. 1965;58(5):295–300.
29. Li Z, McNally L, Hilder L, Sullivan EA. Australia's mothers and babies 2009. Perinatal statistics series no. 25. Cat. no. PER 52. Sydney: AIHW National Perinatal Epidemiology and Statistics Unit; 2011.
30. AIHW. Australia's mothers and babies 2013—in brief. Perinatal statistics series no. 31. Cat. no. PER 72. Canberra: AIHW; 2015.
31. Australian Orthopaedic Association. National Joint Replacement Registry. Annual Report. Adelaide: AOA; 2015.
32. Hussain SM, Wang Y, Wluka AE, Shaw JE, Magliano DJ, Graves S, Cicuttini FM. Association of low birth weight and preterm birth with the incidence of knee and hip arthroplasty for osteoarthritis. Arthritis Care Res (Hoboken). 2015;67(4):502–8.
33. Peel TN, Cheng AC, Liew D, Buising KL, Lisik J, Carroll KA, Choong PF, Dowsey MM. Direct hospital cost determinants following hip and knee arthroplasty. Arthritis Care Res (Hoboken). 2015;67(6):782–90.
34. Clynes MA, Parsons C, Edwards MH, Jameson KA, Harvey NC, Sayer AA, Cooper C, Dennison EM. Further evidence of the developmental origins of

osteoarthritis: results from the Hertfordshire Cohort Study. J Dev Orig Health Dis. 2014;5(6):453–8.

35. Chan A, KA MC, Cundy PJ, Haan EA, Byron-Scott R. Perinatal risk factors for developmental dysplasia of the hip. Arch Dis Child Fetal Neonatal Ed. 1997; 76(2):F94–100.

36. Davis PM, Robinson R, Harris L, Cartlidge PH. Persistent mild hip deformation in preterm infants. Arch Dis Child. 1993;69(5):597–8.

37. Orak MM, Onay T, Gumustas SA, Gursoy T, Muratli HH. Is prematurity a risk factor for developmental dysplasia of the hip? A prospective study. Bone Joint J. 2015;97-b(5):716–20.

38. Altman R, Alarcón G, Appelrouth D, Bloch D, Borenstein D, Brandt K, Brown C, Cooke TD, Daniel W, Feldman D, et al. The American College of Rheumatology criteria for the classification and reporting of osteoarthritis of the hip. Arthritis Rheum. 1991;34(5):505–14.

39. Hunter DJ, Guermazi A, Roemer F, Zhang Y, Neogi T. Structural correlates of pain in joints with osteoarthritis. Osteoarthr Cartil. 2013;21(9):1170–8.

40. Kim C, Nevitt MC, Niu J, Clancy MM, Lane NE, Link TM, Vlad S, Tolstykh I, Jungmann PM, Felson DT, et al. Association of hip pain with radiographic evidence of hip osteoarthritis: diagnostic test study. BMJ. 2015;351:h5983.

41. Edwards MH, van der Pas S, Denkinger MD, Parsons C, Jameson KA, Schaap L, Zambon S, Castell MV, Herbolsheimer F, Nasell H, et al. Relationships between physical performance and knee and hip osteoarthritis: findings from the European Project on Osteoarthritis (EPOSA). Age Ageing. 2014; 43(6):806–13.

42. Engesaeter IO, Lie SA, Lehmann TG, Furnes O, Vollset SE, Engesaeter LB. Neonatal hip instability and risk of total hip replacement in young adulthood: follow-up of 2,218,596 newborns from the Medical Birth Registry of Norway in the Norwegian Arthroplasty Register. Acta Orthop. 2008;79(3):321–6.

43. Engesaeter IO, Lehmann T, Laborie LB, Lie SA, Rosendahl K, Engesaeter LB. Total hip replacement in young adults with hip dysplasia: age at diagnosis, previous treatment, quality of life, and validation of diagnoses reported to the Norwegian Arthroplasty Register between 1987 and 2007. Acta Orthop. 2011;82(2):149–54.

44. Eastwood DM. Neonatal hip screening. The Lancet. 2003;361(9357):595-7.

45. Ichiba H, Shintaku H, Fujimaru M, Hirai C, Okano Y, Funato M. Bone mineral density of the lumbar spine in very-low-birth-weight infants: a longitudinal study. Eur J Pediatr. 2000;159(3):215–8.

46. Harris WH. Etiology of osteoarthritis of the hip. Clin Orthop Relat Res. 1986; 213:20–33.

47. Lane NE, Lin P, Christiansen L, Gore LR, Williams EN, Hochberg MC, Nevitt MC. Association of mild acetabular dysplasia with an increased risk of incident hip osteoarthritis in elderly white women: the study of osteoporotic fractures. Arthritis Rheum. 2000;43(2):400–4.

48. Aly H, Moustafa MF, Amer HA, Hassanein S, Keeves C, Patel K. Gestational age, sex and maternal parity correlate with bone turnover in premature infants. Pediatr Res. 2005;57(5 Pt 1):708–11.

49. Durand M, Komarova SV, Bhargava A, Trebec-Reynolds DP, Li K, Fiorino C, Maria O, Nabavi N, Manolson MF, Harrison RE, et al. Monocytes from patients with osteoarthritis display increased osteoclastogenesis and bone resorption: the In Vitro Osteoclast Differentiation in Arthritis study. Arthritis Rheum. 2013;65(1):148–58.

50. Shibakawa A, Yudoh K, Masuko-Hongo K, Kato T, Nishioka K, Nakamura H. The role of subchondral bone resorption pits in osteoarthritis: MMP production by cells derived from bone marrow. Osteoarthr Cartil. 2005;13(8):679–87.

51. Clarke NMP, Reading IC, Corbin C, Taylor CC, Bochmann T. Twenty years experience of selective secondary ultrasound screening for congenital dislocation of the hip. Arch Dis Child. 2012;97(5):423-9.

52. Oden RP, Powell C, Sims A, Weisman J, Joyner BL, Moon RY. Swaddling: will it get babies onto their backs for sleep? Clin Pediatr (Phila). 2012;51(3):254–9.

53. Clarke NMP. Swaddling and hip dysplasia: an orthopaedic perspective. Arch Dis Child. 2014;99(1):5.

54. Cross M, Smith E, Hoy D, Nolte S, Ackerman I, Fransen M, Bridgett L, Williams S, Guillemin F, Hill CL, et al. The global burden of hip and knee osteoarthritis: estimates from the Global Burden of Disease 2010 study. Ann Rheum Dis. 2014;73(7):1323–30.

55. Barros FC, Barros AJ, Villar J, Matijasevich A, Domingues MR, Victora CG. How many low birthweight babies in low- and middle-income countries are preterm? Rev Saude Publica. 2011;45(3):607–16.

56. Yasmin S, Osrin D, Paul E, Costello A. Neonatal mortality of low-birth-weight infants in Bangladesh. Bull World Health Organ. 2001;79(7):608–14.

57. Kadam UT, Blagojevic M, Belcher J. Statin use and clinical osteoarthritis in the general population: a longitudinal study. J Gen Intern Med. 2013; 28(7):943–9.

58. Backstrom MC, Kuusela AL, Maki R. Metabolic bone disease of prematurity. Ann Med. 1996;28(4):275–82.

59. Li Z, Zeki R, Hilder L, Sullivan EA. Australia's mothers and babies 2010. Perinatal statistics series no. 27. Cat. no. PER 57. Canberra: AIHW National Perinatal Epidemiology and Statistics Unit; 2012.

9

Targeted designed variants of alpha-2-macroglobulin (A2M) attenuate cartilage degeneration in a rat model of osteoarthritis induced by anterior cruciate ligament transection

Yang Zhang[1], Xiaochun Wei[1], Shawn Browning[2], Gaetano Scuderi[2], Lewis S. Hanna[2] and Lei Wei[1,3*]

Abstract

Background: The study was performed to evaluate whether targeted alpha-2-macroglobulin (A2M) variants have a similar or enhanced function at wild-type (wt)-A2M to attenuate cartilage degeneration in vivo.

Methods: In and ex-vivo experiment, bovine cartilage explants (BCE) were incubated with TNF-α and IL-1β with or without wt-A2M or A2M variants. Cartilage catabolism was measured in culture supernatant by sulfated glycosaminoglycan (sGAG). In an in-vivo experiment, 2-month-old male Wistar rats (n = 77) were randomly divided into seven groups and treated with different doses of A2M or its variants by intra-articular injection at 24 hours and day 14 after anterior cruciate ligament transection (ACLT), receiving (1) ACLT/PBS; (2) ACLT/wt-A2M (0.153 mg); (3) ACLT/CYT-108 A2M (0.153 mg); (4) ACLT/CYT-108 A2M (0.077 mg); (5) ACLT/CYT-98 A2M (0.153 mg); (6) ACLT/CYT-98 A2M (0.077 mg); or (7) sham/PBS. The joints and synovial lavage were collected 8 weeks after surgery. Fluorescence molecular tomography was used to monitor inflammation in vivo using probes ProSense and MMPSense at 24 hours, and weeks 2, 4, and 6 after surgery. The cartilage damage was quantified using Osteoarthritis Research Society International score and matrix metalloproteinase (MMP)-3, -13, collagen (Col) X, Col 2, Runx2, and aggrecan (Acan) were detected by immunohistochemical analysis (IHC), ELISA, and RT-PCR.

Results: A2M variants inhibited catabolism in the BCE model by up to 200% compared with wt-A2M. ProSense and MMPSense were dramatically increased in all groups after surgery. Supplemental A2M or its variants reduced ProSense and MMPSense compared with the PBS treatment. Less cartilage damage, lower MMP-13 and Col 2 degraded product, and stronger Col 2 synthesis were detected in animals treated with A2M or its variants compared with PBS-treated animals. A2M and its variants enhanced Col 2 and Acan synthesis, and suppressed MMP-3, MMP-13, Runx2, and Col X production. A2M-108 variant demonstrated less cartilage damage compared with wt-A2M and A2M-98 variant.

Conclusion: The targeted variants of A2M have a chondroprotective effect similar to wt-A2M. However, A2M-108 variant has enhanced function to attenuate cartilage degeneration compared with wt-A2M.

Keywords: Targeted designed variants of A2M, PTOA, Rat ACLT OA model

* Correspondence: Lei_Wei@brown.edu
[1]Department of Orthopedics, the second hospital of the Shanxi Medical University, Taiyuan, China
[3]Department of Orthopedics, Alpert Medical School of Brown University/ Rhode Island Hospital, Providence, RI, USA
Full list of author information is available at the end of the article

Background

Although osteoarthritis (OA) affects over 40 million Americans, its pathogenesis remains undefined. OA progression is due, at least in part, to the upregulation of inflammation mediators and proteases [1–4]. Since collected evidence has demonstrated that elevated levels of catabolic enzymes in synovial fluid (SF) induce chondrocyte death and cartilage matrix degeneration within one week of joint injury [5–9], early intervention strategies should focus on reducing these cartilage-degrading proteases within a similar time frame. Previous studies have indicated that catabolic proteases and cytokines reach their peak within 48 h after joint injury, which initiates cell death and cartilage matrix degeneration [1]. Thus, early intervention to reduce these catabolic proteases and cytokines is critical to prevent or delay cartilage degeneration.

Evidence from our group [4, 10–12] and others [1, 13] suggests that new molecular interventions targeting these catabolic enzymes can potentially arrest these adverse events and preserve joint health. It is unlikely, however, that blocking only one of these catabolic factors would be enough to repress the multi-catabolic inflammation factors after joint injury.

Our laboratory and others have demonstrated that serum alpha-2-macroglobulin (A2M) is a promising bioinhibitor for most of these catabolic enzymes, though it is not adequately present in the joint due to the large molecular weight of A2M, which prevents it from migrating into the SF [5, 14–16]. Recently, we have shown that supplemental intra-articular injection of A2M shortly after joint injury provides chondral protection in anterior cruciate ligament (ACL) injury of the knee by reducing these catabolic enzymes [5]. However, administering serum A2M from patients is time-consuming and complex, which may limit clinical application. We designed targeted variants of A2M to enhance A2M inhibitory function to overcome the purification/concentration burden associated with utilizing circulatory wild-type A2M.

Cytonics scientists have synthesized more than 100 variants and tested their inhibition against 12 proteases mostly implicated in cartilage digestion. The two variants that demonstrated the highest inhibitory characteristics toward largest number of proteases were selected; these were variants 98 and 108 (data not shown). In this study, we used bovine articular cartilage explants (BCE) to screen targeted designed A2M variants in vitro, fluorescence molecular tomography (FMT), a new advanced method for measuring certain catabolic protease levels in vivo, histological and immunohistochemical analyses, and RT-PCR, to compare the efficacy of wild-type-A2M (wt-A2M) and two A2M variants in vivo using our established rat anterior cruciate ligament transection (ACLT) OA model. We have clearly shown that cartilage-degrading

proteases, such as elastase, Cathepsin G, B, L and S, and matrix metalloproteinase (MMP)-3, MMP-9, and MMP-13, and ADAMTS 4 and 5 are potently inhibited by A2M and its targeted variants in both the BCE model and a surgically induced OA rat model. Supplemental A2M and its variants attenuate cartilage degeneration and inhibit MMP-13 compared with rats treated by PBS. Our evidence suggests that these molecular variants of A2M, especially 108 variant, have a potentially enhanced function relative to wt-A2M to block multiple catabolic proteases and attenuate OA development in the rat ACLT-OA model.

Methods

BCE model and treatment

BCE were isolated from heifers 1.0–1.5 years old and were equilibrated for 3 days in culture medium. To degrade cartilage by cytokine treatment, BCE are incubated for 3 days in DMEM containing 10% fetal bovine serum with or without TNF-α 80 ng/ml and IL-1β 8 ng/ml. Cartilage degradation is inhibited with the addition of either a twofold serial dilution standard curve of wt-A2M (2.0–0.13 mg/ml) or A2M variants (0.25 mg/ml) designed to potently inhibit OA. Cartilage catabolism is measured in culture supernatant by sulfated glycosaminoglycan (sGAG) compared to a standard curve of chondroitin sulfate using di-methylmethylamine staining [4, 11, 17].

The bait region of A2M variants was optimized by placing specific sequences around the cleavage sites from the native substrates for ADAMTS 5 and 4, MMPs, elastase and cathepsin. The difference between variables was mainly the order of these sequences. The size of the bait region was the same as the wt and care was taken that the variant sequences maintained a random coil structure similar to the wt sequence (NCBI Reference Sequence: NM_000014.4). Hek293 cells were transiently transfected with plasmid containing the sequence for the new A2M using the Transit Pro Transfection Reagent (Mirus, MIR5700) according to manufacturer's protocols. Following incubation the conditioned medium was harvested and centrifuged first at 150 rcf for 5 minutes then at 5850 rcf for 20 minutes, to remove cells and debris. High-performance liquid chromatography (HPLC) and ion exchange chromatography were used for initial purification steps. The eluted A2M from the ion exchange column was further purified using cobalt affinity chromatography. The purified A2M was diluted with PBS.

Rat ACLT OA model and treatment with supplemental intra-articularA2M or injection of its variants

Two-month-old male Wistar rats (n = 77) were purchased from Charles River and randomly divided into seven groups (n = 11/per group) and treated with different doses of A2M and its variants (provided by Cytonics

Corp.): (1) ACLT + PBS; (2) ACLT + wt-A2M (0.153 mg); (3) ACLT + CYT-108 A2M (0.153 mg); (4) ACLT + CYT-108 A2M (0.077 mg); (5) ACLT + CYT-98 A2M (0.153 mg); (6) ACLT + CYT-98 A2M (0.077 mg); or (7) sham + PBS. ACLT (groups 1–6) or sham surgery (group 7) were performed on the left knee and the right knee served as an internal control, as published previously [18, 19]. A2M and its variants dissolved in 20 μl of PBS were intra-articularly injected 24 h and 14 days after ACLT. Animals in groups 1 and 7 received an equivalent volume of PBS at identical time points to the experimental groups (2–6) in their left knees to control for any procedural effects. Previous research has demonstrated that there is no statistical difference between ACLT + PBS injection and ACLT without PBS injection in the rat ACLT model. Therefore, we did not compare ACLT + PBS treatment with ACLT without PBS injection in this study. All animals were euthanized at week 8 after the operation.

Monitoring inflammation dynamically in vivo
FMT is a new, advanced, sensitive, non-ionizing radiation method used to monitor certain catabolic proteases level in real time in vivo [12]. A mix of fluorescent imaging probes ProSense (10 μl, 13.3 μM) and MMPSense (10 μl, 13.3 μM) were injected intra-articularly 24 h after each A2M injection. The fluorescent imaging probes were also injected at weeks 4 and week 6 after surgery on both the right (control) and left knees, respectively. FMT was used to monitor the levels of inflammation in vivo 24 h after injection of ProSense 750 for the detection of plasmin, cathepsin B, L, and S, and MMPSense 680 was used for the detection of MMP-3, MMP-9, and MMP-13. The picomolar concentrations of probes in the knee joint were determined using region of interest analysis. Data are reported as mean ± SE, with 11 animals per group.

Histologic assessment
The proximal tibiae were removed from the harvested joints and immersed in 10% formalin for 72 h. The specimens were decalcified in 20% ethylenediaminetetraacetic acid solution (pH 7.2). Frontal sectioning was performed. The tibial plateau was cut into two approximately equal pieces, an anterior and a posterior one, along the medial collateral ligament in the frontal plane. The two resulting tissue pieces (anterior and posterior half) were then both embedded in a single paraffin block with the cut planes facing down. The blocks were trimmed to expose the cartilage. Ten adjacent sections were collected at intervals of 0 μm, 200 μm, and 400 μm. Two serial 6-μm-thick sections from each interval were stained with Safranin O. Cartilage degradation was quantified using the Osteoarthritis Research Society

International (OARSI) grading system [20]. Three independent observers scored each section blinded, and the scores from the tibial plateau sections were averaged for each individual animal before comparing groups. Our previous study has demonstrated that A2M attenuates cartilage degeneration [5, 17]. In this study, our pre-specified primary outcome measure was to repeat the comparison between the wt-A2M with PBS and then test whether these targeted designed A2M variants can achieve a similar result or even better result than wt using the microscopic OARSI score system [20].

Immunohistochemical analysis
To detect the distribution of MMP-13, Col 2, Col 2 breakdown product, and Col X in cartilage, 6-μm sections were collected on positively charged glass slides (Thermo Fisher Scientific, Asheville, NC, USA). The sections were dried on a hotplate to increase adherence to the slides. Immunohistochemical (IHC) analysis was carried out using the 3,3'-diaminobenzidine (DAB) streptavidin-peroxidase (SP) DAB Histostain-SP immunohistochemistry kit (ZYMED Laboratories/Invitrogen, Carlsbad, CA, USA). Sections were deparaffinized and rehydrated using conventional methods. Endogenous peroxidase was blocked by treating the sections with 3% hydrogen peroxide in methanol (Sigma-Aldrich) for 30 minutes. The sections were digested by 5 mg/ml hyaluronidase in PBS (Sigma-Aldrich) for 20 minutes. The sections were incubated with specific antibodies against MMP-13 (1:100) (Santa Cruz Biotechnology), types II (1:10) (Developmental Studies Hybridoma Bank, University of Iowa, Iowa City, IA, USA), Col X (1:50) (EMD Biosciences, Billerica, MA, USA) and Col 2 breakdown product (1:100) (IBEX Technologies, Mont-Royal, QC, Canada), respectively, at 4 °C overnight. The negative control sections were incubated with isotype-matched control serum (2 μg/ml) (R&D Systems, Minneapolis, MN, USA) in PBS. Thereafter the sections were treated sequentially with biotinylated secondary antibody and SP conjugate (ZYMED Laboratories/Invitrogen), then developed in DAB chromogen (ZYMED Laboratories/Invitrogen). The sections were counterstained with hematoxylin (ZYMED Laboratories/Invitrogen). Photomicrographs were taken with a Nikon E800 microscope (Nikon, Melville, NY, USA) [17].

Rat SF lavage collection and analyses
SF lavages were collected from the knees immediately after euthanasia [4]: 100 μl of isotonic saline solution was injected intra-articularly using a 30-gauge insulin syringe inserted through the inferior patellar tendon [2]. With injection the joint capsule was visibly distended. The knee was then manually cycled through flexion and extension 10 times to distribute the fluid within the joint

before collection by joint aspiration. About half of the fluid that was injected was recovered. The SF was centrifuged at 2000 g for 10 minutes to remove cells and debris, and frozen at -80 °C until analysis. MMP-13 was measured in the SF lavage samples by ELISA following the manufacturer's instructions (Rat MMP13 ELISA Kit Catalog NO.LS-F5518, LifeSpan Biosciences, Inc, WA, USA). Briefly, 100 µl of the standard or the sample were added per well and incubated for 2 h at room temperature (RT). The liquid of each well was aspirated. Then, 100 µl of detection reagent A working solution was added to each well and incubated for 1 h at 37 °C. After washing, 100 µl of detection reagent B working solution was added to each well and incubated for 1 h at 37 °C. Then, 90 µl of substrate solution was added to each well for 30 minutes at 37 °C (protected from light) after washing 5 times. Finally, 50 µl of stop solution was added to each well, and the colorimetric density of the developed plates was determined within 30 minutes using a microplate reader set to 450 nm (Spectramax M2^e Multi-Mode Microplate Reader, Molecular Devices, Sunnyvale, CA, USA). The ELISA was performed in duplicate.

Real-time PCR (qPCR)

The femoral condyle cartilage was dissected under dissection microscopy. Three rat cartilage samples were pooled (n = 9 per group). Total RNA was isolated using RNeasy isolation kit (Cat. No. 74104, Qiagen, Valencia, CA, USA) [10]; 1 µg of total RNA was transcribed into complementary DNA (cDNA) using the iScript^{TM} cDNA synthesis Kit (Bio-Rad, Hercules, CA, USA). Of the resulting cDNA, 40 ng/ul was used as the template to quantify the relative content of messenger RNA (mRNA) using QuantiTect SYBR Green PCR kit (QIAGEN, Valencia, CA, USA) with the CFX384 Real-Time PCR Detection System (Bio-Rad Laboratories, Hercules, CA, USA). We used rat Col2a1 forward primer - AAG GGA CAC CGA GGT TTC ACT GG, rat Col2a1 reverse primer - GGG CCT GTT TCT CCT GAG CGT; rat Acan forward primer - CAG TGC GAT GCA GGC TGG CT, rat Acan reverse primer - CCT CCG GCA CTC GTT GGC TG; rat Col10a1 forward primer - CCA GGT GTC CCA GGA TTC CC, rat Col10a1 reverse primer - CAA GCG GCA TCC CAG AAA GC; rat Mmp3 forward primer - TTG TCC TTC GAT GCA GTC AG, rat Mmp3 -3 reverse primer - AGA CGG CCA AAA TGA AGA GA; rat Mmp13 forward primer - GGA CCT TCT GGT CTT CTG GC, rat Mmp13 reverse primer - GGA TGC TTA GGG TTG GGG TC; rat Runx2 forward primer - CCGCAC GAC AAC CGC ACC AT; rat Runx2 reverse primer - CGC TCC GGC CCA CAA ATC TC; 18S RNA forward primer - CGG CTA CCA CAT CCA AGG AA,

18S RNA reverse primer - GCT GGA ATT ACC GCG GCT. Relative transcript levels were calculated as

$$x = 2^{-\Delta\Delta Ct}$$

in which $\Delta\Delta Ct = \Delta Ct\ E - \Delta Ct\ C$, and $\Delta Ct\ E = Ctexp\text{-}Ct18S$, and $\Delta Ct\ C = CtC\text{-}Ct18S$ as previously described [5, 17].

Statistical analysis

One-way analysis of variance (ANOVA) was used to analyze the differences among mean cartilage damage scoreS, synovial hyperplasia scoreS, FMT scan results, MMP-13 levels, and the mRNA levels of Acan, MMP-3, MMP-13, Runx2, Col2a1, and Col X. The least significant difference (LSD) multiple comparisons test was used to perform pairwise comparisons following the ANOVA. Differences were considered statistically significant at $P < 0.05$. Statistical analyses were performed using SPSS 13.0 software.

Results

BCE

The data obtained from BCE culture supernatant demonstrated that wt-A2M (left) and A2M variants CYT-98 and CYT-108 (right) inhibit cartilage catabolism induced by TNFα and IL-1β. The absolute sGAG values were 313.5 µg/ml in the untreated cytokine-stimulated explants, 78.6 µg/ml in the A2M-treated cytokine-stimulated explants, 44.6 µg/ml in the CYT-98 A2M-treated cytokine-stimulated explants, 37.8 µg/ml in the CYT-108-treated cytokine-stimulated explants, and 183.1 µg/ml in the untreated un-stimulated explants, respectively. The soluble GAG levels determined after treatment with wt-A2M were 1.76-fold and 2.08-fold the levels determined after treatment with variant CYT-98 and CYT-108, respectively. The results also demonstrated that A2M variants were more effective in inhibiting cartilage catabolism in the BCE model by up to 200% compared with wt-A2M (Fig. 1, right) ($P < 0.05$). The variant 108 was the most efficacious inhibitor in the BCE model.

FMT

Using in vivo deep-tissue imaging methods, real-time information was gained about MMPs and cathepsin biological processes using probes. The levels of ProSense and MMPSense were dramatically increased in all groups after ACLT or sham surgery. MMPs and cathepsin levels peak 2 days after knee joint injury. The highest levels of MMPs (A and B) and cathepsin (C and D), as detected by FMT after ACLT, were observed 2 days after surgery, indicating an early catabolic response. Supplemental A2M or its variants reduced the level of MMPSense (A and B) and ProSense (C and D) compared with the PBS-treated group (Fig. 2, red line) and

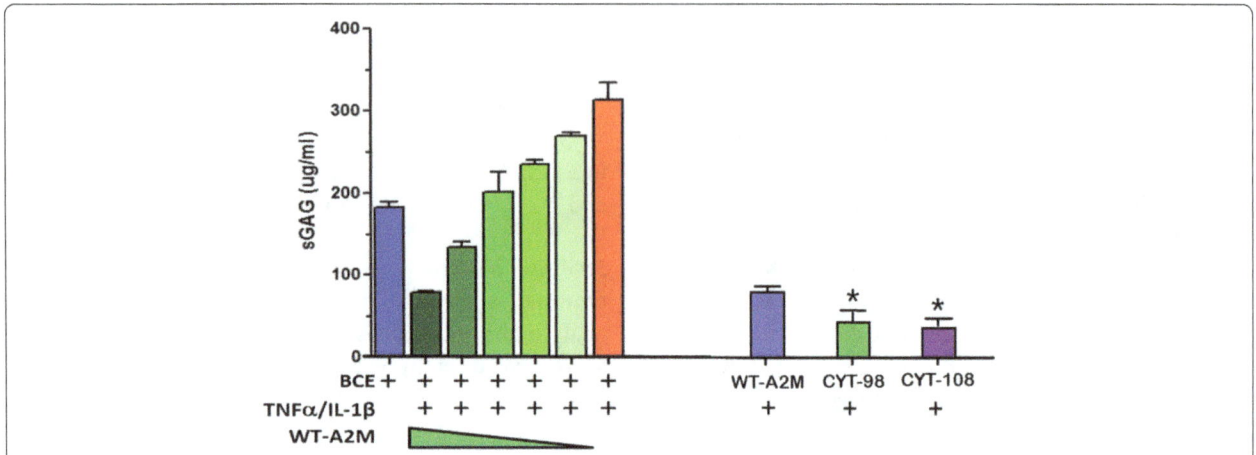

Fig. 1 Wild-type alpha-2-macroglobulin (*WT-A2M*) (*left*) and A2M variants CYT-98 and CYT-108 (*right*) inhibit cartilage catabolism induced by TNFα and IL-1β. *Compared with wt-A2M, $P < 0.05$. *BCE*, bovine articular cartilage explants, *SGAG* sulfated glycosaminoglycan

the sham group (Fig. 2, blue line). This is consistent with our BCE model data. The ProSense remained at a low level at weeks 4 and 6 after surgery even without treatment. Interestingly, at weeks 4 and 6 without treatment, the level of MMPSense was increased again compared with the sham group, but was lower than in the PBS-treated animals. The mean SD region of interest (ROI) signal intensities (n = 11 per group) at each time point over a 6-week period are shown at the bottom (Fig. 2 b and d: *compared with Sham, $P < 0.05$. #compared with PBS, $P < 0.05$).

Supplemental intra-articular injection of wt-A2M and its variants attenuates the severity of OA cartilage degeneration

Histological analysis (OARSI score) showed that the animals treated with A2M and its variants had a significant decrease in OA cartilage damage compared with the rats that underwent ACLT and PBS treatment (Fig. 3). Strong Safranin O staining, more cellularity but less chondrocyte cloning, and less fibrillation were observed in the animals treated with A2M and its variants at either concentration compared with the animals treated with the PBS (Fig. 3a). Cartilage in the rats that were treated with A2M variant 108 at high concentration had stronger staining and more intact surface than cartilage in the rats that were treated with variant 108 at low concentration and others, but had weaker staining than the control rats that underwent sham operation. The OARSI grading score indicated that cartilage damage was most severe in rats that underwent ACLT and PBS treatment and the cartilage in rats that underwent sham operation had the least damage (9.75 ± 0.88 and 0.78 ± 0.11, respectively; $P <0.05$), whereas cartilage damage in the A2M and the A2M-variants-treated group was significantly less than in the PBS group (wt-A2M: 4.43 ± 0.52;

CYT-98-low: 3.36 ± 0.34; CYT-98-high: 3.27 ± 0.32; CYT-108-low: 3.26 ± 0.21; CYT-108-high: 1.98 ± 0.07; respectively; $P < 0.01$) (Fig. 3b). Values are mean ± SD.

The animals treated with wt-A2M and its variants had reduced synovial hyperplasia

Using hematoxylin/eosin staining, we also observed changes in the synovial membrane in the animals treated with A2M and its variants compared with the animals treated with PBS (Fig. 4a). Only one or two layers of synovial membrane existed in the sham animals. Synovial hyperplasia was seen in the PBS-treated animals with the thicker synovial membranes, whereas the animals treated with A2M and its variants had thinner synovial membranes compared with the PBS treated animals. Semi-quantified data are shown in Fig. 4b.

IHC analyses

IHC staining showed that matrix metalloproteinase 13 (MMP-13) (Fig. 5a), type X collagen (Fig. 5b), and type II degraded products staining (Fig. 5c) were significantly elevated in rats that underwent ACLT and PBS treatment, but were lower in the A2M-treated and A2M-variants-treated and sham-operated rats, which is consistent with reduced OA damage in these rats (Fig. 3). In contrast, type II collagen expression in articular cartilage was higher in the A2M and A2M-variants-treated and sham-operated rats than in rats that underwent ACLT and PBS treatment (Fig. 5d). The bottom panels of Fig. 3 are higher-magnification views of the boxed areas in the top panels. ELISA further confirmed that A2M and its variants partially reduce the concentration of MMP-13 (Fig. 5e). In A2M and A2M-ariants-treated rats, the concentration of MMP-13 in SF was significantly lower (A2M: 1.92 ± 0.32 ng/ml; CYT-98 low: 1.49 ± 0.33 ng/ml; CYT-98 high: 1.32 ± 0.17 ng/ml; CYT-108 low: 1.49 ±

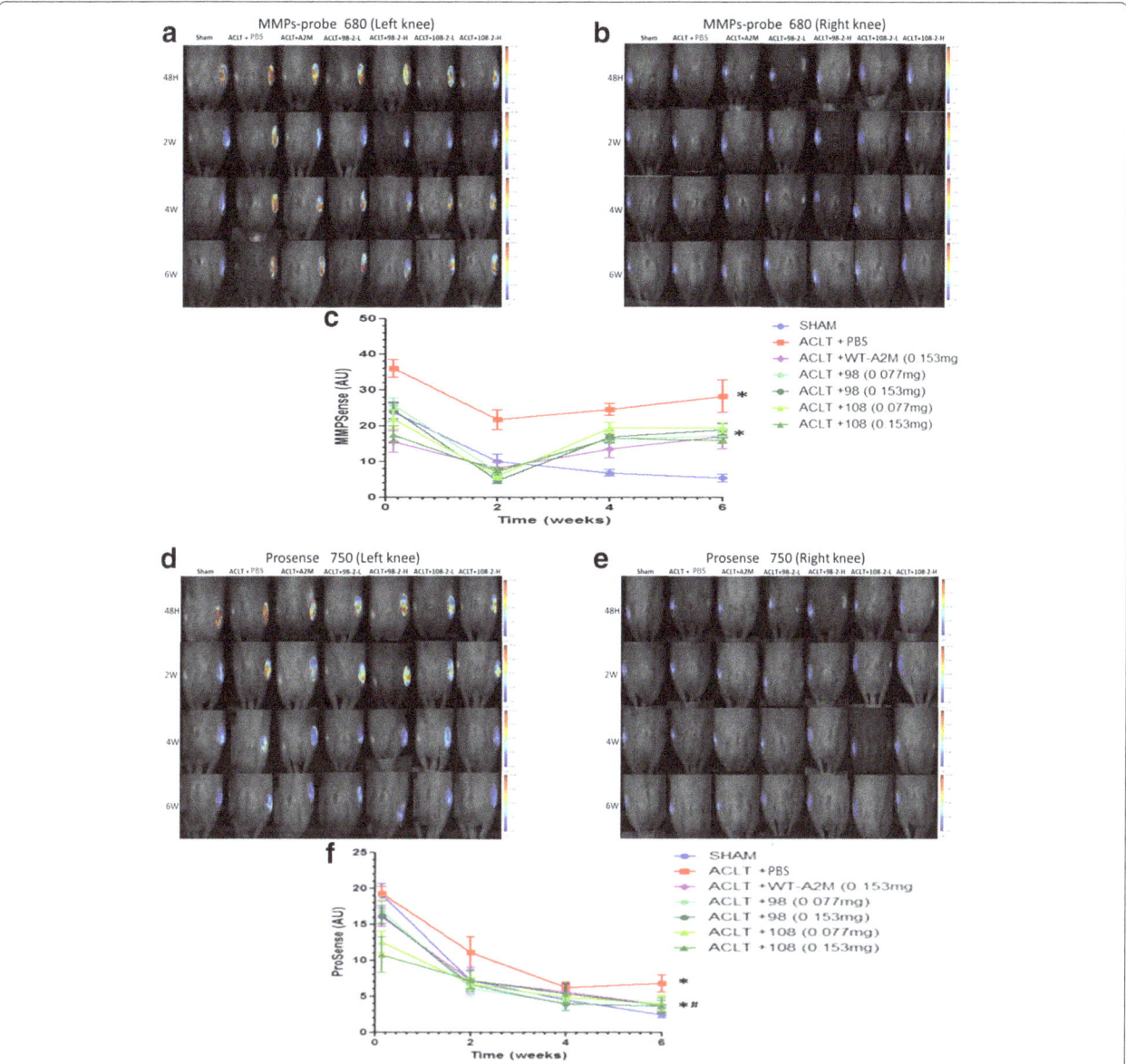

Fig. 2 Wild-type alpha-2-macroglobulin (WT-A2M) and its variants CYT-98 and CYT-108 inhibit matrix. metalloproteinases (MMPs) (**a** and **b**) and cathepsin (**d** and **e**). MMPs and cathepsin levels peak 2 days after knee joint injury. The levels of MMPs (**a**) and cathepsin (**d**), as detected by fluorescence molecular tomography after anterior cruciate ligament transection (ACLT), peaked 2 days after surgery, indicating an early catabolic response that subsided thereafter. The mean SD region of interest signal intensities (n = 11 per group) at each time point over a 6-week period are shown (bottom) (**c** and **f**). *Compared with sham, $P < 0.05$. #Compared with PBS, $P < 0.05$

0.23 ng/ml; CYT-108 high: 1.13 ± 0.10 ng/ml) than that in the rats that underwent ACLT and PBS treatment (3.26 ± 0.40 ng/ml) but it was still higher than that in sham-operated rats (0.92 ± 0.09 ng/ml) ($P < 0.05$). Values are the mean ± SD.

Real-time PCR data indicated that supplemental intra-articular injection of wt-A2M and its variants CYT-98 and CYT-108 reduced cartilage matrix catabolism and enhanced anabolic metabolism in the ACLT rat OA model (Fig. 6). The mRNA levels of the MMP-3, MMP-13, Runx2, and Col X were expressed at a lower level in

rats that were administered A2M and its variants as compared to rats that underwent ACLT and PBS treatment. In contrast, the levels of mRNA for Col X and aggrecan followed the opposite pattern. Both of them were increased in rats that were administered A2M and its variants as compared to rats that underwent ACLT and PBS treatment, suggesting that A2M has a positive impact on cartilage matrix anabolism. Values are the mean ± SEM. # $P < 0.05$ compared with ACLT + PBS; * $P < 0.05$ compared with sham; &Compared with ACLT + A2M, $P < 0.05$, € compared with ACLT + 98-

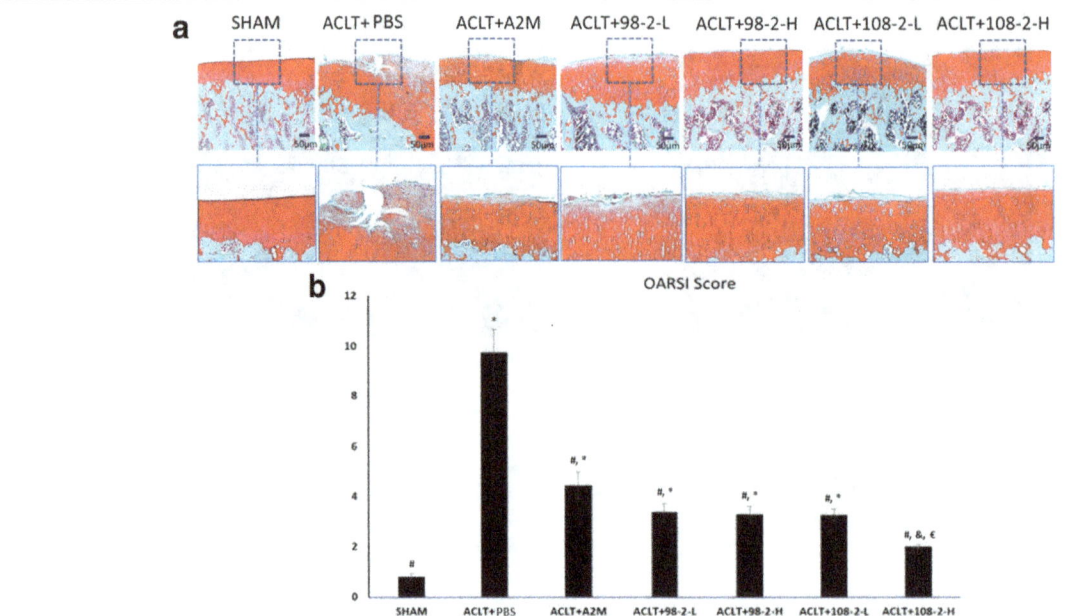

Fig. 3 Supplemental intra-articular injection of wild-type alpha-2-macroglobulin (wt-A2M) and its variants CYT-98 and CYT-108 attenuates cartilage degeneration. **a** Strong Safranin O staining and a relatively smoother surface were detected in the articular cartilage from the animals treated with wt-A2M and its variants as compared to PBS-treated controls. **b** The Osteoarthritis Research Society International grading score indicated that cartilage damage was most severe in rats that underwent anterior cruciate ligament transection (*ACLT*) and PBS treatment, while cartilage in rats that underwent sham operation had the least damage. Cartilage damage was further reduced in the rats that received the high dose of the variants of A2M as compared to the rats that received the low dose of the variants of A2M. Values are the mean ± SD. #Compared with ACLT + PBS, $P < 0.05$; *compared with sham, $P < 0.05$; €compared with ACLT + A2M, $P < 0.05$

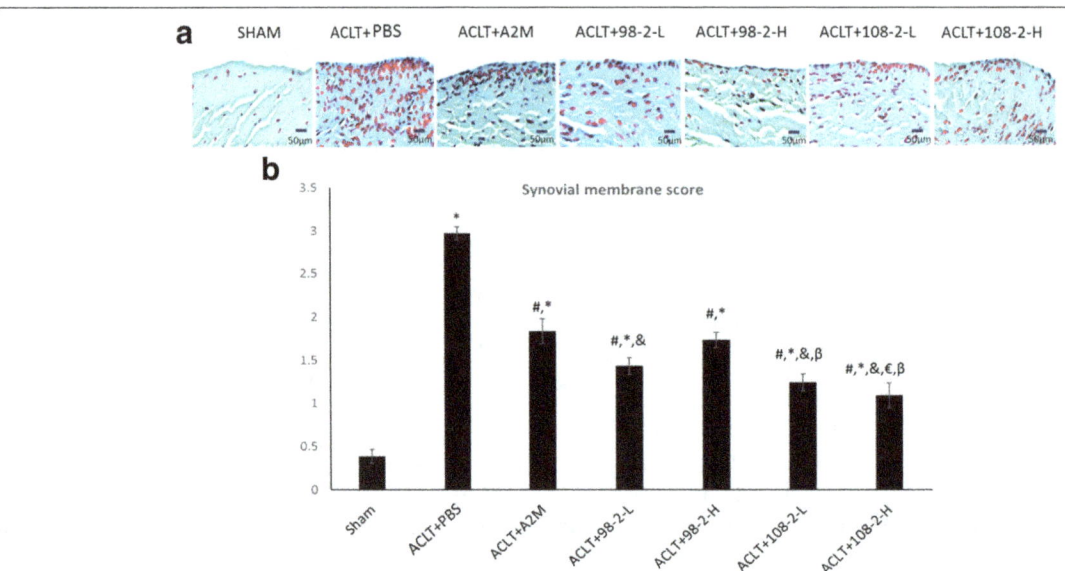

Fig. 4 Intra-articular injection of wild-type alpha-2-macroglobulin (wt-A2M) and its variants CYT-98 and CYT-108 leads to a thinner synovial membrane. **a** Hematoxylin/eosin staining indicates the synovium depicted with 1–2 cell layers of synoviocytes in the sham animals. Synovial hyperplasia is seen in the PBS-treated animals with the thicker synovial membranes, whereas the animals treated with A2M and its variants had thinner synovial membranes compared with the PBS-treated animals. Semi-quantified data are shown (**b**). #Compared with anterior cruciate ligament transection (*ACLT*) + PBS, $P < 0.05$; *compared with sham, $P < 0.05$; &compared with ACLT + A2M, $P < 0.05$; €compared with ACLT + 98-2-L, $P < 0.05$; βcompared with ACLT + 98-2-H, $P < 0.05$; αcompared with ACLT + 108-2-L, $P < 0.05$

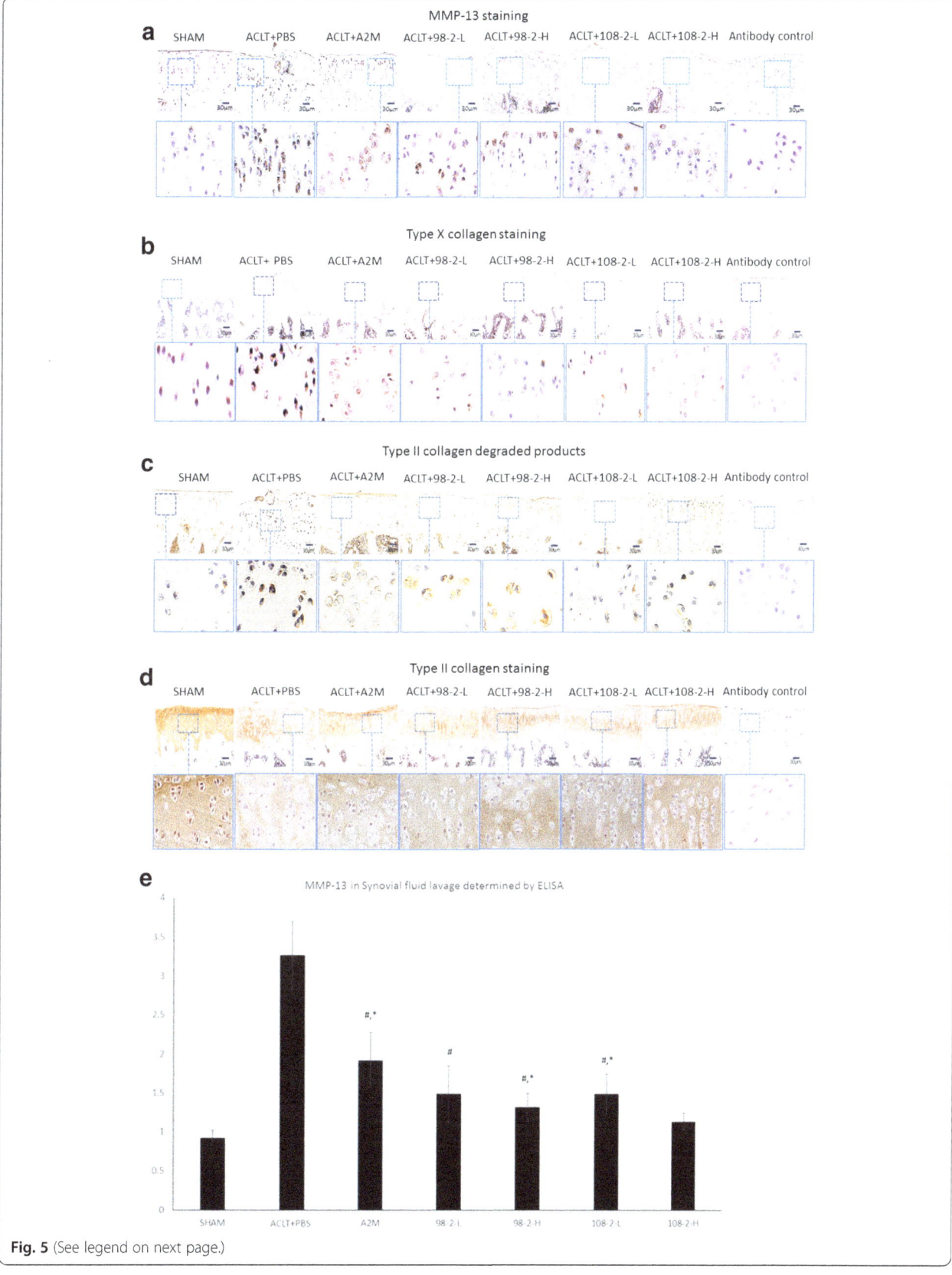

Fig. 5 (See legend on next page.)

(See figure on previous page.)

Fig. 5 Matrix metalloproteinase 13 (MMP-13) (**a**), type X collagen (**b**), and type II degraded products staining (**c**) were elevated in rats that underwent anterior cruciate ligament transection (*ACLT*) and PBS treatment, but was lower in the alpha-2-macroglobulin (*A2M*) and A2M-variants-treated and sham-operated rats, which is consistent with reduced osteoarthritis damage in these rats. In contrast, type II collagen expression in articular cartilage was higher in the A2M and A2M-variants-treated and sham-operated rats than in rats that underwent ACLT and PBS treatment (**d**). The *bottom panels* are higher-magnification views of the *boxed areas* in the *top panels*. ELISA further confirmed that A2M and its variants partially inhibit MMP-13 (**e**). In A2M and A2M-variants-treated rats, the concentration of MMP-13 in SF was lower than that in the rats that underwent ACLT and PBS treatment but it was still higher than that in in sham-operated rats. Values are the mean ± SD. #Compared with ACLT + PBS, *P* < 0.05; *compared with sham, *P* < 0.05; &compared with ACLT + A2M, *P* < 0.05; €compared with ACLT + 108-2-L, *P* < 0.05

2-L, P < 0.05; β Compared with ACLT + 98-2-H, P < 0.05; α Compared with ACLT + 108-2-L, P < 0.05.

Discussion

As A2M inhibits all classes of endoproteases [5, 21, 22], it could be used to mitigate the progression of OA by neutralizing cartilage catabolic factors. Studies have shown that A2M inhibits the activities of ADAMTS-4, ADAMTS-5, ADAMTS-7, and ADAMTS-12 [21, 22], reduces ligament stump resorption following ACL injury [15], and enhances tendon-bone healing of ACL grafts by inhibiting MMP-13 activity [16]. Thus, the balance of the protease/A2M in vivo may play an important role in mediating cartilage destruction by catabolic enzymes. However, A2M is not present in vivo at sufficient levels to counteract the increased concentrations of catabolic factors that appear after joint injury. The level of A2M in serum is 1.53 mg/ml and the level of A2M in OA SF is 0.24 mg/ml as compared to MMP-13 expression in serum of 91.1 ng/ml and MMP-13 expression in SF of 251 ng/ml [5]. Higher A2M concentration is

associated with lower MMP-13 content [5]. The difference is thought to be due to the large molecular weight of A2M, which prevents it's migration from the blood into the SF [14, 15]. Thus, supplemental A2M may be a potential strategy to attenuate cartilage degeneration by reducing these catabolic enzymes induced by joint injury.

Although autologous A2M is an exciting and potential candidate for OA treatment, clinicians may find the time, training, expense, and potential safety concerns of drawing blood and preparing autologous A2M in an outpatient setting burdensome. An off-the-shelf, optimized recombinant form of A2M and its target variants could eliminate these drawbacks. Our FMT and histology results demonstrated that the recombinant target variants of A2M do attenuate OA damage by inhibiting cartilage-degraded enzymes more effectively than wt-A2M.

FMT is a sensitive bio-imaging method providing noninvasive, deep tissue in vivo imaging and it allows for the evaluation of disease progression at multiple time points without sacrifice of the animal [12, 23–25]. In this study,

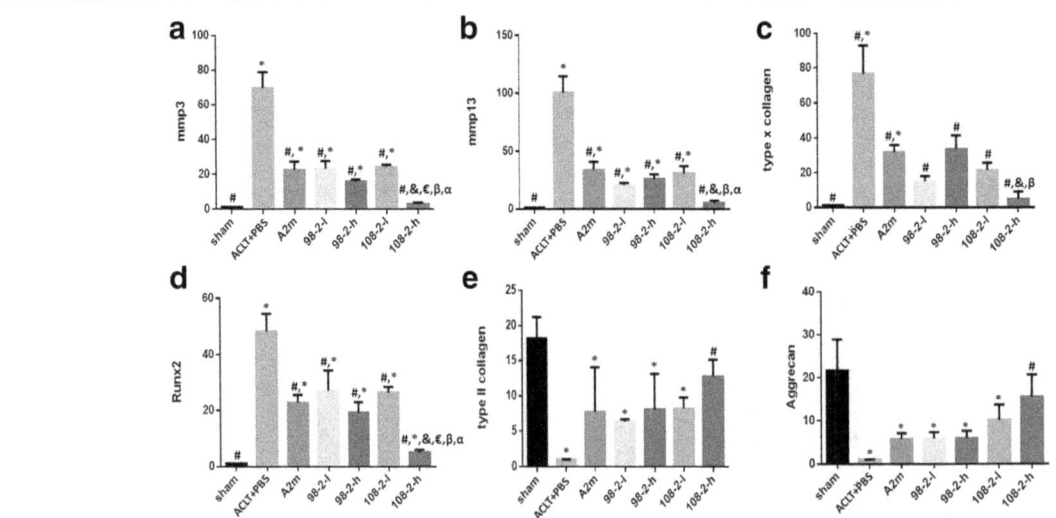

Fig. 6 Supplemental intra-articular wild-type alpha-2-macroglobulin (A2M) and its variants CYT-98 and CYT-108 reduce catabolism and enhance anabolic metabolism in the anterior cruciate ligament transection (ACLT) rat osteoarthritis model. The levels of mRNA of the matrix metalloproteinase (MMP)-3(**a**), MMP-13(**b**), type X collagen(**c**), and Runx2(**d**) were expressed at a lower level in rats that were administered A2M and its variants as compared to the rats that underwent ACLT and PBS treatment. In contrast, the levels of mRNA for type II collagen (**e**) and aggrecan (**f**) followed an opposite pattern. Both of them were increased in rats that were administered A2M and its variants as compared to the rats that underwent ACLT and PBS treatment. Values are the mean ± SEM. #Compared with ACLT + PBS, *P* < 0.05 ; *compared with sham group, *P* < 0.05; &compared with ACLT + A2M, *P* < 0.05; €compared with ACLT + 98-2-L, *P* < 0.05; βcompared with ACLT + 98-2-H, *P* < 0.05; αcompared with ACLT + 108-2-L, *P* < 0.05

we found that A2M and its variants are able to specifically inhibit proteases and MMPs either in ex vivo cartilage or in vivo ACLT rat OA models immediately after injury compared to PBS-treated animals. The targeted variants of A2M were more efficacious than wt-A2M in the BCE experiments. A significant decrease of ProSense and MMPSense detected by FMT was observed immediately in the animals treated by A2M and its variants compared with the animals treated with PBS in vivo in the ACLT rat OA model. The level of the ProSense remained at a low level at weeks 4 and 6 after surgery even without treatment. This suggests that ProSense is an acute indicator of inflammation and not sensitive for late stages of OA. This finding is consistent with previous reports [5]. Furthermore, the level of MMPSense increased again gradually when A2M was not re-dosed at weeks 4 and 6. This indicates that MMPs may have two peaks. The first phase appears after the initial trauma to the joint. The second peak is not related to the acute joint injury but is associated with progressive cartilage degeneration. The gradual increase in protease activity suggests to us that a continuing constant supplemental level of A2M may be necessary to prevent catabolic degeneration after joint injury to prevent development of post traumatic OA.

Our histological and biochemistry data further demonstrated that supplemental A2M and its variants not only attenuate cartilage damage and inhibit catabolic factor MMP-13, but also enhance cartilage matrix Col 2 and aggrecan synthesis. The increase in collagen and aggrecan suggests that A2M may have cartilage repair functions or at least does not interfere with cartilage matrix synthesis to proceed. This finding is consistent with a previous report in which a high dose of A2M did not induce chondrocyte death [5]. The findings strongly indicate that A2M and its variants are promising bioinhibitors for catabolic proteases, and supplemental intra-articular injection of A2M soon after injury may provide a chondral protection effect in vivo in the ACL-injured knee by reducing the presence of local catabolic proteases. Our data also clearly demonstrate these variants of A2M have similar functions compared with wt-A2M. Especially, the targeted 108 variant of A2M has demonstrated a stronger chondroprotective effect to prevent or delay cartilage degeneration compared to wt-A2M and 98 variant.

Collected evidence has demonstrated that A2M has the ability to bind cytokines, such as IL-1b and TNFa and that it also enters cells to regulate cellular responses to other growth factors and cytokines [26–28]. The mechanism by which targeted A2M variants enhance this function is not clear. Since the cytokine binding sites in the A2M variants were not altered, it is very likely these target A2M variants regulate the process through the inhibition of the catabolic enzymes [5, 21, 23–25], but not through binding to the cytokines or altering their function. Further study to explore the strong inhibitory ability of the designed variants to the cytokines compared with wt-A2M is warranted.

One limitation of our study was that the SF samples were obtained from the knees after an injection of 100 μl of saline, and cycling and impartial recovery of diluted fluid. Lavage was required to obtain SF from the rat small joint cavity. All SF measurements should be normalized, i.e. using serum and SF urea. Baseline fluid volume, amongst other factors, might have differed in the SF results. Unfortunately, we did not collect blood samples in this study and were unable to collect enough SF samples, due to the small joint volume, in order to normalize the SF results for the urea experiment. Thus, this MMP-13 data analysis does not preclude other variables such as changes in synovial vascular permeability of protein content with OA onset, although no evidence of joint effusion was noted prior to the lavages.

Conclusion

Our data show that A2M protects cartilage following joint injuries that can progress to OA. Our engineered, recombinant A2M variants are more protective than the wild-type.

Abbreviations
A2M: Alpha-2- macroglobulin; ACAN: Aggrecan; ACL: Anterior cruciate ligament; ACLT: Anterior cruciate ligament transection; ANOVA: analysis of variance; BCE: Bovine articular cartilage explants; cDNA: Complementary DNA; Col: Collagen; Ct: Cycle threshold; DMEM: Dulbecco's modified Eagle's medium; ELISA: Enzyme-linked immunosorbent assay; FMT: Fluorescence molecular tomography; IHC: Immunohistochemical analysis; IL: Interleukin; MMP: Matrix metallopeptidase; mRNA: Messenger RNA; OA: Osteoarthritis; OARSI: Osteoarthritis Research Society International; PBS: Phosphate-buffered saline; ROI: Region of interest; SF: Synovial fluid; SGAG: Sulfated glycosaminoglycan; TNF: Tumor necrosis factor; wt: Wild-type

Acknowledgements
The authors gratefully acknowledge Dr. Sun, C., Du, G., Wang, S., Chen, C., for help with the surgery and animal care.

Funding
The project was supported by a grant from NSFC 81572098, 31271033, 81201435, 8160949, SXNSF 20150313012-6, 201605D211024, NIH/NIAMS R01AR059142, and Cytonics Corp. The content is solely the responsibility of the authors and does not necessarily represent the official view of the NIH.

Authors' contributions
YZ participated in the study design, wrote the manuscript, performed most of the experiments, and analyzed data. XCW, SB, GS, and LSH conceived, designed, and manufactured the recombinant A2M and its variants. They also conceived, designed, and performed the bovine articular cartilage explants in vitro study. They also participated in the interpretation of the data and the revision of the manuscript. Cytonics hold all patents related to the composition of A2M variants and its use. LW conceived the in vivo study and participated in its design and data analysis and revised the manuscript with the Cytonics team. All authors have read and approved the final manuscript.

Competing interests
The authors declare that they have no competing interests.

Consent for publication
Not applicable.

Disclosures
YZ, XW, and LW are associated with Brown University. SB, GS, and LH are employees at Cytonics Corporation.

Author details
[1]Department of Orthopedics, the second hospital of the Shanxi Medical University, Taiyuan, China. [2]Cytonics Corporation, 6917 Vista Pkwy N., Suite 14, West Palm Beach, FL 33411, USA. [3]Department of Orthopedics, Alpert Medical School of Brown University/Rhode Island Hospital, Providence, RI, USA.

References

1. Anderson DD, Chubinskaya S, Guilak F, Martin JA, Oegema TR, Olson SA, Buckwalter JA. Post-traumatic osteoarthritis: improved understanding and opportunities for early intervention. J Orthop Res. 2011;29(6):802–9.

2. Kim KS, Choi HM, Lee Y-A, Choi IA, Lee S-H, Hong S-J, Yang H-I, Yoo MC. Expression levels and association of gelatinases MMP-2 and MMP-9 and collagenases MMP-1 and MMP-13 with VEGF in synovial fluid of patients with arthritis. Rheumatol Int. 2011;31(4):543–7.

3. Kanbe K, Takemura T, Takeuchi K, Chen Q, Takagishi K, Inoue K. Synovectomy reduces stromal-cell-derived factor-1 (SDF-1) which is involved in the destruction of cartilage in osteoarthritis and rheumatoid arthritis. J Bone Joint Surg Br. 2004; 86(2):296–300.

4. Wei L, Fleming BC, Sun X, Teeple E, Wu W, Jay GD, Elsaid KA, Luo J, Machan JT, Chen Q. Comparison of differential biomarkers of osteoarthritis with and without posttraumatic injury in the Hartley guinea pig model. J Orthop Res. 2010;28(7):900–6.

5. Wang S, Wei X, Zhou J, Zhang J, Li K, Chen Q, Terek R, Fleming BC, Goldring MB, Ehrlich MG, et al. Identification of alpha2-macroglobulin as a master inhibitor of cartilage-degrading factors that attenuates the progression of posttraumatic osteoarthritis. Arthritis Rheumatol. 2014;66(7):1843–53.

6. Green DM, Noble PC, Bocell Jr JR, Ahuero JS, Poteet BA, Birdsall HH. Effect of early full weight-bearing after joint injury on inflammation and cartilage degradation. J Bone Joint Surg Am. 2006;88(10):2201–9.

7. Backus JD, Furman BD, Swimmer T, Kent CL, McNulty AL, Defrate LE, Guilak F, Olson SA. Cartilage viability and catabolism in the intact porcine knee following transarticular impact loading with and without articular fracture. J Orthop Res. 2011;29(4):501–10.

8. Borrelli Jr J, Tinsley K, Ricci WM, Burns M, Karl IE, Hotchkiss R. Induction of chondrocyte apoptosis following impact load. J Orthop Trauma. 2003;17(9): 635–41.

9. Tochigi Y, Buckwalter JA, Martin JA, Hillis SL, Zhang P, Vaseenon T, Lehman AD, Brown TD. Distribution and progression of chondrocyte damage in a whole-organ model of human ankle intra-articular fracture. J Bone Joint Surg Am. 2011;93(6):533–9.

10. Wei F, Zhou J, Wei X, Zhang J, Fleming BC, Terek R, Pei M, Chen Q, Liu T, Wei L. Activation of Indian hedgehog promotes chondrocyte hypertrophy and upregulation of MMP-13 in human osteoarthritic cartilage. Osteoarthr Cartil. 2012;20(7):755–63.

11. Wei FMD, Li Y, Zhang G, Wei X, Lee JK, Wei L. Attenuation of osteoarthritis via blockade of the SDF-1/CXCR4 signaling pathway. Arthritis Res Ther. 2012;14(4):R177. [Epub ahead of print](PMCID:PMC3580571).

12. Zhou J, Chen Q, Lanske B, Fleming BC, Terek R, Wei X, Zhang G, Wang S, Li K, Wei L. Disrupting the Indian hedgehog signaling pathway in vivo attenuates surgically induced osteoarthritis progression in Col2a1-CreERT2; Ihhfl/fl mice. Arthritis Res Ther. 2014;16(1):R11.

13. Jay GD, Elsaid KA, Kelly KA, Anderson SC, Zhang L, Teeple E, Waller K, Fleming BC. Prevention of cartilage degeneration and gait asymmetry by lubricin tribosupplementation in the rat following anterior cruciate ligament transection. Arthritis Rheum. 2012;64(4):1162–71.

14. Salvesen G, Enghild JJ. alpha-Macroglobulins: detection and characterization. Methods Enzymol. 1993;223:121–41.

15. Demirag B, Sarisozen B, Durak K, Bilgen OF, Ozturk C. The effect of alpha-2 macroglobulin on the healing of ruptured anterior cruciate ligament in rabbits. Connect Tissue Res. 2004;45(1):23–7.

16. Demirag B, Sarisozen B, Ozer O, Kaplan T, Ozturk C. Enhancement of tendon-bone healing of anterior cruciate ligament grafts by blockage of matrix metalloproteinases. J Bone Joint Surg Am. 2005;87(11):2401–10.

17. Du G, Zhan H, Ding D, Wang S, Wei X, Wei F, Zhang J, Bilgen B, Reginato AM, Fleming BC, et al. Abnormal mechanical loading induces cartilage degeneration by accelerating meniscus hypertrophy and mineralization after ACL injuries in vivo. Am J Sports Med. 2016;44(3):652–63.

18. Jay GD, Fleming BC, Watkins BA, McHugh KA, Anderson SC, Zhang LX, Teeple E, Waller KA, Elsaid KA. Prevention of cartilage degeneration and restoration of chondroprotection by lubricin tribosupplementation in the rat following anterior cruciate ligament transection. Arthritis Rheum. 2010;62(8): 2382–91.

19. Pritzker KPH, Gay S, Jimenez SA, Ostergaard K, Pelletier JP, Revell PA, Salter D, van den Berg WB. Osteoarthritis cartilage histopathology: grading and staging. Osteoarthr Cartil. 2006;14(1):13–29.

20. Gerwin N, Bendele AM, Glasson S, Carlson CS. The OARSI histopathology initiative - recommendations for histological assessments of osteoarthritis in the rat. Osteoarthr Cartil. 2010;18 Suppl 3:S24–34.

21. Tortorella MD, Arner EC, Hills R, Easton A, Korte-Sarfaty J, Fok K, Wittwer AJ, Liu R-Q, Malfait A-M. Alpha2-macroglobulin is a novel substrate for ADAMTS-4 and ADAMTS-5 and represents an endogenous inhibitor of these enzymes. J Biol Chem. 2004;279(17):17554–61.

22. Luan Y, Kong L, Howell DR, Ilalov K, Fajardo M, Bai XH, Di Cesare PE, Goldring MB, Abramson SB, Liu CJ. Inhibition of ADAMTS-7 and ADAMTS-12 degradation of cartilage oligomeric matrix protein by alpha-2-macroglobulin. Osteoarthr Cartil. 2008;16(11):1413–20.

23. Abbink JJ, Kamp AM, Nieuwenhuys EJ, Nuijens JH, Swaak AJ, Hack CE. Predominant role of neutrophils in the inactivation of alpha 2-macroglobulin in arthritic joints. Arthritis Rheum. 1991;34(9):1139–50.

24. Zhang L, Yang M, Yang D, Cavey G, Davidson P, Gibson G. Molecular interactions of MMP-13 C-terminal domain with chondrocyte proteins. Connect Tissue Res. 2010;51(3):230–9.

25. Abbink JJ, Nuijens JH, Eerenberg AJ, Huijbregts CC, van Schijndel RJS, Thijs LG, Hack CE. Quantification of functional and inactivated alpha 2-macroglobulin in sepsis. Thromb Haemost. 1991;65(1):32–9.

26. LaMarre J, Wollenberg GK, Gonias SL, Hayes MA. Cytokine binding and clearance properties of proteinase-activated alpha 2-macroglobulins. Lab Investig. 1991;65(1):3–14.

27. Wollenberg GK, LaMarre J, Rosendal S, Gonias SL, Hayes MA. Binding of tumor necrosis factor alpha to activated forms of human plasma alpha 2 macroglobulin. Am J Pathol. 1991;138(2):265–72.

28. Borth W, Scheer B, Urbansky A, Luger TA, Sottrup-Jensen L. Binding of IL-1 beta to alpha-macroglobulins and release by thioredoxin. J Immunol. 1990; 145(11):3747–54.

10

Adelmidrol, in combination with hyaluronic acid, displays increased anti-inflammatory and analgesic effects against monosodium iodoacetate-induced osteoarthritis in rats

Rosanna Di Paola[1], Roberta Fusco[1], Daniela Impellizzeri[1], Marika Cordaro[1], Domenico Britti[2], Valeria Maria Morittu[2], Maurizio Evangelista[3] and Salvatore Cuzzocrea[1,4*]

Abstract

Background: Osteoarthritis (OA) is a degenerative joint disease produced by a cascade of events that can ultimately lead to joint damage. The aim of this study was to evaluate the effect of adelmidrol, a synthetic palmitoylethanolamide analogue, combined with hyaluronic acid on pain severity and modulation of the inflammatory response in a rat model of monosodium iodoacetate (MIA)-induced osteoarthritis.

Methods: OA was induced by intra-articular injection of MIA in the knee joint. On day 21 post-MIA administration, the knee joint was analyzed. Rats subjected to OA were treated by intra-articular injection of adelmidrol in combination with sodium hyaluronate at different doses and time points after MIA induction. Limb nociception was assessed by the paw withdrawal latency and threshold measurement. Samples were examined macroscopically, histologically, and by immunohistochemistry.

Results: At day 21 post-MIA injection, the MIA + solvent and MIA + 1.0% sodium hyaluronate groups showed irregularities and fibrillation in the surface layer, a decrease in blood cells and multilayering in transition and radial zones, no pannus formation, and modified Mankin scores significantly higher than sham knees. The combination of hyaluronic acid and adelmidrol dose-dependently (adelmidrol 0.6% + 1.0% sodium hyaluronate and adelmidrol 2% + 1.0% sodium hyaluronate) reduced the histological alterations induced by MIA. Moreover, degeneration of articular cartilage, mast cell infiltration, and pro-inflammatory cytokine and chemokine plasma levels were significantly downregulated by treatment with a combination of hyaluronic acid and adelmidrol at the above doses.

Conclusions: Our results clearly demonstrate that the combination of hyaluronic acid and adelmidrol improves the signs of OA induced by MIA.

Keywords: Osteoarthritis, Adelmidrol, Sodium hyaluronate, Inflammation, Cartilage degeneration

* Correspondence: salvator@unime.it
[1]Department of Chemical, Biological, Pharmaceutical and Environmental Sciences, University of Messina, Viale Ferdinando Stagno D'Alcontres, n 31, Messina 98166, Italy
[4]Department of Pharmacological and Physiological Science, Saint Louis University School of Medicine, 1402 South Grand Blvd, St. Louis, MO 63104, USA
Full list of author information is available at the end of the article

Background

Osteoarthritis (OA) is one of the most common joint disabling disorders in adults [1]. It occurs when the protective cartilage on the ends of bones breaks down, causing pain, swelling, and problems in joint articulation [2]. OA is primarily characterized by degeneration of cartilage at the joints but also implicates other pathological changes, including synovial inflammation, osteophyte formation, and subchondral bone sclerosis, in all tissues of joints [3–5]. OA can affect any joint, but the disorder most frequently affects joints in the hands, knees, hips, and spine, where it induces stiffness and joint dysfunction. Current guidelines defined by The Osteoarthritis Research Society International state that OA treatment should be aimed at reducing pain and joint stiffness, maintaining and improving joint mobility, reducing physical disability, and improving patient quality of life by limiting progression of damage [6].

The monosodium iodoacetate (MIA) experimental model is commonly used as an animal model of arthritis pain associated with OA [7]. In particular, the MIA model has been widely used for the pharmacological evaluation of new drug therapy [8]. Nonsteroidal anti-inflammatory drugs (NSAIDs) and steroids reduce the OA symptoms of joint pain and swelling [9]. However, evidence in clinics shows that pharmacological interventions, including acetaminophen, NSAIDS, topical agents, and intra-articular injections (e.g., steroids), and non-pharmacological interventions, such as joint replacement, are both sparse and controversial [10–12]. Glucocorticoids (GCs) have powerful immunosuppressive effects and are widely used in the management of chronic inflammatory diseases. Long-term therapy with GCs is often necessary to control the symptoms of osteoarthritis [13]. Important evidence shows that GCs are also used in association with hyaluronic acid (HA) and partially show an ability to reduce pain as well as the progression of disease [14]. A number of studies suggest that HA associated with GCs might have a beneficial effect partially related to a viscoelastic lubricant effect [15, 16].

A major drawback in the use of HA relates to the ability of the intra-articular environment to depolymerize the polysaccharide with a speed directly proportional to the degree of intra-articular inflammation. The correct degradation of HA is therefore essential to maintain the integrity of tissues and, in particular, joint homeostasis. Moreover, an important question mark remains about therapeutic management of long-term pathologies, with steroids often linked to a series of unwanted side effects [17].

Adelmidrol is a semisynthetic derivative of azelaic acid and analogue of the anti-inflammatory compound palmitoylethanolamide (PEA), an aliamide and member of the family of fatty acid amide signaling molecules with cannabimimetic properties. The anti-inflammatory and antinociceptive effects of the aliamides PEA and adelmidrol have been demonstrated in numerous preclinical studies, both in vitro and in vivo [18–20]. Their actions are thought to be due, at least in part, to their ability to down-modulate mast cell activation and mast cell mediator release in pathophysiological and pathological conditions [21].

The aim of the present study was to demonstrate that adelmidrol in association with HA is able to control depolymerization of exogenous HA, by bringing about a viscoelastic-type lubricating action and consequent modulation of inflammatory processes and pain in a rat model of MIA-induced OA.

Methods

Animals

Forty male Lewis rats (Sprague-Dawley, 200–230 g; Harlan, Nossan Milan, Italy) were maintained in a monitored environment and provided with standard rodent chow and water. The study was authorized by the University of Messina Review Board for the care of animals (Protocol number 8/U-apr16). Animal care was in conformity with Italian regulations for the protection of experimental animals (DM 116192) and with European Economic Community regulations (OJ of EC L 358/1 12/18/1986).

Experimental protocol

OA was induced by intra-articular injection of MIA in the knee joint [22]. On day 0, rats were anesthetized with 5.0% isoflurane (Baxter International). A volume of 25 µl sterile saline solution + 3 mg MIA was injected into the knee joint through the right infrapatellar ligament. The left knee received an equal volume of 0.9% sterile saline. MIA was prepared in sterile conditions and injected using a 50-µl Hamilton syringe with a 27-gauge needle that was inserted into the joint to about 2–3 mm. On day 21 post-MIA administration, knee joints were inspected in detail to determine histopathological changes. Cartilage was stained to verify the presence of OA or not.

Experimental groups

Rats were randomly divided into the following groups:

MIA + vehicle (solvent solution)

Rats were subjected to induction of OA as described above, and received 25 µl of the solvent solution in the infrapatellar area of the right knee at days 3, 7, 14, and 21 (n = 10) by intra-articular injection.

MIA adelmidrol 0.6% + 1.0% sodium hyaluronate

Rats were subjected to induction of OA as described above, and were treated by intra-articular injection of adelmidrol 0.6% + sodium hyaluronate 1.0% (sodium hyaluronate with high molecular weight, between 1.5 and 2.0 million daltons) at a dose of 150 µg/25 µl on days 3, 7, 14, and 21 after MIA induction ($n = 10$)

MIA adelmidrol 2% + sodium hyaluronate 1.0%
Rats were subjected to induction of OA as described above, and were treated by intra-articular injection of adelmidrol 2% + sodium hyaluronate 1.0% (sodium hyaluronate with high molecular weight, between 1.5 and 2.0 million daltons) at a dose of 150 µg/25 µl on days 3, 7, 14, and 21 after MIA induction ($n = 10$)

MIA + sodium hyaluronate 1.0%
Rats were subjected to induction of OA as described above, and were treated by intra-articular injection of sodium hyaluronate 1.0% (sodium hyaluronate with high molecular weight, between 1.5 and 2.0 million daltons) at a dose of 150 µg/25 µl on days 3, 7, 14, and 21 after MIA induction ($n = 10$)

Sham group
Rats were administered by intra-articular injection with 0.9% saline (25 µl) instead of MIA and were treated with either vehicle or different formulations on days 3, 7, 14, and 21 ($n = 10$)

Pain measurement
Mechanical sensitivity was evaluated using a dynamic plantar aesthesiometer (Ugo Basile, Comerio, Italy). The rats were placed on a metal mesh surface in a chamber in a room with a controlled temperature (22 °C) and they were allowed to adapt for 15 min before the testing began. The touch stimulator part was oriented under the animal. When the aesthesiometer was activated, a plastic monofilament touched the paw in the proximal metatarsal region. The filament exercised a gradually increasing force on the plantar, starting below the threshold of detection and increasing until the stimulus became painful and the rat removed its paw. The force required to produce a paw withdrawal reflex was recorded automatically and measured in grams. A maximum force of 50 g and a ramp speed of 20 s were used for all the aesthesiometry tests.

Analysis of motor function (Walking Track Analysis)
The rat was placed in a walking track with a dark end. White office paper of the appropriate size was placed on the bottom of the track. Hind limbs of the rat were dipped in ink, and the rat was allowed to walk along the track, leaving paw prints on the paper. The test was performed before induction on day 0 and at days 3, 7, 14, and 21 after induction [23]. The functionality index of the sciatic nerve (SFI), calculated by Walking Track Analysis, was evaluated at 60 min after the injection on days 3, 7, 14, and 21: values close to 0 indicate normal functioning, and values tending to −100 indicate an alteration of sciatic nerve functionality [24].

Micro-computed tomography analysis
In order to evaluate the bone mass and microarchitecture parameters, including the fraction of bone volume, the proximal and distal parts of the right tibiae were scanned using micro-computed tomography (Micro-CT; Skyscan, Belgium) The scan conditions were as follows: an aluminum filter of 0.5 mm, X-ray voltage of 50Kv, X-ray current of 200 mA, and an exposure time of 360 ms. After scanning, the cross-sectional slices were reconstructed and three-dimensional analyses were performed using CTAn SkyScan software.

Histological analysis
On day 21 after MIA administration, rats were sacrificed by anesthetic overdose and perfused with 4% paraformaldehyde solution. Tibiofemoral joints were collected and post-fixed in neutral buffered formalin (containing 4% formaldehyde), decalcified in EDTA, and processed as following described. After decalcification, the specimens were embedded in paraffin. Mid-coronal tissue sections (5 µm) were stained for evaluation; all histomorphometric analyses were performed by an observer blinded to the treatment groups. Sections were stained with hematoxylin and eosin and observed by light microscopy (Dialux 22 Leitz; Leica Microsystems SpA, Milan, Italy). Histopathological analysis of the cartilage was assessed by the modified score of Mankin [14] (score range 0 to 12, from normal to complete disorganization and hypocellularity).

Cartilage degeneration was assessed by staining with toluidine blue and analyzed using the following criteria described by Janusz et al. [25]: 1 = mild into the surface region; 2 = slightly extended in the upper center; 3 = moderate in the median area; 4 = extended area deep; and 5 = severe degeneration.

Mast cell staining
Identification of mast cells was performed as described previously [26]. Knee sections were cut at 5-µm thickness and stained with 0.25% toluidine blue, pH 2.5, for 45 min at room temperature. The sections were then dehydrated and mounted for viewing. Three nonsequential sections were chosen by a block at random from each paw for examination. All sections were evaluated at 200×, while some sections were photographed at 400× using a Nikon inverted microscope. The density of mast cells is expressed as the number of mast cells per unit area of bone tissue.

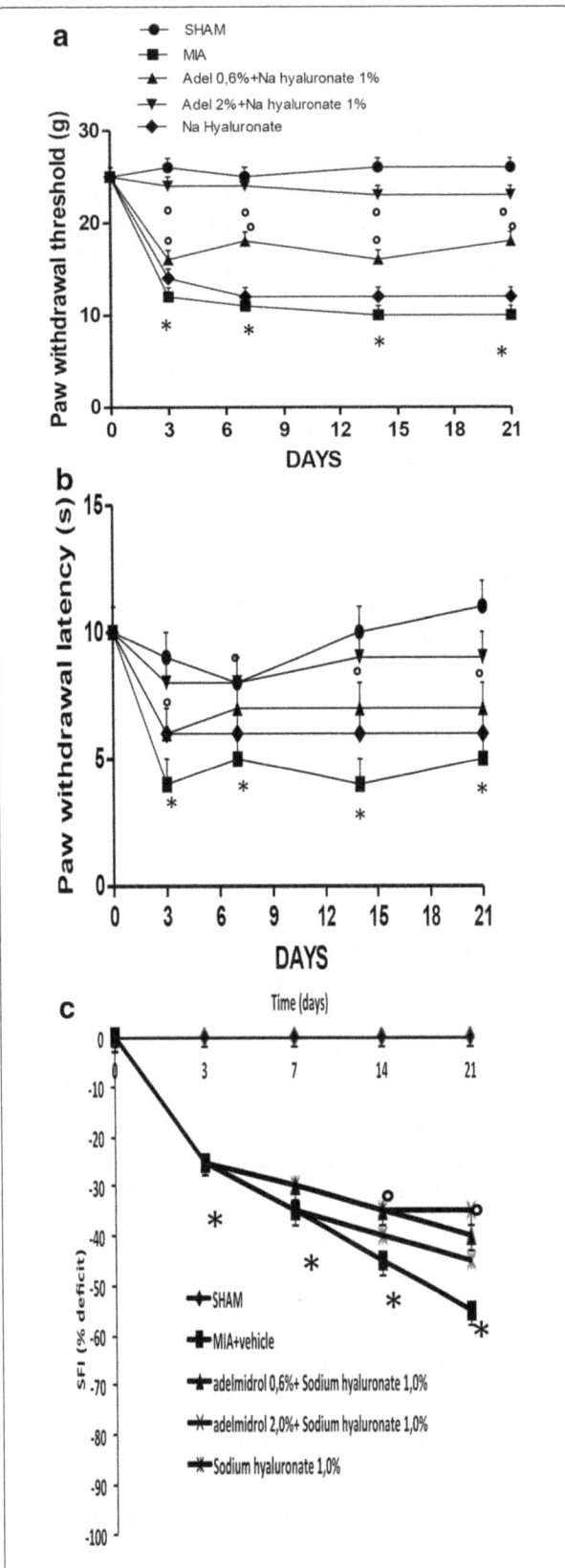

Fig. 1 Effects of sodium hyaluronate (*Na hyaluronate*) and adelmidrol (*Adel.*) combination on OA pain production and motor function. In the von Frey hair assessment test, the paw withdrawal threshold (PWT) (**a**) and the paw withdrawal latency (PWL) (**b**) were prolonged significantly in the inflamed hind paw of the rats given 0.6% adelmidrol + 1.0% sodium hyaluronate and 2% adelmidrol + 1.0% sodium hyaluronate compared with the monosodium iodoacetate (*MIA*) + solvent group and MIA + sodium hyaluronate 1.0% group. The sham group showed no obvious change. **c** In the MIA + vehicle and 1.0% sodium hyaluronate groups, the sciatic nerve functionality index (*SFI*) values were significantly lower than in sham animals. Treatment with a combination of HA acid and adelmidrol improved motor function in a dose-dependent manner. Data are means ± S.E.M. of 10 rats for each group. *$P < 0.05$ versus sham, °$P < 0.05$ versus MIA + vehicle

Measurement of cytokines, metalloproteinases, and nerve growth factor

The levels of tumor necrosis factor (TNF)-α, interleukin (IL)-1β, nerve growth factor (NGF), and matrix metalloproteinase (MMP)-1, MMP-3, and MMP-9 were measured in serum. Assays were performed using commercial colorimetric enzyme-linked immunosorbent assay (ELISA) kits (TNF-α, IL-1β, and NGF: Thermo Fisher Scienfic; MMP-1, MMP-3, and MMP-9: Cusabio).

Reagents

Unless otherwise stated, all compounds were obtained from Sigma-Aldrich Co. All other chemicals were of the highest commercial grade available. All stock solutions were prepared in non-pyrogenic saline (0.9% NaCl; Baxter Healthcare Ltd., Thetford, Norfolk, UK).

Data analysis

All values in the figures and text are expressed as mean ± standard error of the mean (SEM) of *n* observations. For in vivo studies, *n* represents the number of animals studied. In experiments involving histology, the figures shown are representative of at least three experiments performed on different days. The results were analyzed by one-way analysis of variance (ANOVA) followed by a Bonferroni post-hoc test for multiple comparisons. Non-parametric data were analyzed with the Fisher's exact test. A *P* value less than 0.05 is considered significant.

Results

Effects of the HA and adelmidrol combination on OA pain production and motor function

Because pain is the predominant symptom of OA, the secondary tactile allodynia in MIA-induced OA rats was assessed. In the von Frey hair assessment test, the paw withdrawal latency (PWL) (Fig. 1b) and the paw withdrawal threshold (PWT) (Fig. 1a) were significantly prolonged in the inflamed hind paw of the rats given 0.6% adelmidrol + 1.0% sodium hyaluronate and 2% adelmidrol + 1.0% sodium hyaluronate compared with the MIA

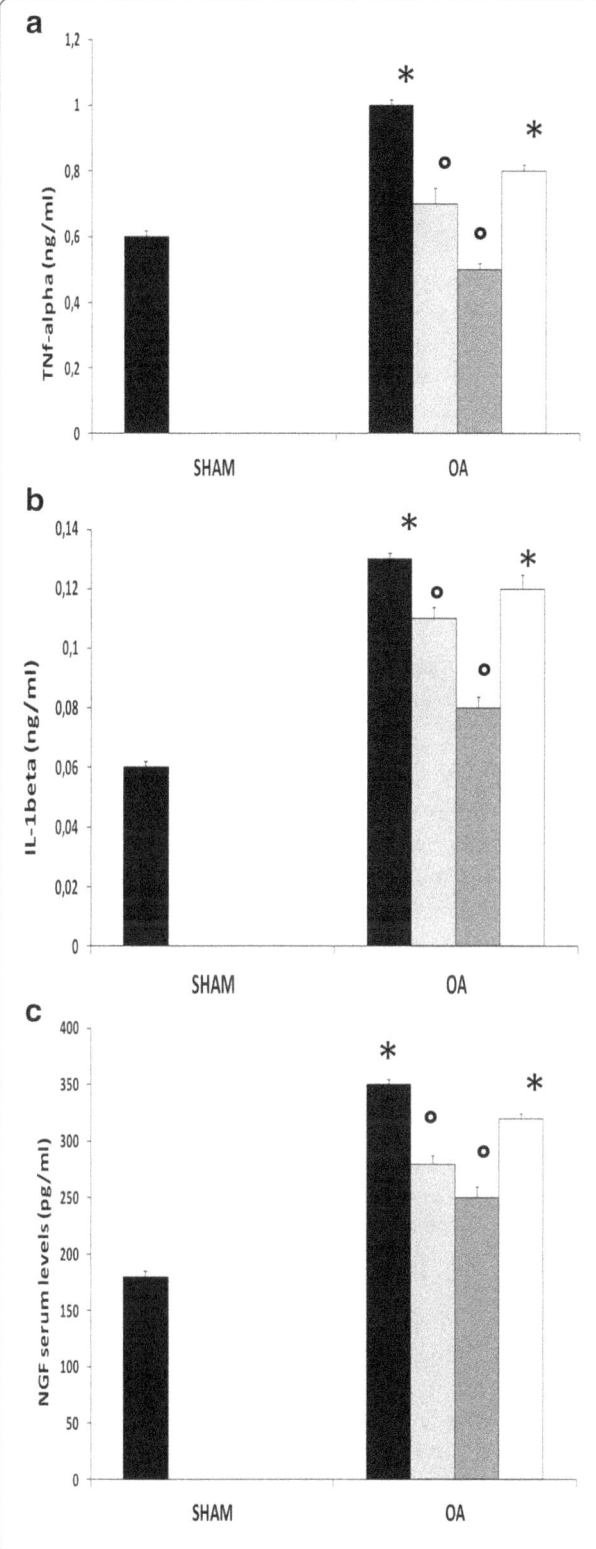

Fig. 2 Effects of the combination of hyaluronic acid and adelmidrol on plasma cytokines and nerve growth factor (*NGF*) in osteoarthritis (*OA*) rats. MIA-induced OA and tissue sample processing were carried out as detailed in the Methods section. Increased tumor necrosis factor alpha (*TNF-α*) (**a**), interleukin-1beta (*IL-1β*) (**b**), and NGF (**c**) plasma levels were detected in the MIA + solvent and MIA + 1.0% sodium hyaluronate groups after MIA administration. OA rats treated with the indicated doses of adelmidrol and HA exhibited a dose-dependent reduction in the plasma levels of all the measured parameters. Values are shown as mean ± SEM of 10 animals for each group. *$P < 0.05$ versus sham, °$P < 0.05$ versus MIA + vehicle.

+ solvent group and the MIA + sodium hyaluronate 1.0% group, demonstrating the antinociceptive property of adelmidrol in a dose-dependent manner. The sham group showed no obvious change (Fig. 1a and b).

Moreover, we tested motor function using a walking track in order to demonstrate that the association of adelmidrol with sodium hyaluronate treatment may improve joint mobility and reduce physical disability. Analysis was performed on days 3, 7, 14, and 21 after induction of OA. As shown in Fig. 1c, the SFI in the sham group was normal throughout the experiment, with SFI approximating 0. In the MIA + vehicle and 1.0% sodium hyaluronate groups, SFI values on post-MIA administration on days 3, 7, 14, and 21 were significantly lower than those observed in the sham group. The combination of HA and adelmidrol (0.6% adelmidrol + 1.0% sodium hyaluronate and 2% adelmidrol + 1.0% sodium hyaluronate) dose-dependently improved motor function (Fig. 1c).

Effects of the HA and adelmidrol combination on plasma levels of pro-inflammatory cytokines and NGF

To test whether the association of adelmidrol with sodium hyaluronate treatment may modulate the secretion of pro-inflammatory cytokines, we analyzed plasma levels of TNF-α, IL-1β, and NGF. A significant increase in serum levels of TNF-α (Fig. 2a), IL-1β (Fig. 2b), and NGF (Fig. 2c) was observed in the MIA + vehicle and 1% sodium hyaluronate groups compared to sham animals. In contrast, the HA and adelmidrol combination (0.6% adelmidrol + 1.0% sodium hyaluronate and 2% adelmidrol + 1.0% sodium hyaluronate) dose-dependently reduced the increase in serum levels of TNF-α (Fig. 2a), IL-1β (Fig. 2b), and NGF (Fig. 2c) after administration of MIA.

Effects of the HA and adelmidrol combination on mast cell infiltration

An important source of cytokines, specifically TNF-α and IL-1β, is characterized by mast cell activation. Mast cell infiltration after OA induction was studied by staining knee joint tissues with toluidine blue. Degranulated mast cells were not seen in knee sections from the sham group (Fig. 3a; mast cell density in Fig. 3f). On the contrary, significant mast cell infiltration was observed in the MIA + solvent (Fig. 3b) and MIA + 1.0% sodium hyaluronate (Fig. 3c) groups in joint tissue near the subchondral bone taken 21 days after the induction of OA. The combination of HA and adelmidrol (0.6% adelmidrol + 1.0% sodium hyaluronate and 2% adelmidrol + 1.0% sodium hyaluronate) (Fig. 3d and e) dose-dependently reduced mast cell infiltration induced by administration of MIA.

Effects of the HA and adelmidrol combination on plasma levels of metalloproteinases

The progressive destruction of articular cartilage is caused by a number of matrix-degrading enzymes produced by the chondrocytes and synovium. Among the various biomarkers associated with OA, MMPs play a primary role in the downstream signaling pathways in OA and cartilage degradation. The MIA + vehicle and 1% sodium hyaluronate group showed a markedly higher expression of MMP-1 (Fig. 4a), MMP-3 (Fig. 4b), and

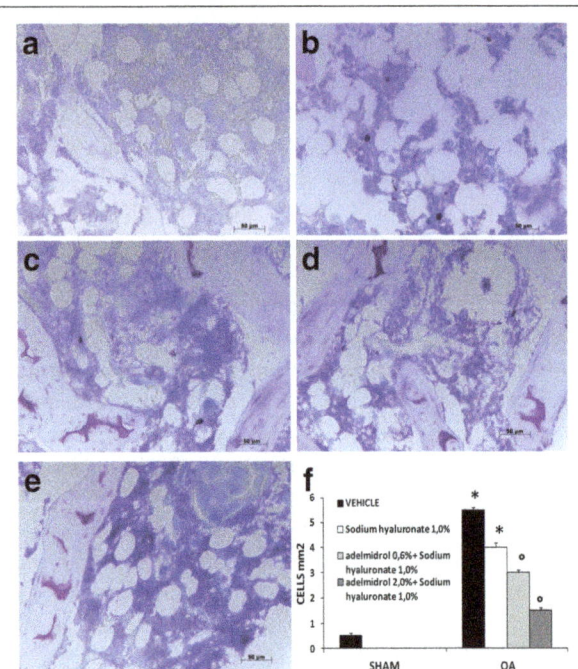

Fig. 3 Effects of the combination of hyaluronic acid and adelmidrol on mast cell staining in osteoarthritis (*OA*) knee tissue. Compared with sham knees (**a**), the MIA + solvent (**b**) and MIA + 1.0% sodium hyaluronate (**c**) groups displayed significant increases in the numerical density of toluidine blue-positive cells. In contrast, the combination of HA and adelmidrol at the doses indicated (0.6% adelmidrol + 1.0% sodium hyaluronate (**d**), and 2% adelmidrol + 1.0% sodium hyaluronate (**e**)) produced a dose-dependent reduction in mast cell infiltration in the knees of MIA-treated rats. (**f**) Number of mast cells per unit area of muscle parenchyma (mast cell density). Data are means ± SEM of 10 rats for each group. *$P < 0.05$ versus sham, °$P < 0.05$ versus MIA + vehicle

MMP-9 (Fig. 4c). However, compared to the MIA group, the group treated with 0.6% adelmidrol + 1.0% sodium hyaluronate and, in particular, 2% adelmidrol + 1.0% sodium hyaluronate showed a decrease in MMP-1, MMP-3, and MMP-9 expression (Fig. 4a, b and c, respectively).

Effects of the HA and adelmidrol combination on OA articular cartilage degeneration

As indicated by toluidine blue O staining (Fig. 5), MIA intra-articular injection induced articular cartilage degeneration on the medial tibia platform in the MIA + solvent (Fig. 5b; cartilage degeneration scores in Fig. 5f) and MIA + 1.0% sodium hyaluronate (Fig. 5c) groups. Compared with knee joints in the MIA + solvent group, knees in the 0.6% adelmidrol + 1.0% sodium hyaluronate (Fig. 5d) group exhibited moderate cartilage degeneration; matrix and chondrocyte loss affected the middle to deep zone. The group with the higher treatment dose of 2% adelmidrol + 1.0% sodium hyaluronate showed no statistical improvement in cartilage degeneration (Fig. 5e). Sham knee joints (Fig. 5a) showed no obvious changes.

Effects of the HA and adelmidrol combination on OA subchondral bone

In order to demonstrate the crucial role of subchondral bone in the pathogenesis and progression of OA, knee sections 21 days after MIA induction were examined for the number of osteoclasts and bone volume. In the MIA + solvent (Fig. 6b; cell number per joint in Fig. 6f) and MIA + 1.0% sodium hyaluronate (Fig. 6c) groups, the number of osteoclasts was increased after MIA injection. Compared with knee joints in the MIA + solvent group, knees in the 0.6% adelmidrol + 1.0% sodium hyaluronate (Fig. 6d) group exhibited a moderately increased number of osteoclasts. The higher treatment dose of 2% adelmidrol + 1.0% sodium hyaluronate showed no statistical improvement in cell numbers (Fig. 6e). There is no variation in cell numbers in Sham knee joints (Fig. 6a).

Moreover, to quantity the structural changes in the subchondral bone in MIA-induced OA, each rat was scanned for bone volume density (mm^3) (Fig. 6g). Compared with the MIA + solvent and MIA + 1.0% sodium hyaluronate groups, 0.6% adelmidrol + 1.0% sodium hyaluronate and the higher treatment dose of 2% adelmidrol + 1.0% sodium hyaluronate showed a marked increase in bone volume (Fig. 6g). Thus, treatment with 0.6% adelmidrol + 1.0% sodium hyaluronate and the higher treatment dose of 2% adelmidrol + 1.0% sodium hyaluronate showed significant and dose-dependent effects on MIA-induced deterioration of the subchondral bone.

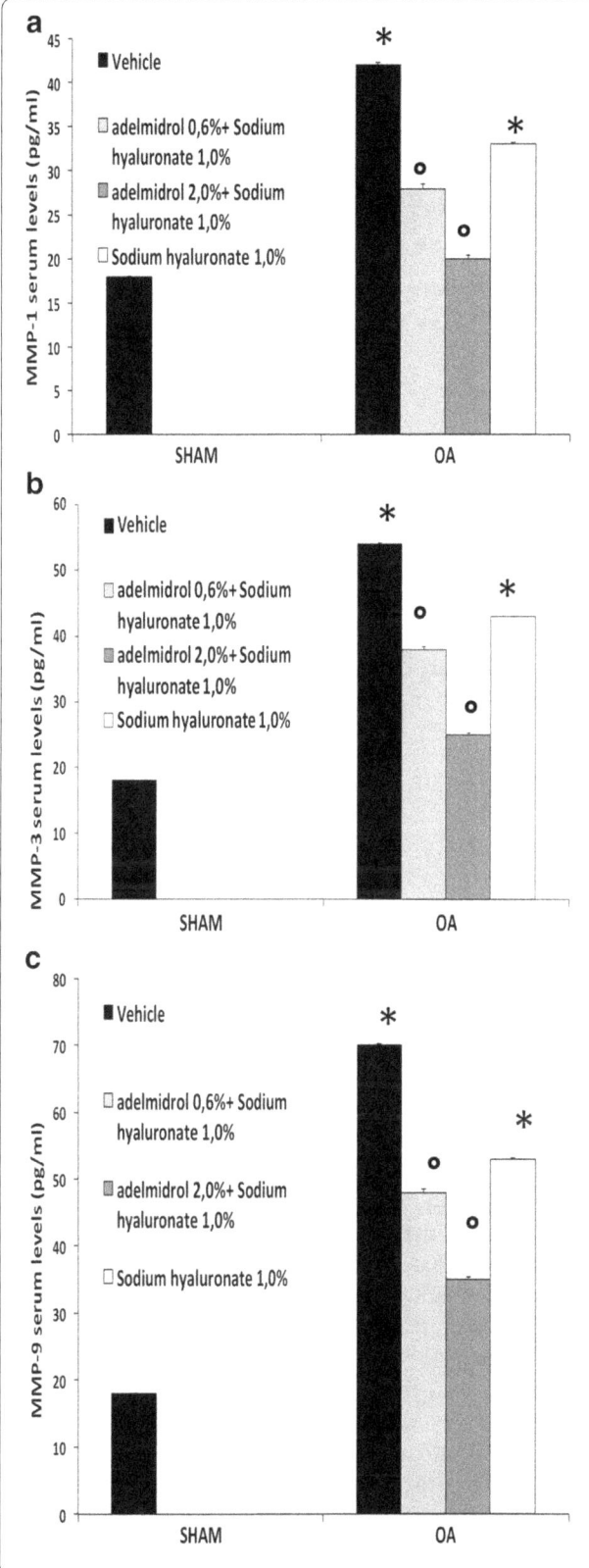

Fig. 4 Effects of HA and adelmidrol combination on plasma levels of matrix metalloproteinases (*MMPs*). MMPs play a primary role in the downstream signaling pathways in osteoarthritis (*OA*) and cartilage degradation. The MIA + vehicle and 1% sodium hyaluronate group showed a markedly higher expression of MMP-1 (**a**), MMP-3 (**b**), and MMP-9 (**c**). Compared to the MIA group, the group treated with 0.6% adelmidrol + 1.0% sodium hyaluronate and, in particular, with 2% adelmidrol + 1.0% sodium hyaluronate showed a decrease in MMP-1, MMP-3, and MMP-9 expression (**a–c**, respectively). Data are means ± SEM of 10 rats for each group. $*P < 0.05$ versus sham, $°P < 0.05$ versus MIA + vehicle

Effects of the HA and adelmidrol combination on OA histopathology

In order to demonstrate that adelmidrol promotes the beneficial and lubricant action of HA, knee sections were stained with hematoxylin and eosin 21 days after intra-articular injection of MIA. Histological examination by light microscopy showed irregularities and fibrillation in the surface layer, a decrease in blood cells and multilayering in transition and radial zones, no pannus formation, and modified Mankin scores (Fig. 7f) in the MIA + solvent and MIA + sodium hyaluronate 1.0% knees groups (Fig. 7b and c, respectively; see Mankin scores in Fig. 7f) compared to sham knees. The combination of HA and adelmidrol (0.6% adelmidrol + 1.0% solium hyaluronate (Fig. 7d) and 2% adelmidrol + 1.0% sodium hyaluronate (Fig. 7e)) reduced, in a dose-dependent manner, the histological alterations induced by administration of MIA.

Discussion

OA is a complex disease with inflammatory mediators released by cartilage, bone, and synovium [27]. Numerous inflammatory mediators contribute to both degradative and nociceptive pathways associated with the progression of pathology. Inflammatory stimuli initiate a cascade of events, including the release of cytokines by chondrocytes, leading to complex biochemical and mechanical interplay with other biological mediators to induce OA and promote pain [27, 28].

Although the role of cytokines in the pathogenesis of OA is not yet clear, several in vitro studies support an elevated catabolic role for cytokines in the OA joint. IL-1β and TNF-α signaling, culminating in the activation of nuclear factor-κB and activator protein 1 transcription factors, can induce autocrine production of IL-1β and TNF-α as well as expression of other critical inflammatory and chrondrolytic mediators, including MMP1, MMP9, MMP13, nitric oxide, prostaglandin E2, IL-6, and pain [29].

Moreover it has been demonstrated that IL-1β induces an increase in levels of NGF [30]. NGF is a key factor in hyperalgesia associated with inflammation, whose protein is detected in OA synovial fluid [31]. NGF synthesis

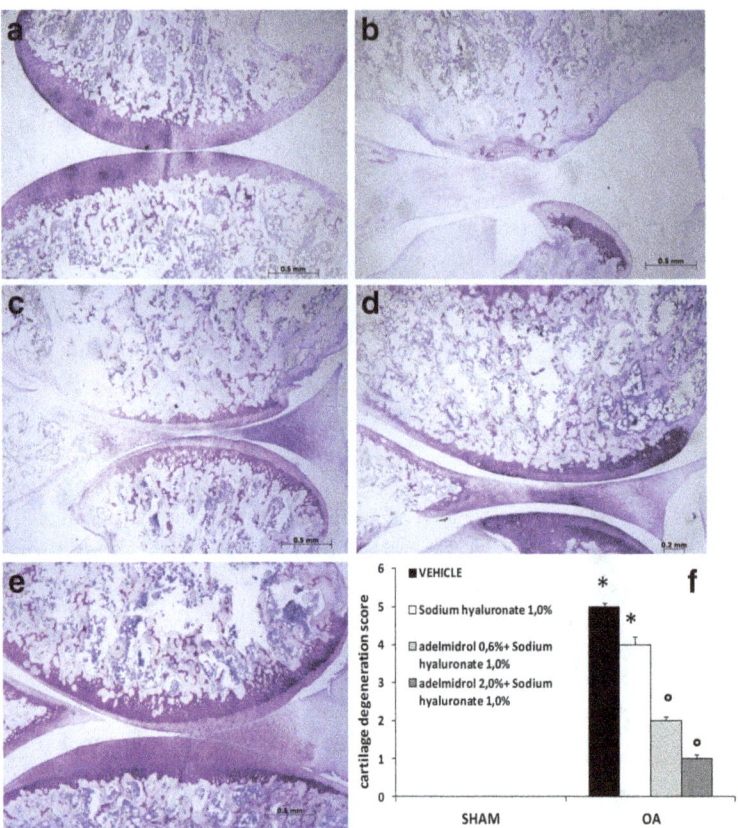

Fig. 5 Effects of the combination of hyaluronic acid and adelmidrol on cartilage degeneration in osteoarthritis (*OA*) knee tissue. MIA-induced OA and tissue sample processing were carried out as detailed in the Methods section. No cartilage degeneration was observed in the sham group (**a**). Significant histopathological changes were evident in the MIA + solvent (**b**) and MIA + 1.0% sodium hyaluronate (**c**) groups, as indicated by surface irregularity, disorganization of articular cartilage with apparent cloning of chondrocytes in the transitional and radial zones, and an intact tidemark. The combination of HA and adelmidrol at the doses indicated (0.6% adelmidrol + 1.0% sodium hyaluronate (**d**), and 2% adelmidrol + 1.0% sodium hyaluronate (**e**)) significantly prevented damage to the cartilage structure, reduced cellular abnormalities, and prevented change of the tidemark induced by administration of MIA. Cartilage degeneration scoring was performed by an independent observer (**f**). Data are means ± SEM of 10 rats for each group. *$P < 0.05$ versus sham, °$P < 0.05$ versus MIA + vehicle

is highly correlated with the degree of cartilage degradation in human OA [32]. Clinical trials have demonstrated that acting against NGF leads to a dramatic reduction in OA pain [33]. In this study, we confirmed an increase in cytokine production and showed that treatment with HA in combination with adelmidrol in increasing doses significantly reduced pro-inflammatory cytokine levels and NGF expression.

The literature indicates that an important source of cytokines, specifically TNF-α and IL-1β, is also characterized by mast cell activation. There is a well-established correlation between mast cell numbers and total inflammatory infiltrate. Mast cells are potent regulators of vascular permeability and have a crucial role in the recruitment of leukocytes to OA joints. Degranulated mast cells have been found in OA synovium [34], and Buckley and Walls [35] reported a selective expansion and higher ratio of mast cell tryptase phenotype in OA synovium, a phenotype consistent with degranulation.

The present study confirms an increased infiltration of mast cells in the knee joint after MIA administration, and their consequent reduction after treatment with HA in combination with adelmidrol in increasing doses. Mast cells in the joint capsule become hyper-reactive due to joint inflammation, a process markedly influenced by the degradation of HA caused by the in situ release of β-hexosaminidase [36, 37]. In fact, OA animals and those treated only with HA displayed a significant degeneration of articular cartilage. Significant restoration of cartilage was achieved after treatment with increasing doses of HA and adelmidrol in combination.

Along with progressive loss of articular cartilage, OA is characterized by increased subchondral bone sclerosis with thickening of the cortical plate, extensive remodeling of the trabeculae, formation of new bone at the joint margins (osteophytes), and the development of subchondral bone cysts. Changes to subchondral bone are due to increased osteoclastic bone resorption and changes in bone density.

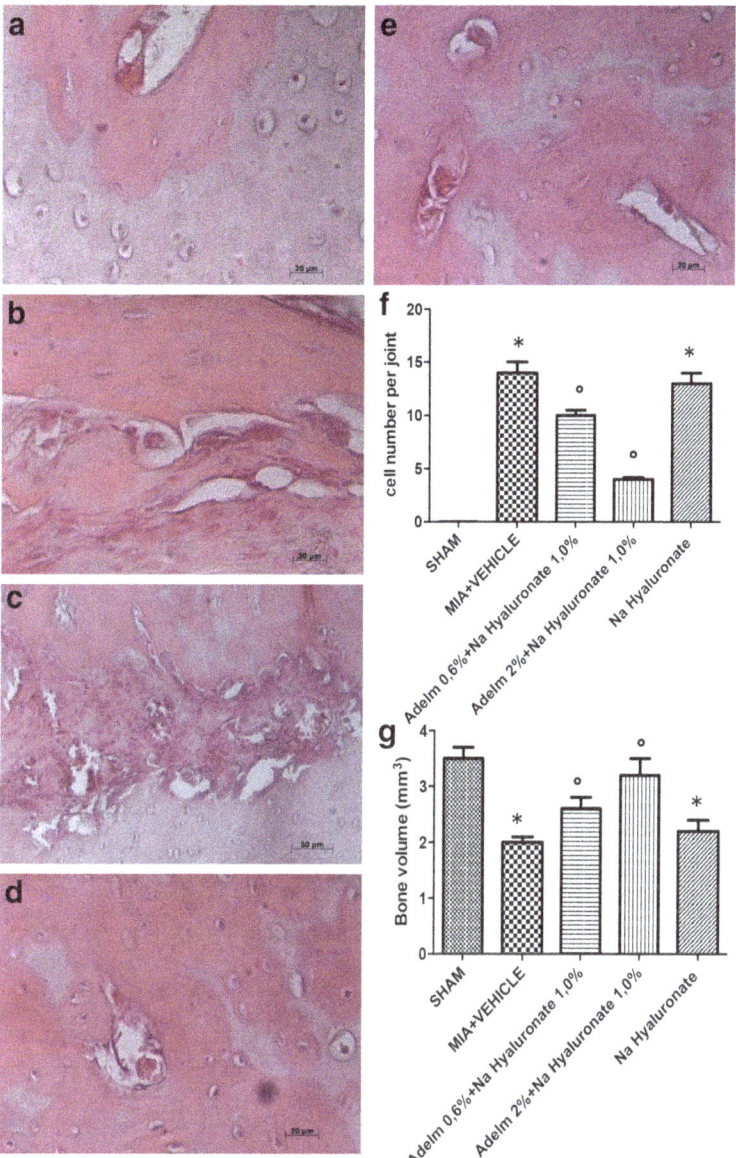

Fig. 6 Effects of hyaluronic acid and adelmidrol combination on the pathogenesis of subchondral bone. In the monosodium iodoacetate (*MIA*) + solvent (**b**) and MIA + 1.0% sodium (*Na*) hyaluronate (**c**) knee groups, the number of osteoclasts was increased after MIA injection. Compared with knee joints in the MIA + solvent group, knees in the 0.6% adelmidrol (*Adelm*) + 1.0% sodium hyaluronate (**d**) group exhibited moderately increased numbers of osteoclasts. The higher treatment dose of 2% adelmidrol + 1.0% sodium hyaluronate showed no statistical improvement in cell numbers (**e**). There is no variation in cell numbers in sham knee joints (**a**). **f** Cell number per joint. **g** Moreover to quantify the structural changes in the subchondral bone in MIA-induced OA, each rat was scanned for bone volume density (mm³). Compared with the MIA + solvent and MIA + 1.0% sodium hyaluronate groups, 0.6% adelmidrol + 1.0% sodium hyaluronate and higher treatment dose of 2% adelmidrol + 1.0% sodium hyaluronate showed a marked increase in bone volume. Thus, treatment with 0.6% adelmidrol + 1.0% sodium hyaluronate and a higher treatment dose of 2% adelmidrol + 1.0% sodium hyaluronate showed significant and dose-dependent effects on MIA-induced deterioration of the subchondral bone. Data are means ± SEM of 10 rats for each group. *$P < 0.05$ versus sham, °$P < 0.05$ versus MIA + vehicle

Our study demonstrated that adelmidrol and hyaluronic acid treatment showed significant and dose-dependent effects on MIA-induced deterioration of the subchondral bone, reducing osteoclastic bone resorption.

Strong evidence associates subchondral bone alterations with cartilage damage and pain severity in OA [38]. In this study, motor functionality was evaluated by Walking Track Analysis. An SFI value of approximately zero indicates normal locomotor function, while a value close to −100 indicates significant impairment of locomotor function. As expected, intra-articular injection of MIA resulted in a significant increase in joint discomfort. Importantly, the combination of HA and adelmidrol, in a dose-dependent fashion, completely restored locomotor functionality.

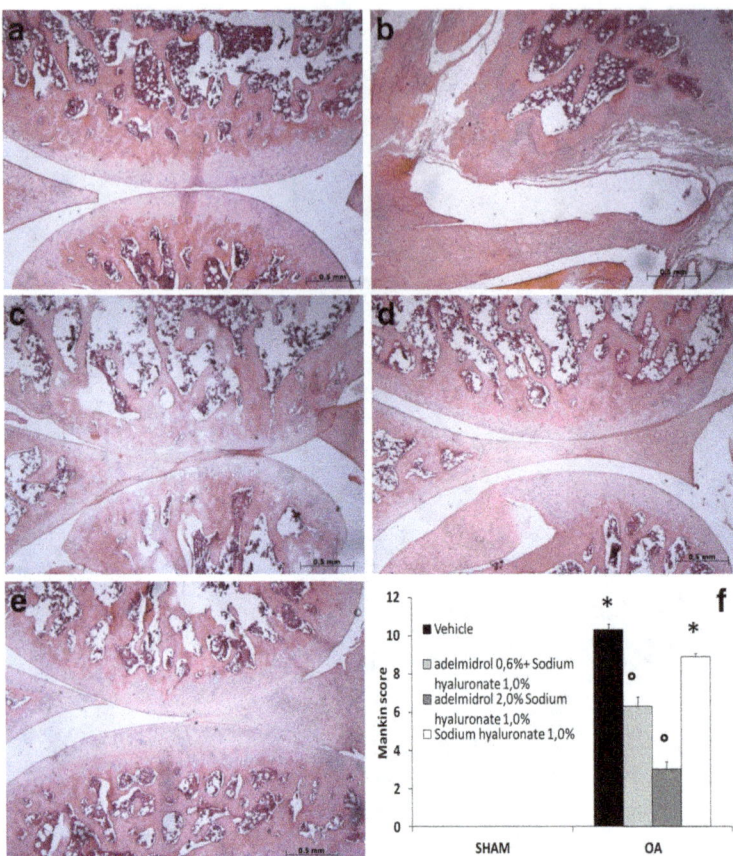

Fig. 7 Effects of hyaluronic acid and adelmidrol combination on histological features of osteoarthritis (*OA*) knee tissue. MIA-induced OA and tissue sample processing were carried out as detailed in the Methods section. Knee sections from sham rats displayed normal architecture of the joint tissue (**a**; see Mankin Score in **f**). The MIA + solvent (**b**) and MIA + 1.0% sodium hyaluronate (**c**) groups showed surface layer fibrillation, a decrease in blood cells, multilayering in transition and radial zones, no pannus formation, and modified Mankin scores. The combination of HA and adelmidrol at the doses indicated (0.6% adelmidrol + 1.0% sodium hyaluronate (**d**), and 2% adelmidrol + 1.0% sodium hyaluronate (**e**)) reduced histological alterations induced by administration of MIA. Histological scoring was performed by an independent observer (**f**). Data are means ± SEM of 10 rats for each group. *$P < 0.05$ versus sham, °$P < 0.05$ versus MIA + vehicle

Conclusions

Our results clearly demonstrated that a combination of HA and adelmidrol dose-dependently produced a significant reduction in: 1) pain severity; 2) OA histopathology; 3) articular cartilage degeneration; 4) mast cell infiltration; 5) pro-inflammatory cytokines, MMPs, and NGF production; and 6) the degree of motor function.

The association of HA with adelmidrol is accompanied by a reduced depolymerization of HA, which would otherwise be promoted by intra-articular inflammation.

Moreover application of infiltrative adelmidrol produces a significant increase in endogenous PEA levels [39], which are found to be significantly reduced in joint inflammation [40]. Several of our works demonstrated the beneficial effects of PEA alone and in combination in different models of inflammation and pain [41, 42], such as in a mouse model of collagen-induced arthritis (CIA) [19]. Thus, local analgesic and anti-inflammatory effects

observed with adelmidrol treatment could be useful in the treatment of inflammatory diseases associated with pain.

Abbreviations

GC: Glucocorticoid; HA: Hyaluronic acid; IL: Interleukin; MIA: Monosodium iodoacetate; MMP: Matrix metalloproteinase; NGF: Nerve growth factor; NSAID: Nonsteroidal anti-inflammatory drug; OA: Osteoarthritis; PEA: Palmitoylethanolamide; PWL: Paw withdrawal latency; PWT: Paw withdrawal threshold; SFI: Sciatic nerve functionality index; TNF: Tumor necrosis factor

Acknowledgements

The authors would like to thank Mrs. Medici Maria Antonietta for excellent technical assistance during this study, Mr. Francesco Soraci for secretarial and administrative assistance, and Miss. Malvagni Valentina for editorial assistance with the manuscript.

Funding

This research did not receive any specific grant from funding agencies in the public, commercial, or not-for-profit sectors.

Authors' contributions

RDP designed the study and drafted the manuscript. RF carried out the immunoassays and revised the manuscript. DI participated in the design of the study. MC helped to revise the manuscript. DB conceived of the study. VMM performed the statistical analysis. ME helped to draft the manuscript. SC drafted and revised the manuscript. All authors read and approved the final manuscript.

Competing interests

SC is co-inventor on patent WO2013121449 A8 (Epitech Group Srl) which deals with methods and compositions for the modulation of amidases capable of hydrolysing N-acylethanolamines employable in the treatment of inflammatory diseases. This invention is wholly unrelated to the present study. Moreover, SC is also, with Epitech Group, a co-inventor on the following patents, EP 2 821 083, MI2014 A001495, and 102015000067344, that are unrelated to the study. The remaining authors declare that they have no competing interests.

Consent for publication

Not applicable.

Author details

[1]Department of Chemical, Biological, Pharmaceutical and Environmental Sciences, University of Messina, Viale Ferdinando Stagno D'Alcontres, n 31, Messina 98166, Italy. [2]Department of Health Science, University of Catanzaro, Viale Europa, Campus S. Venuta, Germaneto, Catanzaro 88100, Italy. [3]Institute of Anaesthesiology and Reanimation, Catholic University of the Sacred Heart, Rome, Italy. [4]Department of Pharmacological and Physiological Science, Saint Louis University School of Medicine, 1402 South Grand Blvd, St. Louis, MO 63104, USA.

References

1. Duncan R, Peat G, Thomas E, Hay EM, Croft P. Incidence, progression and sequence of development of radiographic knee osteoarthritis in a symptomatic population. Ann Rheum Dis. 2011;70(11):1944–8.
2. Longo UG, Loppini M, Fumo C, Rizzello G, Khan WS, Maffulli N, Denaro V. Osteoarthritis: new insights in animal models. Open Orthop J. 2012;6:558–63.
3. Bian Q, Wang YJ, Liu SF, Li YP. Osteoarthritis: genetic factors, animal models, mechanisms, and therapies. Front Biosci (Elite Ed). 2012;4:74–100.
4. Loeser RF, Goldring SR, Scanzello CR, Goldring MB. Osteoarthritis: a disease of the joint as an organ. Arthritis Rheum. 2012;64(6):1697–707.
5. Little CB, Hunter DJ. Post-traumatic osteoarthritis: from mouse models to clinical trials. Nat Rev Rheum. 2013;9(8):485–97.
6. Zhang W, Moskowitz RW, Nuki G, Abramson S, Altman RD, Arden N, Bierma-Zeinstra S, Brandt KD, Croft P, Doherty M, et al. OARSI recommendations for the management of hip and knee osteoarthritis. Part II: OARSI evidence-based, expert consensus guidelines. Osteoarthritis Cartilage. 2008;16(2):137–62.
7. Guzman RE, Evans MG, Bove S, Morenko B, Kilgore K. Mono-iodoacetate-induced histologic changes in subchondral bone and articular cartilage of rat femorotibial joints: an animal model of osteoarthritis. Toxicol Pathol. 2003;31(6):619–24.
8. Fernihough J, Gentry C, Malcangio M, Fox A, Rediske J, Pellas T, Kidd B, Bevan S, Winter J. Pain related behaviour in two models of osteoarthritis in the rat knee. Pain. 2004;112(1-2):83–93.
9. Felson DT. Osteoarthritis. Rheum Dis Clin N Am. 1990;16(3):499–512.
10. Dieppe P, Brandt KD. What is important in treating osteoarthritis? Whom should we treat and how should we treat them? Rheum Dis Clin N Am. 2003;29(4):687–716.
11. Dieppe PA, Lohmander LS. Pathogenesis and management of pain in osteoarthritis. Lancet. 2005;365(9463):965–73.
12. Sarzi-Puttini P, Cimmino MA, Scarpa R, Caporali R, Parazzini F, Zaninelli A, Atzeni F, Canesi B. Osteoarthritis: an overview of the disease and its treatment strategies. Semin Arthritis Rheum. 2005;35(1 Suppl 1):1–10.
13. Riis RG, Henriksen M, Klokker L, Bartholdy C, Ellegaard K, Bandak E, Hansen BB, Bliddal H, Boesen M. The effects of intra-articular glucocorticoids and exercise on pain and synovitis assessed on static and dynamic magnetic resonance imaging in knee osteoarthritis: exploratory outcomes from a randomized controlled trial. Osteoarthritis Cartilage.2016
14. Kaluzynski K, Trybek G, Smektala T, Masiuk M, Mysliwiec L, Sporniak-Tutak K. Effect of methylprednisolone, hyaluronic acid and pioglitazone on histological remodeling of temporomandibular joint cartilage in rabbits affected by drug-induced osteoarthritis. Postepy Hig Med Dosw. 2016;70:74–9.
15. Morgan TK, Jensen E, Lim J, Riggs R. Image-guided hyaluronic acid injection and knee bracing significantly improve clinical outcomes for high-grade osteoarthritis. Sports Med Open. 2015;1(1):31.
16. Galluccio F, Barskova T, Cerinic MM. Short-term effect of the combination of hyaluronic acid, chondroitin sulfate, and keratin matrix on early symptomatic knee osteoarthritis. Eur J Rheumatol. 2015;2(3):106–8.
17. Richette P. Pharmacological therapies for osteoarthritis. Therapie. 2011; 66(5):383–90.
18. De Filippis D, D'Amico A, Cinelli MP, Esposito G, Di Marzo V, Iuvone T. Adelmidrol, a palmitoylethanolamide analogue, reduces chronic inflammation in a carrageenin-granuloma model in rats. J Cell Mol Med. 2009;13(6):1086–95.
19. Impellizzeri D, Esposito E, Di Paola R, Ahmad A, Campolo M, Peli A, Morittu VM, Britti D, Cuzzocrea S. Palmitoylethanolamide and luteolin ameliorate development of arthritis caused by injection of collagen type II in mice. Arthritis Res Ther. 2013;15(6):R192.
20. Di Paola R, Impellizzeri D, Torre A, Mazzon E, Cappellani A, Faggio C, Esposito E, Trischitta F, Cuzzocrea S. Effects of palmitoylethanolamide on intestinal injury and inflammation caused by ischemia-reperfusion in mice. J Leukoc Biol. 2012;91(6):911–20.
21. Re G, Barbero R, Miolo A, Di Marzo V. Palmitoylethanolamide, endocannabinoids and related cannabimimetic compounds in protection against tissue inflammation and pain: potential use in companion animals. Vet J. 2007;173(1):21–30.
22. Vonsy JL, Ghandehari J, Dickenson AH. Differential analgesic effects of morphine and gabapentin on behavioural measures of pain and disability in a model of osteoarthritis pain in rats. Eur J Pain. 2009;13(8):786–93.
23. Wong KH, Naidu M, David P, Abdulla MA, Abdullah N, Kuppusamy UR, Sabaratnam V. Peripheral nerve regeneration following crush injury to rat peroneal nerve by aqueous extract of medicinal mushroom Hericium erinaceus (Bull.: Fr) Pers. (Aphyllophoromycetideae). Evid Based Complement Alternat Med. 2011;2011:580752.
24. Sarikcioglu L, Demirel BM, Utuk A. Walking track analysis: an assessment method for functional recovery after sciatic nerve injury in the rat. Folia Morphol (Warsz). 2009;68(1):1–7.
25. Janusz MJ, Little CB, King LE, Hookfin EB, Brown KK, Heitmeyer SA, Caterson B, Poole AR, Taiwo YO. Detection of aggrecanase- and MMP-generated catabolic neoepitopes in the rat iodoacetate model of cartilage degeneration. Osteoarthr Cartil. 2004;12(9):720–8.
26. Ahmad A, Crupi R, Impellizzeri D, Campolo M, Marino A, Esposito E, Cuzzocrea S. Administration of palmitoylethanolamide (PEA) protects the neurovascular unit and reduces secondary injury after traumatic brain injury in mice. Brain Behav Immun. 2012;26(8):1310–21.
27. Schaible HG. Mechanisms of chronic pain in osteoarthritis. Curr Rheumatol Rep. 2012;14(6):549–56.
28. Read SJ, Dray A. Osteoarthritic pain: a review of current, theoretical and emerging therapeutics. Expert Opin Investig Drugs. 2008;17(5):619–40.
29. Attur MG, Patel IR, Patel RN, Abramson SB, Amin AR. Autocrine production of IL-1 beta by human osteoarthritis-affected cartilage and differential regulation of endogenous nitric oxide, IL-6, prostaglandin E2, and IL-8. Proc Assoc Am Physicians. 1998;110(1):65–72.
30. Manni L, Aloe L. Role of IL-1 beta and TNF-alpha in the regulation of NGF in experimentally induced arthritis in mice. Rheumatol Int. 1998;18(3):97–102.
31. Aloe L, Tuveri MA, Carcassi U, Levi-Montalcini R. Nerve growth factor in the synovial fluid of patients with chronic arthritis. Arthritis Rheum. 1992;35(3):351–5.
32. Iannone F, De Bari C, Dell'Accio F, Covelli M, Patella V, Lo Bianco G, Lapadula G. Increased expression of nerve growth factor (NGF) and high affinity NGF receptor (p140 TrkA) in human osteoarthritic chondrocytes. Rheumatology. 2002;41(12):1413–8.
33. Lane NE, Schnitzer TJ, Birbara CA, Mokhtarani M, Shelton DL, Smith MD, Brown MT. Tanezumab for the treatment of pain from osteoarthritis of the knee. N Engl J Med. 2010;363(16):1521–31.

34. Dean G, Hoyland JA, Denton J, Donn RP, Freemont AJ. Mast cells in the synovium and synovial fluid in osteoarthritis. Br J Rheumatol. 1993;32(8):671–5.

35. Buckley M, Walls AF. Identification of mast cells and mast cell subpopulations. Methods Mol Med. 2008;138:285–97.

36. Masuko K, Murata M, Yudoh K, Kato T, Nakamura H. Anti-inflammatory effects of hyaluronan in arthritis therapy: not just for viscosity. Int J Gen Med. 2009;2:77–81.

37. Guo N, Baglole CJ, O'Loughlin CW, Feldon SE, Phipps RP. Mast cell-derived prostaglandin D2 controls hyaluronan synthesis in human orbital fibroblasts via DP1 activation: implications for thyroid eye disease. J Biol Chem. 2010;285(21):15794–804.

38. Li G, Yin J, Gao J, Cheng TS, Pavlos NJ, Zhang C, Zheng MH. Subchondral bone in osteoarthritis: insight into risk factors and microstructural changes. Arthritis Res Ther. 2013;15(6):223.

39. Petrosino S, Puigdemont A, Della Valle MF, Fusco M, Verde R, Allara M, Aveta T, Orlando P, Di Marzo V. Adelmidrol increases the endogenous concentrations of palmitoylethanolamide in canine keratinocytes and down-regulates an inflammatory reaction in an in vitro model of contact allergic dermatitis. Vet J. 2016;207:85–91.

40. Richardson D, Ortori CA, Chapman V, Kendall DA, Barrett DA. Quantitative profiling of endocannabinoids and related compounds in rat brain using liquid chromatography-tandem electrospray ionization mass spectrometry. Anal Biochem. 2007;360(2):216–26.

41. Paterniti I, Impellizzeri D, Di Paola R, Navarra M, Cuzzocrea S, Esposito E. A new co-ultramicronized composite including palmitoylethanolamide and luteolin to prevent neuroinflammation in spinal cord injury. J Neuroinflammation. 2013;10:91.

42. Impellizzeri D, Bruschetta G, Cordaro M, Crupi R, Siracusa R, Esposito E, Cuzzocrea S. Micronized/ultramicronized palmitoylethanolamide displays superior oral efficacy compared to nonmicronized palmitoylethanolamide in a rat model of inflammatory pain. J Neuroinflammation. 2014;11:136.

11

Osteoarthritis-associated basic calcium phosphate crystals activate membrane proximal kinases in human innate immune cells

Emma M. Corr[1], Clare C. Cunningham[1], Laura Helbert[2], Geraldine M. McCarthy[2] and Aisling Dunne[1*]

Abstract

Background: Osteoarthritis (OA) is a chronic debilitating joint disorder of particularly high prevalence in the elderly population. Intra-articular basic calcium phosphate (BCP) crystals are present in the majority of OA joints and are associated with severe degeneration. They are known to activate macrophages, synovial fibroblasts, and articular chondrocytes, resulting in increased cell proliferation and the production of pro-inflammatory cytokines and matrix metalloproteases (MMPs). This suggests a pathogenic role in OA by causing extracellular matrix degradation and subchondral bone remodelling. There are currently no disease-modifying drugs available for crystal-associated OA; hence, the aim of this study was to explore the inflammatory pathways activated by BCP crystals in order to identify potential therapeutic targets to limit crystal-induced inflammation.

Methods: Primary human macrophages and dendritic cells were stimulated with BCP crystals, and activation of spleen tyrosine kinase (Syk), phosphoinositide-3 kinase (PI3K), and mitogen-activated protein kinases (MAPKs) was detected by immunoblotting. Lipopolysaccharide (LPS)-primed macrophages were pre-treated with inhibitors of Syk, PI3K, and MAPKs prior to BCP stimulation, and cytokine production was quantified by enzyme-linked immunosorbent assay (ELISA). Aa an alternative, cells were treated with synovial fluid derived from osteoarthritic knees in the presence or absence of BCP crystals, and gene induction was assessed by real-time polymerase chain reaction (PCR).

Results: We demonstrate that exposure of primary human macrophages and dendritic cells to BCP crystals leads to activation of the membrane-proximal tyrosine kinases Syk and PI3K. Furthermore, we show that production of the pro-inflammatory cytokines interleukin (IL)-1α and IL-1β and phosphorylation of downstream MEK and ERK MAPKs is suppressed following treatment with inhibitors of Syk or PI3K. Finally, we demonstrate that treatment of macrophages with BCP crystals induces the production of the damage-associated molecule S100A8 and MMP1 in a Syk-dependent manner and that synovial fluid from OA patients together with BCP crystals exacerbates these effects.

Conclusions: We identify Syk and PI3K as key signalling molecules activated by BCP crystals prior to inflammatory cytokine and DAMP expression and therefore propose that Syk and PI3K represent potential targets for the treatment of BCP-related pathologies.

Keywords: BCP crystals, Inflammation, Syk, PI3K, S100 proteins

---

* Correspondence: aidunne@tcd.ie
[1]School of Biochemistry & Immunology and School of Medicine, Trinity Biomedical Sciences Institute, Trinity College Dublin, Dublin, Ireland
Full list of author information is available at the end of the article

Background

It is well established that intra-articular deposition of particulates, such as gout-associated monosodium urate (MSU) crystals and osteoarthritis (OA)-associated basic calcium phosphate (BCP) crystals, drives joint degeneration through the production of pro-inflammatory cytokines and cartilage-degrading proteases. BCP crystals are a heterogeneous group of ultramicroscopic crystalline substances composed mainly of hydroxyapatite (HA), along with smaller proportions of its precursor forms octacalcium phosphate (OCP) and tricalcium phosphate [1, 2]. The concentration of BCP crystals found in the synovial fluid is reported to be between 20 and 100 µg/ml [3–5]. Furthermore, a 3-year prospective analysis of synovial fluid (SF) samples obtained from 330 patients with knee OA showed that the initial presence of BCP crystals was associated with worsening of radiographic lesions [6]. The concentration in the tissues is more difficult to quantify; however, Fuerst and colleagues demonstrated that human knee and hip cartilage specimens ($n = 120$ and $n = 80$, respectively), harvested at the time of total joint arthroplasty for primary OA, contained BCP crystals in 100% of cases [7, 8]. Sun et al. have also reported calcium deposition in all eight OA menisci harvested at the time of joint replacement surgery and that calcium crystal formation could be generated by both the meniscal and cartilage cells of patients with end-stage OA [9]. As crystal deposition does not occur in healthy cartilage, it is becoming more widely accepted that cartilage calcification plays a pathogenic role in OA and that BCP crystals are not the "innocent bystanders" that they were once believed to be. Indeed, the crystals are now considered to be a damage-associated molecular pattern (DAMP) as they can activate fibroblasts through a variety of signalling pathways involving protein kinase C (PKC), ERK1/2 mitogen-activated protein kinases (MAPKs), and transcription factors such as NFκB which, in turn, leads to the production of tumour necrosis factor (TNF)α, interleukin (IL)-6, and IL-1β [10, 11]. Cytokine induction has also been observed in BCP-activated chondrocytes [12] and macrophages [13–16], with IL-1β, in particular, implicated as a key player in the inflammatory and degradative responses observed in OA joints. It is induced early on in the disease and has the ability to upregulate matrix metalloproteases (MMPs) and aggrecanases, induce cell infiltration into the joints, promote osteoclastogenesis, and suppress the biosynthesis of type II collagen and aggrecan, crucial components of cartilage [17–20]. We have recently demonstrated that BCP crystals can inhibit anti-osteoclastogenic cytokine signalling, and therefore the crystals may also contribute to joint destruction by promoting the differentiation of bone-resorbing osteoclasts [21]. Together, these events lead to an imbalance in the production of anabolic versus catabolic mediators and, in many cases, total joint replacement is eventually required.

Current therapies for OA focus merely on pain relief and improvement of joint function rather than halting disease progression. While much progress has been made in elucidating the cellular and molecular events contributing to OA, the complex nature of the disease has hampered the development of a successful disease-modifying drug despite a multitude of potential targets. We and others have previously reported that BCP crystals activate the NLRP3 inflammasome in vitro leading to potent IL-1β production. However, conflicting results from in vivo models have called into question the relevance of these findings to a clinical setting, and additional targets are currently being sought [14, 16, 22]. Another potential target of interest in particulate-mediated disease is the membrane-proximal kinase, spleen tyrosine kinase (Syk). Belonging to the tyrosine kinase family, Syk is activated during phagocytosis and following Fc receptor engagement on immune cells [23]. Syk has been implicated in both the internalisation of MSU crystals and subsequent MSU-induced signalling in neutrophils and dendritic cells (DC) [24, 25]. In addition to MSU crystals, alum particles and cholesterol crystals have also been reported to activate Syk in a receptor-independent manner, by a process known as membrane affinity-triggered signalling (MATS). This involves direct binding of the particulates to the cell membrane which results in lipid raft formation and aggregation of immunoreceptor tyrosine-based activation motif (ITAM)-containing molecules which mediate the recruitment of Syk to the plasma membrane and its subsequent activation [26, 27]. We have previously demonstrated that BCP crystals activate Syk and its downstream interacting partner, phosphoinositide-3 kinase (PI3K), in murine macrophages [16]. Therefore, the aim of this study was to determine whether BCP crystals activate similar pathways in human macrophages and DC and to examine the downstream effect of inhibiting these pathways in order to identify potential therapeutic targets to treat crystal-induced inflammation in OA.

Methods

Reagents

Ultrapure lipopolysaccharide (LPS) and the PI3K inhibitor, LY294002, were from Invivogen (Toulouse, France). The Syk inhibitor, R788, was from AdooQ BioScience (Irvine, CA, USA). Recombinant human M-CSF was from PeproTech (Rocky Hill, NJ, USA). Recombinant human IL-4 and GM-CSF were from Immunotools (Friesoythe, Germany). Lymphoprep was from Stemcell Technologies (Grenoble, France). Primary antibodies were obtained from Cell Signaling Technology (Beverly,

MA, USA). The Syk inhibitor, piceatannol, methyl-β-cyclodextrin (M-βCD), secondary antibodies, cell culture reagents and all other chemicals were from Sigma Aldrich (St. Louis, MO, USA). Human FcR binding inhibitor was from eBioscience. BCP crystals were synthesized by alkaline hydrolysis of brushite as described previously [28] and contain partially carbonate-substituted hydroxyapatite in addition to octacalcium phosphate. OA synovial fluid was obtained with permission from The Mater Misericordiae Hospital Research Ethics Committee.

Cell culture and differentiation

Peripheral blood mononuclear cells (PBMCs) were isolated by means of density gradient centrifugation from leukocyte-enriched buffy coats from anonymous healthy donors, obtained with permission from the Irish Blood Transfusion Board, St. James's Hospital, Dublin. CD14+ cells were positively selected using anti-CD14 magnetic beads (Miltenyi Biotech, Germany) and shown to be >90% pure, as determined by flow cytometry. Cells were cultured for 6 days in six-well plates (for immunoblotting assays) or 24-well plates (for real-time polymerase chain reaction (PCR) and enzyme-linked immunosorbent assay (ELISA)) in RPMI 1640 medium supplemented with 1% penicillin-streptomycin and 10% foetal bovine serum. Cells were treated on days 0 and 3 with M-CSF (50 ng/ml) for macrophage differentiation or IL-4 (40 ng/ml) and GM-CSF (50 ng/ml) for DC differentiation (as adapted from [29, 30]). Cells were shown to be >95% pure as determined by flow cytometry, using CD14 and CD11b as macrophage markers and CD14 and CD209 as DC markers [31, 32].

Kinase activation

Primary macrophages or DC (2×10^6/well) were stimulated with BCP crystals (50 µg/ml) over the course of 30 min. Alternatively, cells were pre-treated with piceatannol, R788, or LY294002 for 30 min prior to crystal stimulation. Cells were lysed by the addition of RIPA buffer (Tris 50 mM; NaCl 150 mM; SDS 0.1%; sodium deoxycholate 0.5%; Triton X 100) containing phosphatase inhibitor cocktail 3 (Sigma-Aldrich). Samples were electrophoresed on a 12% SDS-polyacrylamide gel and transferred to PVDF membranes prior to detection with anti-phospho-Syk, anti-phospho-PI3K, anti-phospho-MEK, or anti-phospho-ERK.

Cytokine measurements

Primary macrophages (5×10^5/well) were primed with a known TLR4 activator, LPS (100 ng/ml), for 2 h prior to treatment with piceatannol, LY294002, M-βCD, or a human FcR binding inhibitor for 1 h and stimulation with BCP crystals (50 µg/ml) for 6 h. Supernatants were harvested and cytokine concentrations were quantified by ELISA (R&D Systems). S100A8 is also capable of activating TLR4; therefore, in order to determine whether this DAMP could be used to facilitate pro-IL-1β induction, in place of LPS, primary macrophages (5×10^5/well) were primed with endotoxin-free recombinant S100A8 (1 µg/ml) for 3 h prior to stimulation with BCP crystals (50 µg/ml) for 6 h, and cytokine concentrations were quantified by ELISA.

Real-time PCR

Human macrophages (5×10^5/well) were treated with BCP crystals alone for 3, 6, or 24 h or were pre-treated with piceatannol (50 µM, 100 µM) or LY294002 (25 µM, 50 µM) prior to BCP crystal treatment for 6 h. Alternatively, human macrophages were treated with OA synovial fluid alone or in combination with BCP crystals for 24 h. RNA was extracted using High Pure RNA Isolation Kits (Roche) and assessed for concentration and purity using the NanoDrop 2000c UV-Vis spectrophotometer. RNA was equalised and reverse transcribed using the Applied Biosystems High-Capacity cDNA reverse transcription kit. Real-time PCR was carried out on triplicate cDNA samples with the use of the CFX96 Touch Real-Time PCR Detection System (Bio-Rad Laboratories, CA, USA). Reactions included TaqMan fast universal PCR Master Mix (Applied Biosystems), cDNA and predesigned TaqMan S100A8, and MMP1 and TIMP1 gene expression probes (Applied Biosystems). mRNA expression data were normalised to the housekeeping gene, 18S ribosomal RNA, and relative gene expression levels were analysed using the $2^{-\Delta\Delta CT}$ method.

Statistical analysis

All experiments were run at least three times. For real-time PCR and ELISA, three technical replicates, per donor, were obtained and the mean for each donor $\pm$ SEM was then plotted for $n \geq 3$ healthy donors. Statistical analysis was performed by one-way analysis of variance (ANOVA) with Tukey post-test where applicable or Student's t test when comparing only two observations. All experiments were run at least three times and analysed on GraphPad Prism 6 software. A P value ≤ 0.05 was deemed statistically significant.

Results

BCP crystals activate Syk and PI3K in primary human macrophages and DC

We have previously demonstrated that BCP crystals activate the membrane-proximal tyrosine kinase Syk in murine bone marrow-derived macrophages (BMDM) [16]. It is also reported to be activated by MSU crystals, alum particles, and cholesterol crystals [24–27]. In order to determine if BCP crystals can induce the activation of

Syk in human innate immune cells, primary macrophages and DC were stimulated with BCP crystals (50 µg/ml) over the course of 30 min. This concentration of BCP crystals was chosen as it is within the range used in previously published studies [14, 15, 22] and is considered to be physiologically relevant as the concentration in OA synovial fluid ranges between 20 and 100 µg/ml [3–5]. Activation of Syk, as indicated by phosphorylation, was examined by immunoblotting. Phosphorylation of Syk was detected in both macrophages (Fig. 1a) and DC (Fig. 1b) within 2 min of BCP crystal treatment and increased in the first 10 min. Densitometric analysis of three Western blots revealed that maximal phosphorylation occurs at 10 min post-stimulation in both cell types (Fig. 1c and d).

Having demonstrated that BCP crystals are capable of activating Syk in both primary human macrophages and DC, we next sought to determine whether PI3K (a known interacting partner) is activated by BCP crystals downstream of Syk. Robust phosphorylation of the regulatory p85 and p55 subunits of the enzyme was detected in both macrophages (Fig. 1e) and DC (Fig. 1f) within 10 min of crystal treatment, with densitometric analysis of three Western blots revealing that maximal phosphorylation occurs at between 10 and 30 min in both cell types (Fig. 1g and h).

BCP crystals drive IL-1 production by primary macrophages in a Syk- and PI3K-dependent manner

BCP crystals are known to drive IL-1β production in murine macrophages that have been primed, for example, with a TLR agonist such as LPS [14–16]. Priming serves to induce pro-IL-1β expression within the cell while subsequent treatment of cells with the crystals leads to IL-1β processing and secretion. In an in vitro setting, this event is mediated by the NLRP3 inflammasome and active caspase-1, whereas it is likely to be mediated by alternative enzymes such as granzymes in the diseased joint [15]. In order to investigate if Syk is involved in BCP crystal-induced IL-1 production, primary human macrophages were primed with LPS (100 ng/ml) for 2 h prior to treatment with piceatannol, a pharmacological inhibitor of Syk, for 1 h and stimulation with BCP crystals for 6 h. Treatment with the Syk inhibitor resulted in a dose-dependent reduction in BCP crystal-induced IL-1β production, while having no effect on LPS-induced TNF-α which occurs independently of caspase-1 activation (Fig. 2a and c). Syk inhibition also significantly reduced IL-1α secretion (Fig. 2b) which is known to coincide with IL-1β release during pyroptosis. Similar results were obtained with an additional Syk inhibitor, R788, which is orally available (data not shown).

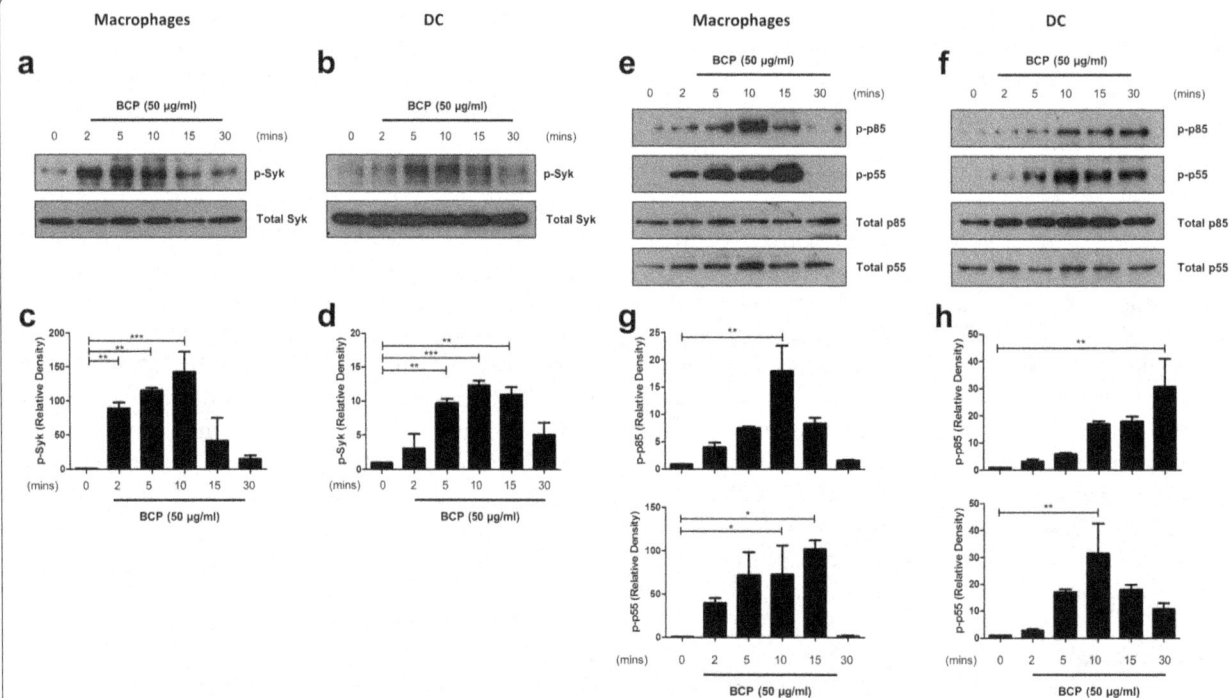

Fig. 1 BCP crystals activate Syk and PI3K in primary macrophages and DC. **a, e** Human macrophages and **b, f** DC (2×10^6 cells/well) were stimulated with BCP crystals (50 µg/ml) for the indicated time points, and phosphorylation of Syk and PI3K was detected by immunoblotting using phospho-specific antibodies. Representative blots of three independent experiments are shown. **c, d, g, h** Densitometric analysis of three blots was performed using ImageJ software. Bar graphs illustrate the mean (± SEM) increase in phosphorylation, relative to the untreated sample (0) and normalised to total Syk/PI3K protein. *$P \leq 0.05$, **$P \leq 0.01$, ***$P \leq 0.001$

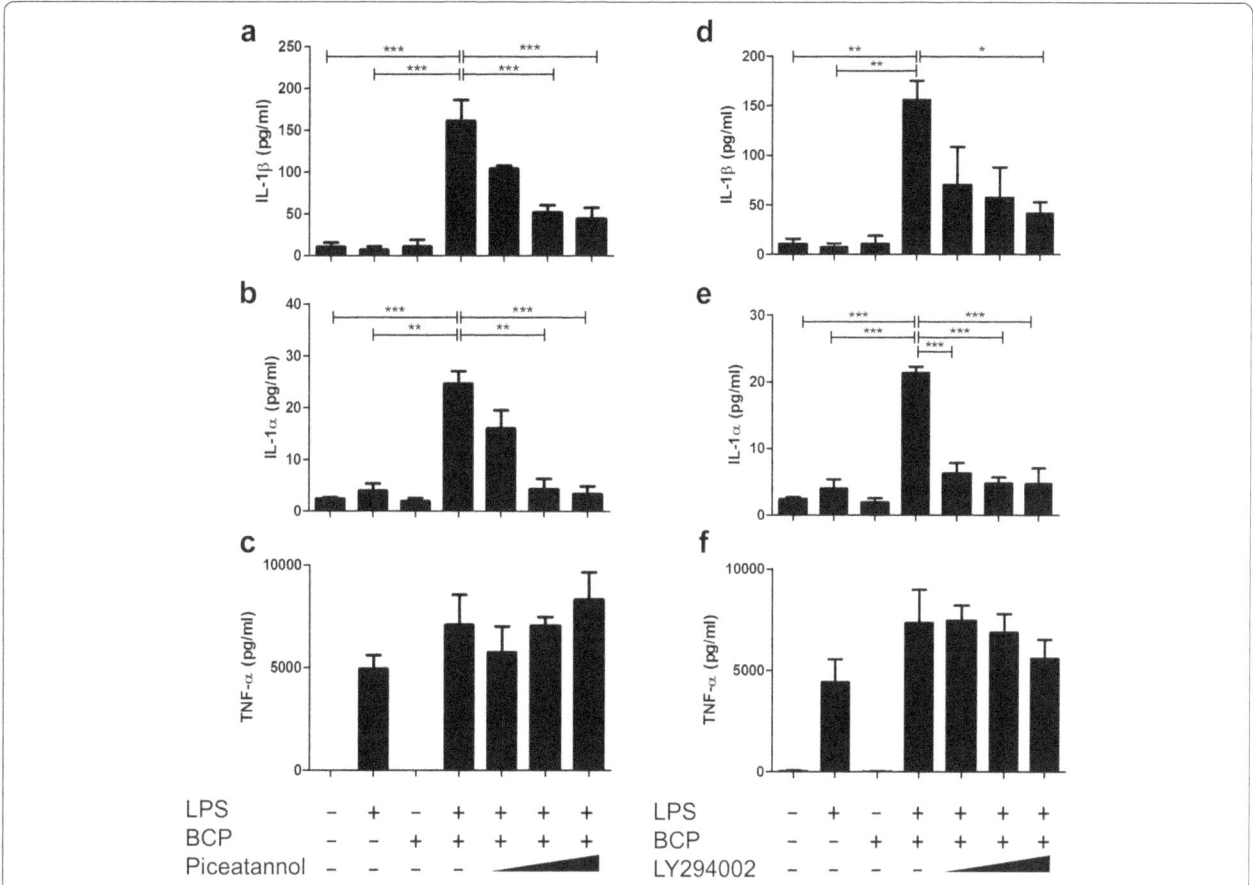

Fig. 2 Inhibition of Syk and PI3K reduces BCP crystal-induced IL-1 production in primary macrophages. Human macrophages (0.5 × 10⁶ cells/well) were primed with LPS (100 ng/ml) for 2 h prior to treatment with **a–c** piceatannol (10 μM, 25 μM, and 50 μM) or **d–f** LY294002 (10 μM, 25 μM, and 50 μM) for 1 h and stimulation with BCP crystals (50 μg/ml) for 6 h. Cell supernatants were assessed for IL-1β, IL-1α, and TNF-α by ELISA. Results indicate mean (± SEM) of three independent experiments. *$P \leq 0.05$, **$P \leq 0.01$, ***$P \leq 0.001$ vs LPS + BCP

In order to determine the effect of PI3K inhibition on BCP crystal-induced IL-1 production, LPS-primed human macrophages were pre-treated with the PI3K inhibitor, LY294002, for 1 h prior to BCP crystal stimulation. Similar to Syk inhibition, PI3K inhibition significantly reduced both IL-1α and IL-1β secretion, once again having no effect on LPS-induced TNFα production (Fig. 2d–f). This suggests that activation of Syk and PI3K is directly coupled to BCP crystal-induced cytokine production.

BCP crystal-induced IL-1 production occurs via lipid raft formation in primary human macrophages

Syk is typically activated following FcγR engagement which induces ITAM phosphorylation [23]; however, recent studies have demonstrated that MSU crystals, cholesterol crystals, and alum particles are capable of directly binding to the plasma membrane and activating Syk in a receptor-independent manner via MATS [24–27]. In order to ascertain whether MATS or FcγR activation is involved in BCP crystal-induced IL-1

production, LPS-primed human macrophages were either treated with an FcγR neutralising antibody or depleted of membrane cholesterol with M-βCD (10 mM) to prevent lipid sorting, prior to stimulation with BCP crystals. Blockade of the FcγR had no effect on BCP crystal-induced IL-1 production (Fig. 3a and b) whereas treatment with M-βCD significantly reduced BCP crystal-induced IL-1β production (Fig. 3d) and, while not statistically significant, also reduced IL-1α (Fig. 3e). Neither FcγR blockade nor M-βCD treatment affected LPS-induced TNFα (Fig. 3c and f). These results suggest that, like alum particles, MSU, and cholesterol crystals, BCP crystals may activate cell signalling pathways and drive cytokine production by primary macrophages through direct interaction with the plasma membrane.

BCP crystals activate MEK and ERK MAPK in primary human macrophages and DC

It well known that MEK and ERK MAPK are activated downstream of Syk and PI3K [33]. In addition, BCP crystals have been shown to activate MAPKs in human fibroblasts and osteoclast precursor cells [16, 21, 34]. In order to determine whether BCP crystals can activate MAPKs in human innate immune cells, and to determine if this is associated with the activation of membrane-proximal kinases, primary macrophages and DC were stimulated with BCP crystals over the course of 30 min and MEK/ERK activation, as indicated by phosphorylation, was assessed by immunoblotting. Robust BCP crystal-induced phosphorylation of MEK and ERK was evident after 2 min in macrophages (Fig. 4a and b; corresponding densitometry is also shown). While basal phosphorylation of MEK and ERK was higher in DC than in macrophages, densitometric analysis of three Western blots from individual donors revealed that phosphorylation of both kinases was significantly increased following BCP treatment (Fig. 4c and d; corresponding densitometry is also shown).

In order to confirm that BCP crystal-induced MEK/ERK activation occurs downstream of Syk and PI3K, primary human macrophages and DC were pre-treated for 30 min with one of two Syk inhibitors, piceatannol (50 μM or 100 μM) or R788 (5 μM), or the PI3K inhibitor, LY294002 (50 μM), prior to stimulation with BCP crystals for 15 min. As previously observed, BCP crystals induced the phosphorylation of MEK and ERK in primary macrophages (Fig. 4e and f; corresponding densitometry is also shown) and DC (Fig. 4g and h; corresponding densitometry is also shown) and this was reduced when either Syk or PI3K were inhibited, which demonstrates that BCP crystals activate MAPKs in a Syk- and PI3K-dependent manner.

BCP crystals upregulate the damage-associated molecules, S100A8, S100A12, and MMP1 in primary macrophages in a Syk- and PI3K-dependent manner

The calgranulins, specifically S100A8 and S100A9, have been implicated in both rheumatoid arthritis and OA and are considered potent damage-associated molecules which exacerbate inflammation following their release under conditions of cellular stress or injury [35, 36]. In a collagenase-induced OA model, S100A8 and S100A9

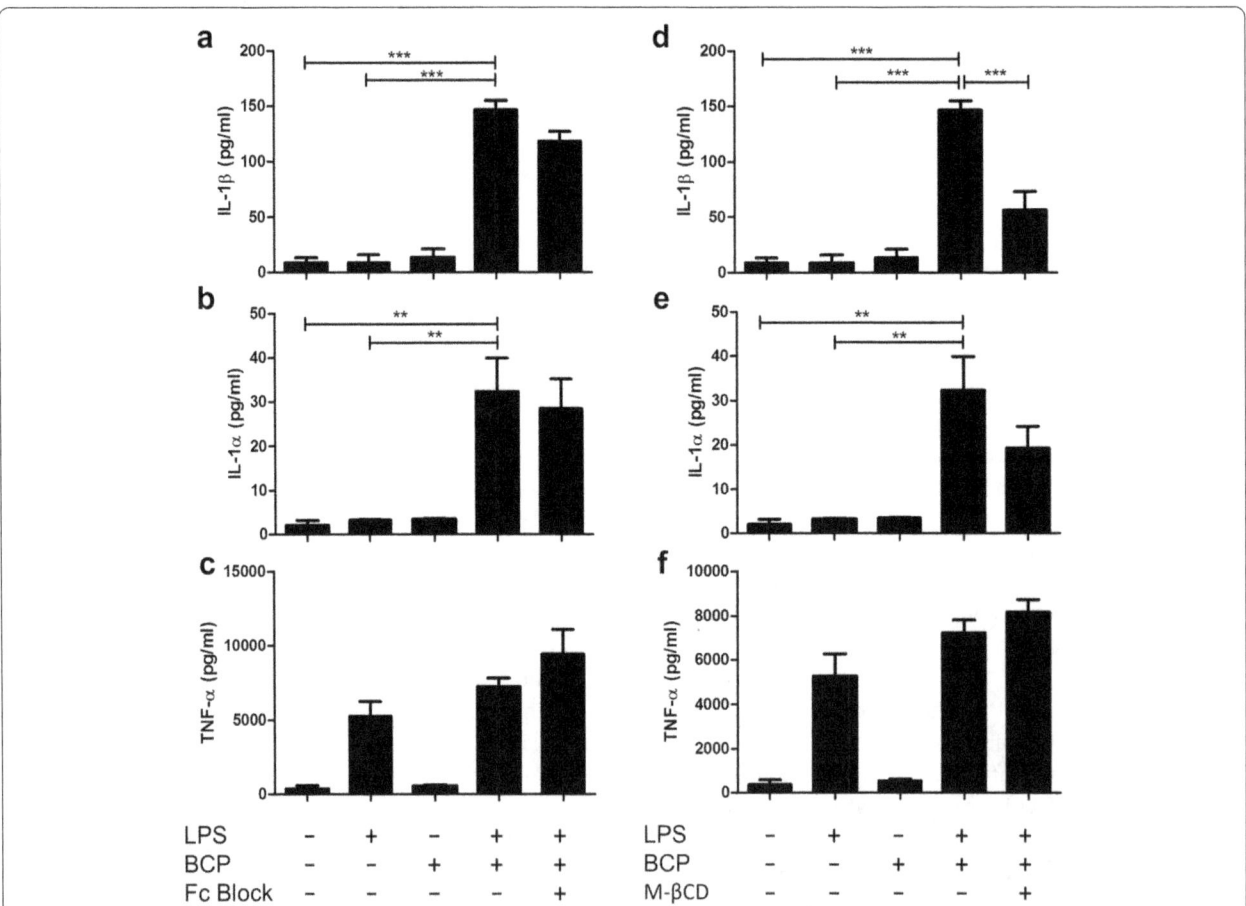

Fig. 3 BCP crystal-induced IL-1 production occurs via lipid raft formation in primary macrophages. LPS-primed human macrophages were treated with **a–c** an Fc receptor blocking antibody (5 μg/ml) or **d–f** M-βCD (10 mM) for 1 h prior to BCP crystal stimulation for 6 h. Cell supernatants were assessed for IL-1β, IL-1α, and TNF-α by ELISA. Results indicate mean (± SEM) of three independent experiments. ***P < 0.001

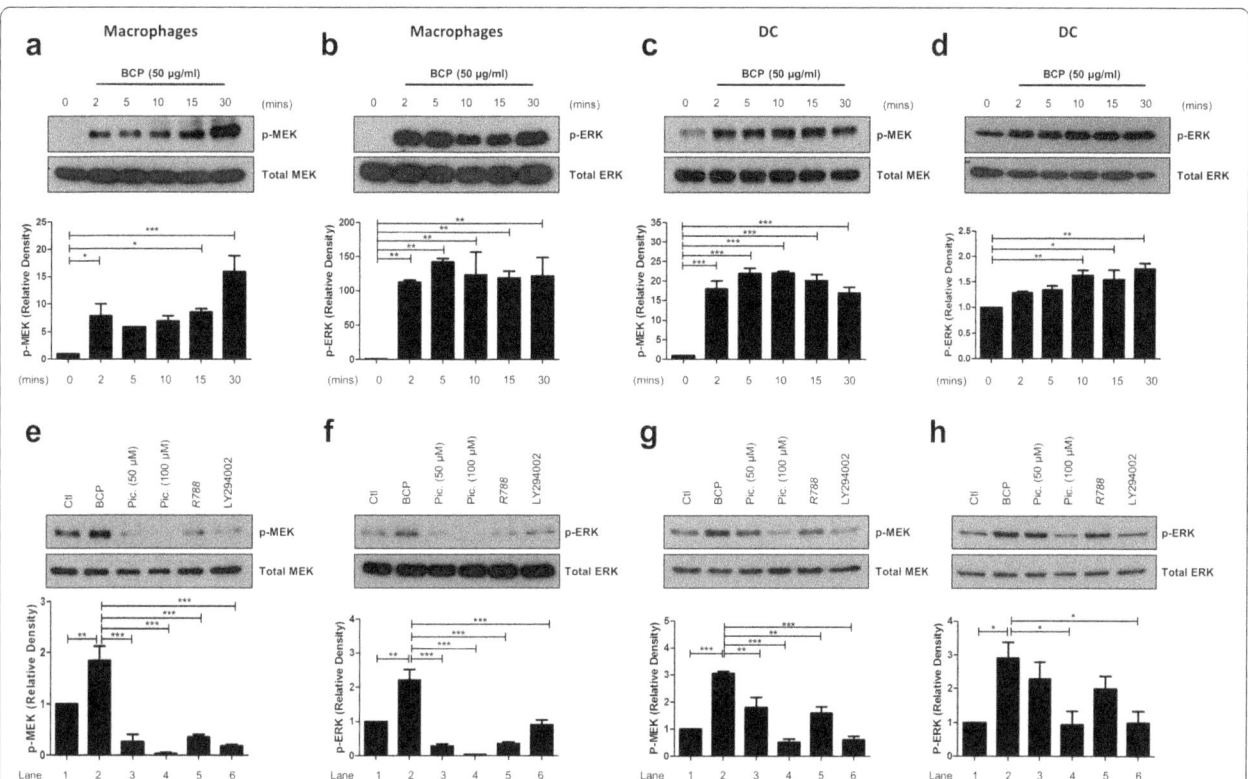

Fig. 4 BCP crystals activate MEK and ERK downstream of Syk/PI3K in primary macrophages and DC. **a,b** Human macrophages and **c, d** DC (2×10^6 cells/well) were stimulated with BCP crystals (50 μg/ml) for the indicated time points. Phosphorylation of MEK and ERK was detected by immunoblotting using phospho-specific antibodies. **e,f** Human macrophages and **g,h** DC were pre-treated with piceatannol (50 μM, 100 μM; lanes 3, 4), R788 (5 μM; lane 5), or LY294002 (50 μM; lane 6) for 30 min prior to stimulation with BCP crystals for 15 min. Phosphorylation of MEK and ERK was detected by immunoblotting. Representative blots of three independent experiments are shown. Densitometric analysis of three blots was performed using ImageJ software. Bar graphs illustrate the mean (± SEM) increase in phosphorylation, relative to the untreated sample (0) and normalised to total MEK/ERK protein. *$P \leq 0.05$, **$P \leq 0.01$, ***$P \leq 0.001$

expression remained elevated long after inflammatory cytokine levels had subsided, while in a BCP crystal-induced peritonitis model, both peritoneal and serum concentrations of S100A8 and S100A9 were increased [35–37]. Studies from our laboratory have demonstrated that BCP crystals can directly induce the upregulation of S100A8 in murine macrophages [16]; therefore, experiments were next carried out in order to determine whether these crystals also induce the expression of this DAMP in human immune cells. We also examined expression of the DAMP, S100A12, which, although not as widely studied as S100A8, has also been implicated in OA [38]. Primary human macrophages were stimulated with BCP crystals for 3, 6, and 24 h, and expression of S100A8 and S100A12 was analysed by real-time PCR. A time-dependent increase in S100A8 and S100A12 mRNA was observed in response to BCP crystal treatment, with significant induction observed at 24 h post-stimulation (Fig. 5a and b). We also examined the expression of MMP1, MMP2, and MMP9 given their known association with cartilage destruction in OA [39, 40]. As with the S100 proteins, MMP1 mRNA was

significantly elevated after 24 h of crystal treatment (Fig. 5c). There was also a modest increase in MMP2 (Fig. 5d), whereas there was no significant effect on MMP9 or the MMP inhibitor, TIMP1 (Fig. 5e and f). An increase in S100A8 protein expression was also detected in cell lysates after 3 h, suggesting a rapid mRNA turnover (Fig. 5g), while a time-dependent increase in the secreted and active forms of MMP1 and S100A12 was detected in the cell supernatants (Fig. 5h and i), which may further exacerbate damage at a site of inflammation.

We next examined the effect of Syk, PI3K, and MAPK inhibition on the induction of S100A8, S100A12, and MMP1 by BCP crystals. Macrophages were pre-treated with the Syk inhibitor, piceatannol, the PI3K inhibitor, LY294002, or the ERK/MEK inhibitor, PD98059, for 30 min prior to BCP crystal treatment for 24 h, and expression of S100A8, S100A12, MMP1, and TIMP1 was analysed by real-time PCR. All three inhibitors significantly reduced BCP crystal-induced S100A8, S100A12, and MMP1 expression (Fig. 6a–c) suggesting that all three signalling molecules are involved in their

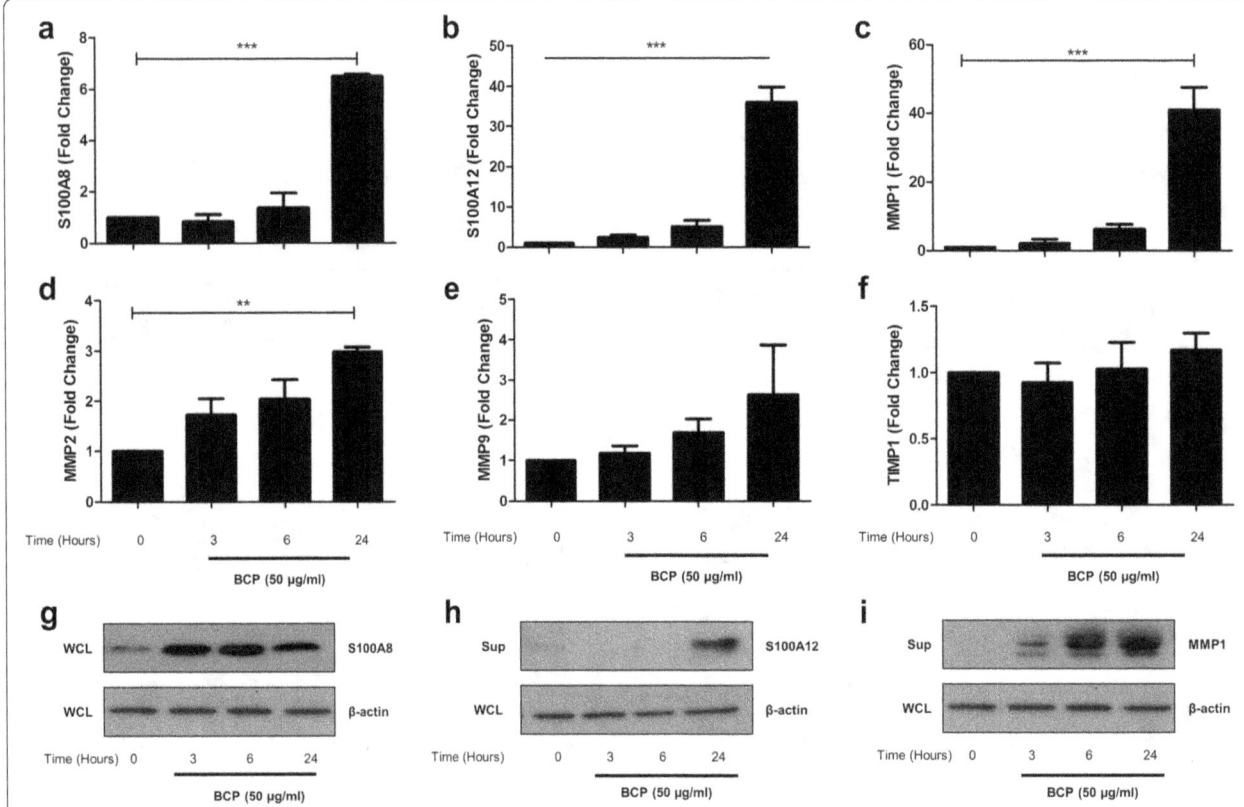

Fig. 5 BCP crystals induce expression of damage-associated molecules and MMPs in primary human macrophages in a Syk- and PI3K-dependent manner. Human macrophages (0.5×10^6 cells/well) were stimulated with BCP crystals (50 µg/ml) for 3, 6, and 24 h, and mRNA levels of **a** S100A8, **b** S100A12, **c** MMP1, **d** MMP2, **e** MMP9, and **f** TIMP1 were analysed by real-time PCR. Alternatively, supernatants were harvested; whole cell lysates (WCL) were prepared and both were analysed for the presence of **g** S100A8, **h** S100A12, and **i** MMP1 protein by immunoblotting. Representative blots of three independent experiments are shown. *$P \leq 0.05$, **$P \leq 0.01$, ***$P \leq 0.001$

induction. The ERK inhibitor reduced basal TIMP1 expression; however, this was not significant, while the PI3K inhibitor appeared to enhance the expression of TIMP1 which reflects previous reports that inhibition of PI3K correlated with induction of TIMP1 [41, 42].

As mentioned previously, an initial priming signal is required to drive pro-IL-1β expression prior to its subsequent proteolytic processing and release. The standard in vitro system utilises LPS for priming cells; however, this is unlikely to act as signal 1 in the context of OA and it has been suggested that DAMPs released at the site of injury can assume this role in vivo. Given that S100A8 is capable of activating TLR4 and is shown here to be induced by BCP crystals, we next examined if substitution of endotoxin-free recombinant S100A8 for LPS was sufficient to facilitate pro-IL-1β induction prior to BCP-induced processing in vitro. Primary human macrophages were primed with S100A8 for 3 h and then stimulated with BCP crystals for 6 h, and cytokine production was quantified. Both IL-1β and IL-1α were found to be significantly elevated following S100A8

priming and BCP stimulation (Fig. 7), suggesting that the DAMP can indeed induce pro-IL-1β expression. As expected, given that S100A8 is a TLR4 ligand, TNFα was also induced following S100A8 treatment (data not shown). Taken together, these results suggest that, in addition to pro-inflammatory cytokine production, Syk and PI3K are involved in BCP crystal-induced S100A8, S100A12, and MMP1 induction, making them attractive therapeutic targets.

OA synovial fluid enhances BCP crystal-induced S100A8 and MMP1 production in a Syk-dependent manner

Having observed that OA-associated BCP crystals drive S100A8, S100A12, and MMP1 expression in human innate immune cells, we next sought to examine 1) whether synovial fluid from OA patients exerts a similar effect to the crystals, and 2) whether BCP crystals and OA synovial fluid synergise to promote cartilage damage. Primary human macrophages from healthy donors were treated with synovial fluid from one of three OA patients (A, B, or C) either alone or in the presence of BCP crystals for 24 h, and expression of S100A8 and

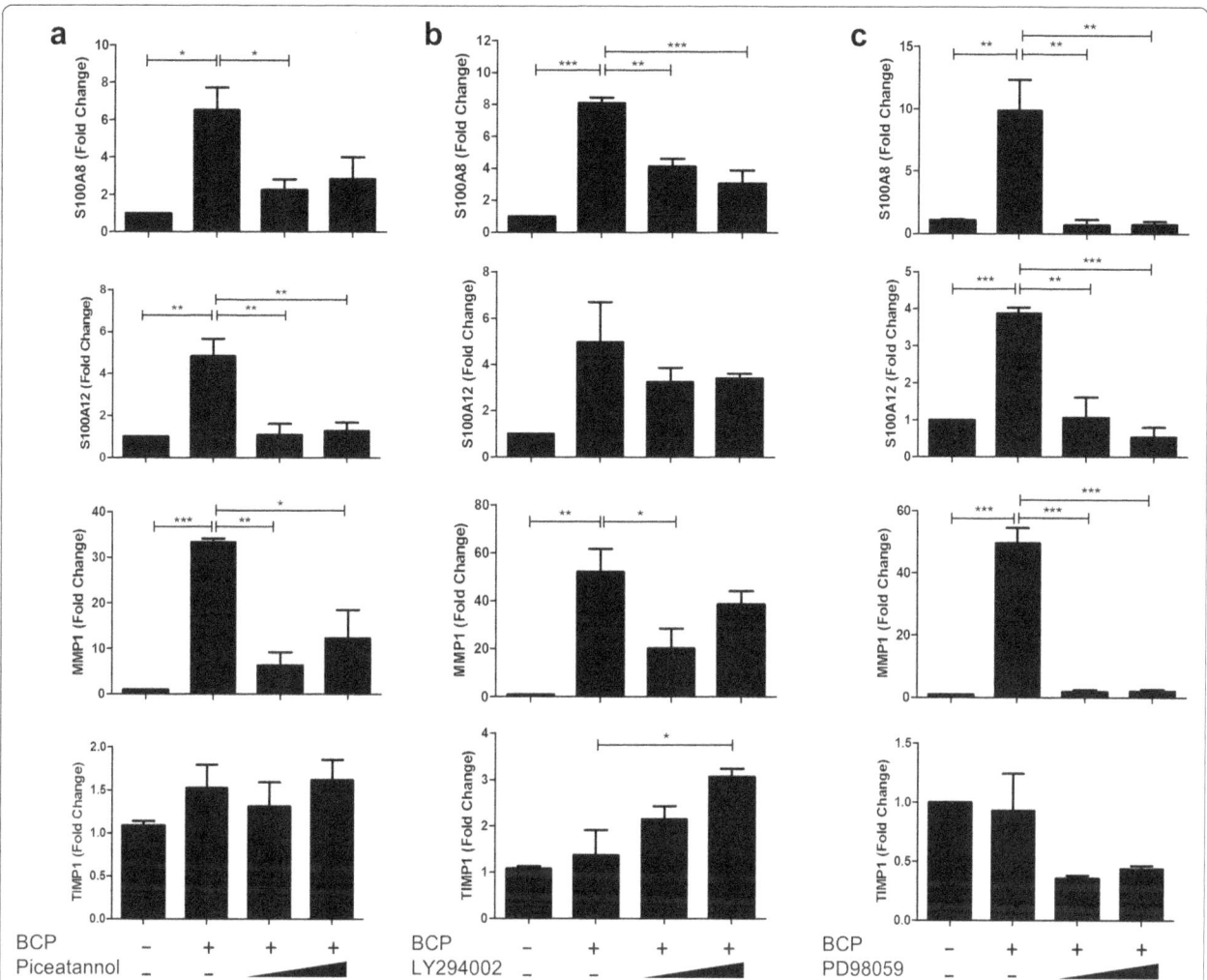

Fig. 6 BCP crystals induce expression of S100A8, S100A12, and MMP1 in primary macrophages in a Syk-, PI3K-, and ERK-dependent manner. Human macrophages were pre-treated with **a** piceatannol (50 μM, 100 μM), **b** LY294002 (25 μM, 50 μM), or **c** PD98059 (5 μM, 10 μM) for 30 mins prior to stimulation with BCP crystals for 24 h. mRNA levels of S100A8, S100A12, MMP1, and TIMP1 were analysed by real-time PCR. Results indicate mean (± SEM) of three independent experiments. *$P \leq 0.05$, **$P \leq 0.01$, ***$P \leq 0.001$

MMP1 was analysed by real-time PCR (Fig. 8a–c). As previously observed, BCP crystals alone upregulated the expression of both S100A8 and MMP1. Using a Student's paired t test to analyse the effect of OA synovial fluid alone versus no treatment, expression of S100A8 was significantly increased as previously observed; P values: A = 0.04, B = 0.06, C = 0.02. Interestingly, co-treatment with OA synovial fluid and BCP crystals led to higher levels of both S100A8 and MMP1 when compared with either synovial fluid or BCP crystals alone. Furthermore, pre-treatment of macrophages with the Syk inhibitor R788 dampened the synergistic effects observed following co-treatment, suggesting that R788 is effective in the presence of synovial fluid, which is important when considering the optimum method of administration of an OA drug.

Discussion

BCP crystals are associated with a number of rheumatic syndromes, and particularly with OA where the HA form of these crystals is most prevalent and is found to be deposited in the joints of 70% of total OA cases and in 100% of knee and hip osteoarthritic joints requiring arthroplasty. The crystals can be found in the synovial fluid and cartilage and are thought to form as a result of dysregulated ossification processes. They are known to play a pathogenic role in OA through the activation of macrophages, synovial fibroblasts, and articular chondrocytes [3, 7, 22, 43–45]. This study provides further insight into the mechanism by which BCP crystals activate intracellular signalling pathways in human innate immune cells and induce pro-inflammatory cytokine production. We report that BCP crystals activate the

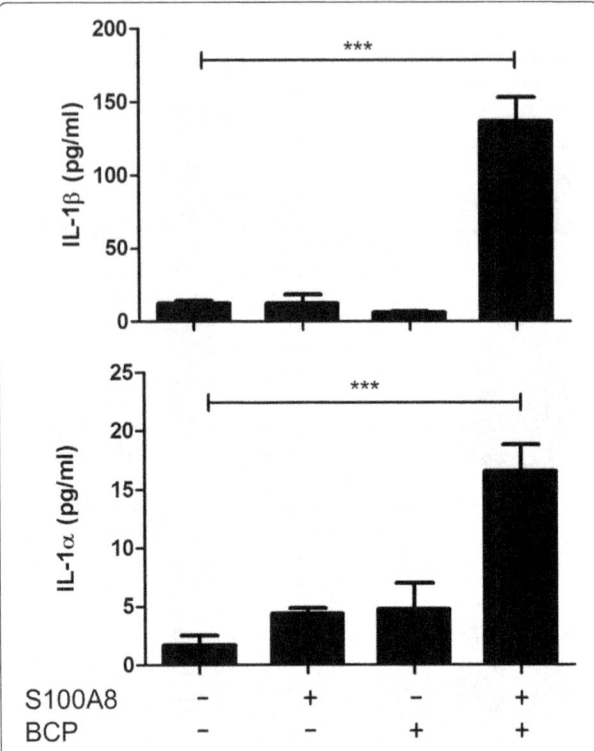

Fig. 7 S100A8 primes human macrophages for BCP-induced IL-1β production. Human macrophages were primed with recombinant human S100A8 (1 μg/ml) for 3 h prior to stimulation with BCP for 6 h. Cell supernatants were assessed for IL-1β, IL-1α, and TNF-α by ELISA. Results indicate mean (± SEM) of three independent experiments. ***$P \leq 0.001$

membrane-proximal kinase Syk and its interacting partner PI3K, and demonstrate that pharmacological inhibition of these enzymes abrogates BCP-induced IL-1α and IL-1β production. We demonstrate that, like gout-associated MSU crystals, alum particles, and cholesterol crystals, BCP crystals also activate Syk by MATS. In all cases, disruption of lipid rafts with M-βCD prevents the ITAM phosphorylation which normally ensues following the direct binding of the particulates to the cell membrane and thus prevents the recruitment and activation of Syk [24–27]. Furthermore, this results in a significant impairment of IL-1 production. Atomic Force Microscopy could be used for a more in-depth analysis to confirm that BCP crystals are, indeed, mediating their effects on macrophages through a direct interaction with the cell membrane. In addition to driving cell activation, this interaction is likely to cause cell damage, leading to the release of DAMPs which may propagate the initial inflammatory response. Interestingly, phosphorylation of the two subunits of PI3K appears to be regulated differently by BCP crystals, and further study is required to determine if these events are mutually exclusive. We have also shown that BCP crystals activate MEK and ERK MAPK downstream of Syk and PI3K, thus providing a link between the initial immune cell activation and subsequent gene expression. The PI3K pathway is a potential target for OA treatment as it can regulate gene expression through its target proteins which include NF-κB, a transcription factor that is reported to regulate MMP production [46, 47]. We demonstrate that BCP

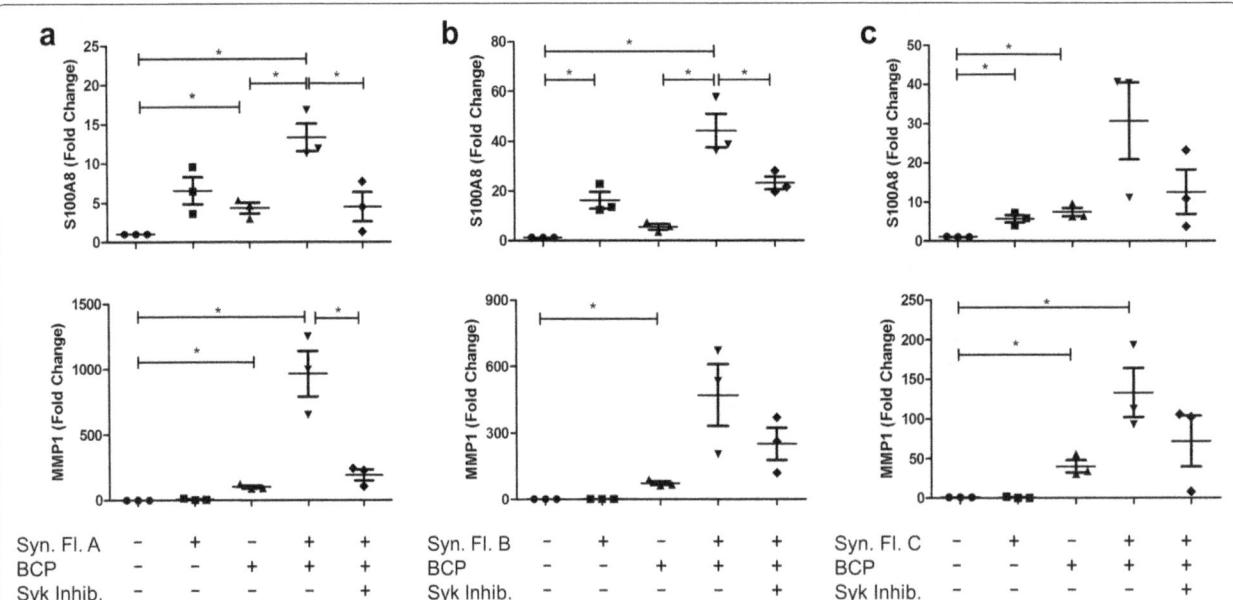

Fig. 8 BCP crystals exert synergistic effects with OA synovial fluid on primary macrophages. Human macrophages (0.5 × 10⁶ cells/well) were pre-treated with R788 (2.5 μM) prior to treatment with BCP crystals alone, synovial fluid from one of three OA patients (**a**, **b** or **c**), or OA synovial fluid and BCP crystals together for 24 h. Expression of (*upper panel*) S100A8 and (*lower panel*) MMP1 were analysed by real-time PCR. Results indicate mean (± SEM) of at least three healthy macrophage donors treated with synovial fluid from one OA patient. *$P \leq 0.05$, **$P \leq 0.01$

crystals directly induce the upregulation of the calgranulins S100A8 and S100A12 as well as the cartilage-degrading protease MMP1 in a Syk- and PI3K-dependent manner, and report that the presence of OA synovial fluid exacerbates the effects of BCP crystals on macrophages.

S100A8 was first identified in the context of RA where both the serum and synovial concentration of it and its binding partner, S100A9, were found to be elevated in patient samples [48]. Recent studies using the collagenase-induced OA model subsequently revealed a potential catabolic role for these proteins in OA-associated inflammation, revealing that S100A8 was abundant in the synovium of both early-stage and late-stage OA patients [35]. Of particular interest was the observation that serum levels of S100A8 were markedly higher in patients showing progression of OA, rather than those without progression, suggesting that these proteins may also be useful markers of disease advancement. Interestingly, analysis of cartilage from OA patients revealed that the protein is found only in areas of proteoglycan loss, suggesting a correlation between the presence of S100A8/A9 and MMP activity leading to aggrecan degradation [49]. The same study demonstrated that stimulation of cartilage explants with S100A8 and S100A9, or a combination of the two, led to increased mRNA levels of MMPs 1, 9, and 13, as well as IL-6, IL-8, and monocyte chemotactic protein-1, while it significantly downregulated the expression of aggrecan and type II collagen. A role for S100A12 has also been implicated in OA, where immunohistochemical analyses revealed that S100A12 expression was markedly increased in OA cartilage compared to non-OA cartilage. The same study also demonstrated that mRNA expression of S100A12 was significantly upregulated in OA chondrocytes in vitro by IL-1β stimulation and that treatment of OA chondrocytes with recombinant human S100A12 resulted in a significant increase in MMP13 mRNA expression [38]. This suggests that S100 proteins may amplify the inflammatory response and induce the degradation of cartilage, while also preventing its repair and regeneration. TLR4 has been identified as the key receptor for S100A8/9 activity, and we have demonstrated that S100A8 can act as a priming signal for BCP crystal-induced IL-1β maturation (at least in an in vitro context). Hence, small molecule inhibitors or biologics targeting TLR4 and/or relevant S100 proteins may be of benefit to OA patients. Furthermore, Syk and PI3K appear to be activated upstream of gene transcription as pharmacological inhibition of these molecules reduces BCP crystal-induced S100A8 and MMP1 mRNA. Therefore, Syk and PI3K may also represent potential therapeutic targets. Indeed, preventing the actual deposition of calcium crystals, as recently demonstrated in a murine OA model by Nasi et al. [50], could limit these responses in the first instance and prevent

crystal-associated cell inflammation. Expression of Syk and PI3K has been detected in the intimal lining of OA synovial tissues at similar levels to those detected in healthy synovial tissue, though the degree of activation compared to healthy synovial tissue has not been investigated in any detail [51, 52]. Furthermore, Syk is also known to be expressed by osteoclasts and is crucial to osteoclastic bone resorption [53]; therefore, further studies are required to determine if Syk activation is heightened in OA joints.

Conclusions

The studies presented here demonstrate that BCP crystals are capable of activating specific intracellular signalling pathways which drive inflammation and the production of cartilage-degrading enzymes and DAMPs that promote disease initiation and exacerbate progression in OA. Patients are currently treated with intra-articular corticosteroids and non-steroidal anti-inflammatory drugs to provide symptomatic relief. Corticosteroids have previously been demonstrated to reduce early OA changes such as osteophyte formation and cartilage lesion in a canine OA model [54] and to reduce cartilage degradation when administered early after anterior cruciate ligament injury in a porcine model [55]; however, they do not entirely halt disease progression. Clinical trials are currently underway to examine the effect of intra-articular administration of a synthetic glucocorticoid on pain, joint function, inflammation, and cartilage degradation (ClinicalTrials.gov identifier: NCT01692756). Anti-cytokine, anti-MMP therapies, and anti-S100A8/A9 therapies are promising candidates for new disease-modifying OA drugs. However, preventing the expression and/or release of degradative mediators rather than inhibiting their activity may prove more efficient. Membrane-proximal kinases such as Syk and PI3K require consideration not just in the context of OA but also for other crystal-mediated diseases such as gout and atherosclerosis, and in vivo studies are required in order to fully implicate these kinases in crystal-induced responses. The orally available Syk inhibitor R788 that was used in this study has previously shown efficacy in clinical trials for rheumatoid arthritis; however, reports of side effects during phase III trials led to trial termination [56]. Nevertheless, a modification on the current drug or, indeed, an alternate method of administration, such as direct injection into the joint, may still prove to be effective as a treatment for OA. Indeed, Syk inhibitors are currently in development by a number of pharmaceutical companies.

Abbreviations
BCP: Basic calcium phosphate; DAMP: Damage-associated molecular pattern; DC: Dendritic cells; ELISA: Enzyme-linked immunosorbent assay; HA: Hydroxyapatite; LPS: Lipopolysaccharide; MAPK: Mitogen-activated protein kinase; MATS: Membrane affinity-triggered signalling; M-βCD: Methyl-

β-cyclodextrin; MMP: Matrix metalloprotease; MSU: Monosodium urate; OA: Osteoarthritis; PCR: Polymerase chain reaction; PI3K: Phosphoinositide-3 kinase; Syk: Spleen tyrosine kinase; TIMP: Tissue inhibitor of metalloprotease

Acknowledgements

This work was funded by the Health Research Board, Ireland. We would also like to thank Dr Trudy McGarry and Professor Ursula Fearon for critically reviewing this manuscript.

Funding

This work was funded by the Health Research Board, Ireland.

Authors' contributions

EMC contributed to the conception and design of the study, the acquisition, analysis and interpretation of the data, and the drafting of the article. AD contributed to the conception and design of the study, analysis and interpretation of the data, and drafting of the article. CCC contributed to the analysis and interpretation of the data, and drafting of the article. GMM contributed to the analysis and interpretation of the data, drafting of the article, collection of patient samples, and provision of study materials. LH contributed to the collection of patient samples. All authors read and approved the final manuscript.

Competing interests

The authors declare that they have no competing interests.

Consent for publication

All authors have read the journal's authorship agreement, and the manuscript has been reviewed and approved by all named authors.

Author details

[1]School of Biochemistry & Immunology and School of Medicine, Trinity Biomedical Sciences Institute, Trinity College Dublin, Dublin, Ireland. [2]Mater Misericordiae University Hospital, Dublin, Ireland.

References

1. Ea HK, Nguyen C, Bazin D, Bianchi A, Guicheux J, Reboul P, Daudon M, Liote F. Articular cartilage calcification in osteoarthritis: insights into crystal-induced stress. Arthritis Rheum. 2011;63:10–8.
2. Molloy ES, McCarthy GM. Hydroxyapatite deposition disease of the joint. Curr Rheumatol Rep. 2003;5:215–21.
3. Rachow JW, Ryan LM, McCarty DJ, Halverson PC. Synovial fluid inorganic pyrophosphate concentration and nucleotide pyrophosphohydrolase activity in basic calcium phosphate deposition arthropathy and Milwaukee shoulder syndrome. Arthritis Rheum. 1988;31:408–13.
4. Cheung HS, Story MT, McCarty DJ. Mitogenic effects of hydroxyapatite and calcium pyrophosphate dihydrate crystals on cultured mammalian cells. Arthritis Rheum. 1984;27:668–74.
5. McCarthy GM, Cheung HS, Abel SM, Ryan LM. Basic calcium phosphate crystal-induced collagenase production: role of intracellular crystal dissolution. Osteoarthritis Cartilage. 1998;6:205–13.
6. Nalbant S, Martinez JA, Kitumnuaypong T, Clayburne G, Sieck M, Schumacher Jr HR. Synovial fluid features and their relations to osteoarthritis severity: new findings from sequential studies. Osteoarthritis Cartilage. 2003; 11:50–4.
7. Fuerst M, Bertrand J, Lammers L, Dreier R, Echtermeyer F, Nitschke Y, Rutsch F, Schafer FK, Niggemeyer O, Steinhagen J, et al. Calcification of articular cartilage in human osteoarthritis. Arthritis Rheum. 2009;60:2694–703.
8. Fuerst M, Niggemeyer O, Lammers L, Schafer F, Lohmann C, Ruther W. Articular cartilage mineralization in osteoarthritis of the hip. BMC Musculoskelet Disord. 2009;10:166.
9. Sun Y, Mauerhan DR, Honeycutt PR, Kneisl JS, Norton HJ, Zinchenko N, Hanley Jr EN, Gruber HE. Calcium deposition in osteoarthritic meniscus and meniscal cell culture. Arthritis Res Ther. 2010;12:R56.
10. McCarthy GM, Augustine JA, Baldwin AS, Christopherson PA, Cheung HS, Westfall PR, Scheinman RI. Molecular mechanism of basic calcium phosphate crystal-induced activation of human fibroblasts. Role of nuclear factor kappa b, activator protein 1, and protein kinase C. J Biol Chem. 1998; 273:35161–9.
11. Reuben PM, Brogley MA, Sun Y, Cheung HS. Molecular mechanism of the induction of metalloproteinases 1 and 3 in human fibroblasts by basic calcium phosphate crystals. Role of calcium-dependent protein kinase C alpha. J Biol Chem. 2002;277:15190–8.
12. Nasi S, So A, Combes C, Daudon M, Busso N. Interleukin-6 and chondrocyte mineralisation act in tandem to promote experimental osteoarthritis. Ann Rheum Dis. 2016;75:1372–9.
13. Nadra I, Mason JC, Philippidis P, Florey O, Smythe CD, McCarthy GM, Landis RC, Haskard DO. Proinflammatory activation of macrophages by basic calcium phosphate crystals via protein kinase C and MAP kinase pathways: a vicious cycle of inflammation and arterial calcification? Circ Res. 2005;96:1248–56.
14. Jin C, Frayssinet P, Pelker R, Cwirka D, Hu B, Vignery A, Eisenbarth SC, Flavell RA. NLRP3 inflammasome plays a critical role in the pathogenesis of hydroxyapatite-associated arthropathy. Proc Natl Acad Sci U S A. 2011;108: 14867–72.
15. Pazar B, Ea HK, Narayan S, Kolly L, Bagnoud N, Chobaz V, Roger T, Liote F, So A, Busso N. Basic calcium phosphate crystals induce monocyte/macrophage IL-1beta secretion through the NLRP3 inflammasome in vitro. J Immunol. 2011;186:2495–502.
16. Cunningham CC, Mills E, Mielke LA, O'Farrell LK, Lavelle E, Mori A, McCarthy GM, Mills KH, Dunne A. Osteoarthritis-associated basic calcium phosphate crystals induce pro-inflammatory cytokines and damage-associated molecules via activation of Syk and PI3 kinase. Clin Immunol. 2012;144:228–36.
17. Benito MJ, Veale DJ, FitzGerald O, van den Berg WB, Bresnihan B. Synovial tissue inflammation in early and late osteoarthritis. Ann Rheum Dis. 2005;64:1263–7.
18. Daheshia M, Yao JQ. The interleukin 1beta pathway in the pathogenesis of osteoarthritis. J Rheumatol. 2008;35:2306–12.
19. Pujol JP, Chadjichristos C, Legendre F, Bauge C, Beauchef G, Andriamanalijaona R, Galera P, Boumediene K. Interleukin-1 and transforming growth factor-beta 1 as crucial factors in osteoarthritic cartilage metabolism. Connect Tissue Res. 2008;49:293–7.
20. Moon SJ, Ahn IE, Jung H, Yi H, Kim J, Kim Y, Kwok SK, Park KS, Min JK, Park SH, et al. Temporal differential effects of proinflammatory cytokines on osteoclastogenesis. Int J Mol Med. 2013;31:769–77.
21. Cunningham CC, Corr EM, McCarthy GM, Dunne A. Intra-articular basic calcium phosphate and monosodium urate crystals inhibit anti-osteoclastogenic cytokine signalling. Osteoarthritis Cartilage. 2016;24(12):2141–52.
22. Ea HK, Chobaz V, Nguyen C, Nasi S, van Lent P, Daudon M, Dessombz A, Bazin D, McCarthy G, Jolles-Haeberli B, et al. Pathogenic role of basic calcium phosphate crystals in destructive arthropathies. PLoS One. 2013;8, e57352.
23. Sedlik C, Orbach D, Veron P, Schweighoffer E, Colucci F, Gamberale R, Ioan-Facsinay A, Verbeek S, Ricciardi-Castagnoli P, Bonnerot C, et al. A critical role for Syk protein tyrosine kinase in Fc receptor-mediated antigen presentation and induction of dendritic cell maturation. J Immunol. 2003;170:846–52.
24. Ng G, Sharma K, Ward SM, Desrosiers MD, Stephens LA, Schoel WM, Li T, Lowell CA, Ling CC, Amrein MW, Shi Y. Receptor-independent, direct membrane binding leads to cell-surface lipid sorting and Syk kinase activation in dendritic cells. Immunity. 2008;29:807–18.
25. Desaulniers P, Fernandes M, Gilbert C, Bourgoin SG, Naccache PH. Crystal-induced neutrophil activation. VII. Involvement of Syk in the responses to monosodium urate crystals. J Leukoc Biol. 2001;70:659–68.
26. Flach TL, Ng G, Hari A, Desrosiers MD, Zhang P, Ward SM, Seamone ME, Vilaysane A, Mucsi AD, Fong Y, et al. Alum interaction with dendritic cell membrane lipids is essential for its adjuvanticity. Nat Med. 2011;17:479–87.
27. Corr EM, Cunningham CC, Dunne A. Cholesterol crystals activate Syk and PI3 kinase in human macrophages and dendritic cells. Atherosclerosis. 2016; 251:197–205.
28. Evans RW, Cheung HS, McCarty DJ. Cultured human monocytes and fibroblasts solubilize calcium phosphate crystals. Calcif Tissue Int. 1984;36:645–50.
29. Hiasa M, Abe M, Nakano A, Oda A, Amou H, Kido S, Takeuchi K, Kagawa K, Yata K, Hashimoto T, et al. GM-CSF and IL-4 induce dendritic cell differentiation and disrupt osteoclastogenesis through M-CSF receptor

shedding by up-regulation of TNF-alpha converting enzyme (TACE). Blood. 2009;114:4517–26.

30. Ohradanova-Repic A, Machacek C, Fischer MB, Stockinger H. Differentiation of human monocytes and derived subsets of macrophages and dendritic cells by the HLDA10 monoclonal antibody panel. Clin Transl Immunology. 2016;5, e55.

31. Rehman J, Li J, Orschell CM, March KL. Peripheral blood "endothelial progenitor cells" are derived from monocyte/macrophages and secrete angiogenic growth factors. Circulation. 2003;107:1164–9.

32. Menck K, Behme D, Pantke M, Reiling N, Binder C, Pukrop T, Klemm F. Isolation of human monocytes by double gradient centrifugation and their differentiation to macrophages in teflon-coated cell culture bags. J Vis Exp. 2014;91, e51554.

33. King WG, Mattaliano MD, Chan TO, Tsichlis PN, Brugge JS. Phosphatidylinositol 3-kinase is required for integrin-stimulated AKT and Raf-1/mitogen-activated protein kinase pathway activation. Mol Cell Biol. 1997;17:4406–18.

34. Nair D, Misra RP, Sallis JD, Cheung HS. Phosphocitrate inhibits a basic calcium phosphate and calcium pyrophosphate dihydrate crystal-induced mitogen-activated protein kinase cascade signal transduction pathway. J Biol Chem. 1997;272:18920–5.

35. van Lent PL, Blom AB, Schelbergen RF, Sloetjes A, Lafeber FP, Lems WF, Cats H, Vogl T, Roth J, van den Berg WB. Active involvement of alarmins S100A8 and S100A9 in the regulation of synovial activation and joint destruction during mouse and human osteoarthritis. Arthritis Rheum. 2012;64:1466–76.

36. Chen YS, Yan W, Geczy CL, Brown MA, Thomas R. Serum levels of soluble receptor for advanced glycation end products and of S100 proteins are associated with inflammatory, autoantibody, and classical risk markers of joint and vascular damage in rheumatoid arthritis. Arthritis Res Ther. 2009;11:R39.

37. Narayan S, Pazar B, Ea HK, Kolly L, Bagnoud N, Chobaz V, Liote F, Vogl T, Holzinger D, Kai-Lik So A, Busso N. Octacalcium phosphate crystals induce inflammation in vivo through interleukin-1 but independent of the NLRP3 inflammasome in mice. Arthritis Rheum. 2011;63:422–33.

38. Nakashima M, Sakai T, Hiraiwa H, Hamada T, Omachi T, Ono Y, Inukai N, Ishizuka S, Matsukawa T, Oda T, et al. Role of S100A12 in the pathogenesis of osteoarthritis. Biochem Biophys Res Commun. 2012;422:508–14.

39. Yuan GH, Tanaka M, Masuko-Hongo K, Shibakawa A, Kato T, Nishioka K, Nakamura H. Characterization of cells from pannus-like tissue over articular cartilage of advanced osteoarthritis. Osteoarthritis Cartilage. 2004;12:38–45.

40. Maiotti M, Monteleone G, Tarantino U, Fasciglione GF, Marini S, Coletta M. Correlation between osteoarthritic cartilage damage and levels of proteinases and proteinase inhibitors in synovial fluid from the knee joint. Arthroscopy. 2000;16:522–6.

41. Zhou R, Xu L, Ye M, Liao M, Du H, Chen H. Formononetin inhibits migration and invasion of MDA-MB-231 and 4 T1 breast cancer cells by suppressing MMP-2 and MMP-9 through PI3K/AKT signaling pathways. Horm Metab Res. 2014;46:753–60.

42. Su Y, Wan D, Song W. Dryofragin inhibits the migration and invasion of human osteosarcoma U2OS cells by suppressing MMP-2/9 and elevating TIMP-1/2 through PI3K/AKT and p38 MAPK signaling pathways. Anticancer Drugs. 2016;27:660–8.

43. McCarthy GM, Cheung HS. Point: Hydroxyapatite crystal deposition is intimately involved in the pathogenesis and progression of human osteoarthritis. Curr Rheumatol Rep. 2009;11:141–7.

44. Schumacher Jr HR. Crystals, inflammation, and osteoarthritis. Am J Med. 1987;83:11–6.

45. Anderson HC. Matrix vesicles and calcification. Curr Rheumatol Rep. 2003;5: 222–6.

46. Lin TH, Tang CH, Wu K, Fong YC, Yang RS, Fu WM. 15-deoxy-Delta(12,14) -prostaglandin-J2 and ciglitazone inhibit TNF-alpha-induced matrix metalloproteinase 13 production via the antagonism of NF-kappaB activation in human synovial fibroblasts. J Cell Physiol. 2011;226:3242–50.

47. Chen J, Crawford R, Xiao Y. Vertical inhibition of the PI3K/Akt/mTOR pathway for the treatment of osteoarthritis. J Cell Biochem. 2013;114:245–9.

48. Foell D, Roth J. Proinflammatory S100 proteins in arthritis and autoimmune disease. Arthritis Rheum. 2004;50:3762–71.

49. Schelbergen RF, Blom AB, van den Bosch MH, Sloetjes A, Abdollahi-Roodsaz S, Schreurs BW, Mort JS, Vogl T, Roth J, van den Berg WB, van Lent PL. Alarmins S100A8 and S100A9 elicit a catabolic effect in human osteoarthritic chondrocytes that is dependent on Toll-like receptor 4. Arthritis Rheum. 2012;64:1477–87.

50. Nasi S, Ea HK, Liote F, So A, Busso N. Sodium thiosulfate prevents chondrocyte mineralization and reduces the severity of murine osteoarthritis. PLoS One. 2016;11, e0158196.

51. Cha HS, Boyle DL, Inoue T, Schoot R, Tak PP, Pine P, Firestein GS. A novel spleen tyrosine kinase inhibitor blocks c-Jun N-terminal kinase-mediated gene expression in synoviocytes. J Pharmacol Exp Ther. 2006;317:571–8.

52. Bartok B, Boyle DL, Liu Y, Ren P, Ball ST, Bugbee WD, Rommel C, Firestein GS. PI3 kinase delta is a key regulator of synoviocyte function in rheumatoid arthritis. Am J Pathol. 2012;180:1906–16.

53. Zou W, Kitaura H, Reeve J, Long F, Tybulewicz VL, Shattil SJ, Ginsberg MH, Ross FP, Teitelbaum SL. Syk, c-Src, the alphavbeta3 integrin, and ITAM immunoreceptors, in concert, regulate osteoclastic bone resorption. J Cell Biol. 2007;176:877–88.

54. Pelletier JP, Martel-Pelletier J. Protective effects of corticosteroids on cartilage lesions and osteophyte formation in the Pond-Nuki dog model of osteoarthritis. Arthritis Rheum. 1989;32:181–93.

55. Sieker JT, Ayturk UM, Proffen BL, Weissenberger MH, Kiapour AM, Murray MM. Immediate administration of intraarticular triamcinolone acetonide after joint injury modulates molecular outcomes associated with early synovitis. Arthritis Rheumatol. 2016;68:1637–47.

56. Weinblatt ME, Kavanaugh A, Burgos-Vargas R, Dikranian AH, Medrano-Ramirez G, Morales-Torres JL, Murphy FT, Musser TK, Straniero N, Vicente-Gonzales AV, Grossbard E. Treatment of rheumatoid arthritis with a Syk kinase inhibitor: a twelve-week, randomized, placebo-controlled trial. Arthritis Rheum. 2008;58:3309–18.

12

Cartilage-specific deletion of ephrin-B2 in mice results in early developmental defects and an osteoarthritis-like phenotype during aging in vivo

Gladys Valverde-Franco[1], Bertrand Lussier[1,2], David Hum[1], Jiangping Wu[3], Adjia Hamadjida[4,5], Numa Dancause[4,5], Hassan Fahmi[1], Mohit Kapoor[1,6], Jean-Pierre Pelletier[1] and Johanne Martel-Pelletier[1*]

Abstract

Background: Ephrins and their related receptors have been implicated in some developmental events. We have demonstrated that ephrin-B2 (EFNB2) could play a role in knee joint pathology associated with osteoarthritis (OA). Here, we delineate the in vivo role of EFNB2 in musculoskeletal growth, development, and in OA using a cartilage-specific EFNB2 knockout (EFNB2^{Col2}KO) mouse model.

Methods: EFNB2^{Col2}KO was generated with Col2a1-Cre transgenic mice. The skeletal development was evaluated using macroscopy, immunohistochemistry, histomorphometry, radiology, densitometry, and micro-computed tomography. Analyses were performed at P0 (birth) and on postnatal days P15, P21, and on 8-week- and 1-year-old mice.

Results: EFNB2^{Col2}KO mice exhibited significant reduction in size, weight, length, and in long bones. At P0, the growth plates of EFNB2^{Col2}KO mice displayed increased type X collagen, disorganized hyphertrophic zone, and decreased mineralization. At P15, mutant mice demonstrated a significant reduction in VEGF and TRAP at the chondro-osseous junction and a delay in the secondary ossification, including a decrease in bone volume and trabecular thickness. At P21 and 8 weeks old, EFNB2^{Col2}KO mice exhibited reduced bone mineral density in the total skeleton, femur and spine. One-year-old EFNB2^{Col2}KO mice demonstrated OA phenotypic features in both the knee and hip. By P15, 27 % of the EFNB2^{Col2}KO mice developed a hip locomotor phenotype, which further experiments demonstrated reflected the neurological midline abnormality involving the corticospinal tract.

Conclusion: This in vivo study demonstrated, for the first time, that EFNB2 is essential for normal long bone growth and development and its absence leads to a knee and hip OA phenotype in aged mice.

Keywords: Ephrin-B2, Bone development, Osteoarthritis, Knockout mouse model

Background

Erythropoietin-producing hepatocellular receptors (Eph) are the largest family of cell surface receptor tyrosine kinases, representing about 25 % of known receptor tyrosine kinases [1, 2]. There are a total of 15 Ephs classified by sequence homology into subfamilies A and B, but not all are expressed in a given species [3, 4]. Ephs bind to their ephrin (EFN) ligands, which are also cell surface molecules [2]. There are nine EFNs divided into A and B subfamilies. Generally, type A receptors bind preferentially to EFNA, and type B receptors (EphB1-4 and B6) to EFNB, but there are a few exceptions.

The Eph/EFN system was first demonstrated to be essential in the development of neuronal connections, circuit plasticity and repair. Subsequently, their presence and functions have been shown in many organs and tissues in which they were shown to play a role in a number of biological processes [5]. The receptor/ligand

* Correspondence: jm@martelpelletier.ca
[1]Osteoarthritis Research Unit, University of Montreal Hospital Research Centre (CRCHUM), 900 Saint-Denis, R11.412B, Montreal, QC H2X 0A9, Canada
Full list of author information is available at the end of the article

EphB4/EFNB2 has been shown to be implicated in bone maintenance and repair [6–8]. However, the role of EFNB2 in skeletal growth and development has never been investigated, likely due to the fact that germ-line mutation of EFNB2 in mice leads to embryonic lethality in homozygous nulls [9, 10].

As both EphB4/EFNB2 are present in the growth plate [8], in vivo EphB4 enhances the process of endochondral ossification bone repair [11], and their presence and activity in adult articular chondrocytes have been demonstrated [12], we further investigated the in vivo role of EFNB2 in skeletal growth and development. To this end, we generated a cartilage-specific EFNB2 knockout (KO) mouse model, using Col2a1-Cre transgenic mice (EFNB2^{Col2}KO), as chondrocytes are crucial to bone development.

Moreover, our group previously demonstrated that EFNB2 treatment of human osteoarthritic (OA) chondrocytes positively impacts the abnormal metabolism of these cells [12]. Thus, the present mouse model, in addition to permitting a better understanding of the role of EFNB2 in endochondral bone development, will enable further exploration of the long-term effect of this deletion on knee and hip cartilage in order to substantiate whether this factor could be a new OA therapeutic approach.

Materials and methods
Mouse model
Mice were maintained in accordance with the Canadian Council on Animal Care (CCAC) and protocols reviewed and approved by the Institutional Animal Care Committee (CIPA) of the University of Montreal Hospital Centre (CHUM). All mice were kept in a 12-h light/dark cycle. Food and water were available *ad libitum.*

We have previously reported on the generation of EFNB2 floxed (EFNB2$^{fl/fl}$) mice [13]. They were backcrossed with C57BL/6 for 10 generations and then mated with transgenic mice expressing Cre recombinanse driven by type II collagen promoter (Col2a1-Cre) in the C57BL/6 background [14] to obtain mutant mice with a cartilage-specific deletion of EFNB2 (EFNB2^{Col2}KO).

The generation and characterization of EFNB2^{Col2}KO cartilage conditional mice were as follows. C57BL/6-EFNB2$^{fl/fl}$ mice were mated with C57BL/6 Col2-Cre transgenic mice to generate offspring bearing Col2-Cre and a floxed allele in their germline (genotype: EFNB2$^{fl/+}$, Cre). These mice were backcrossed to homozygote floxed mice in the following cross: EFNB2$^{fl/+}$, Cre X EFNB2$^{fl/fl}$, to generate mice with both alleles inactivated in chondrocytes (genotype: EFNB2$^{fl/fl}$, Cre), and EFNB2$^{fl/fl}$ mice without Cre transgene were used as control mice. Such breeding results in wild type, and heterozygote and homozygote knockout (EFNB2^{Col2}KO) mice. The study used the homozygote EFNB2^{Col2}KO and the EFNB2$^{fl/fl}$ as controls.

The offspring of the breeding animals were genotyped using PCR analysis. The EFNB2^{Col2}KO cartilage conditional mice were born at the expected Mendelian frequencies.

The transgenic mouse genotype was determined by PCR analyses of genomic DNA isolated from ear biopsies as previously described [15, 16]. The EFNB2^{Col2}KO were identified using the following primers: forward 5′-TCATTTCCCAACCACCGCCAGAAA-3′ and reverse 5′-AGATACCACGCCAGGAGAGCAAAT-3′ for EFNB2; forward 5′-GCATTACCGGTCGATGCAACGAGTGAT GAG-3′ and reverse 5′-GAGTGAACGAACCTGGTC GAAATCAGTGCG-3′ for Cre recombinase; and forward 5′-AGATACCACGCCAGGAGAGCAAAT-3′ and reverse 5′-GCGCACGGAGTTGGGTCTCG-3′ for EFNB2 exon 1 deletion. Schematic representation of the EFNB2 knockout construct and primer design are illustrated in Fig. 1a.

The presence of the Cre transgene in postnatal day zero (P0) heterozygous and homozygous knockout mice and its absence in wild type mice were detected by the EFNB2 floxed band at 552 base pairs (bp), the wild type at 450 bp, Cre at 700 bp, and the EFNB2 exon 1 deletion at 550 bp (Fig. 1b). EFNB2$^{fl/fl}$ mice without the Cre transgene were used as control mice. Homozygous mice were compared to control at birth (P0) and on postnatal days P15 and P21, and at 8 weeks and 1 year old.

Skeletal staining
Skeletal staining was processed in newborn mouse cadavers as described [17].

Radiographic, bone mineral density and morphometric determinations
High resolution full body radiographic images were obtained using a Kubtec XPERT 80 Digital Cabinet X-ray System with a geometric magnification of × 1 and a resolution of 5 μm (KUB Technologies Inc., Milford, CT, USA). The mouse radiographs were obtained in the ventrodorsal projection with the limbs in abduction (frog-legged position) and a standard ventrodorsal projection with the limbs extended.

The bone mineral density (BMD) was determined using a Lunar PixiMUS 1.46 (GE Lunar Corporation, Madison, WI, USA). The morphometric analyses, including the bone length and hip bone measurements, were performed directly on the acquired images using a calibrated program of the BIOQUANT OSTEO II Image Analysis Software (BIOQUANT Image Analysis Corporation, Nashville, TN, USA).

Other analyses included mouse weight and length at P0, P15 and P21, and long bone measurements of the tibia, femur and humerus at P0 and P15. These measurements were performed directly on freshly dissected

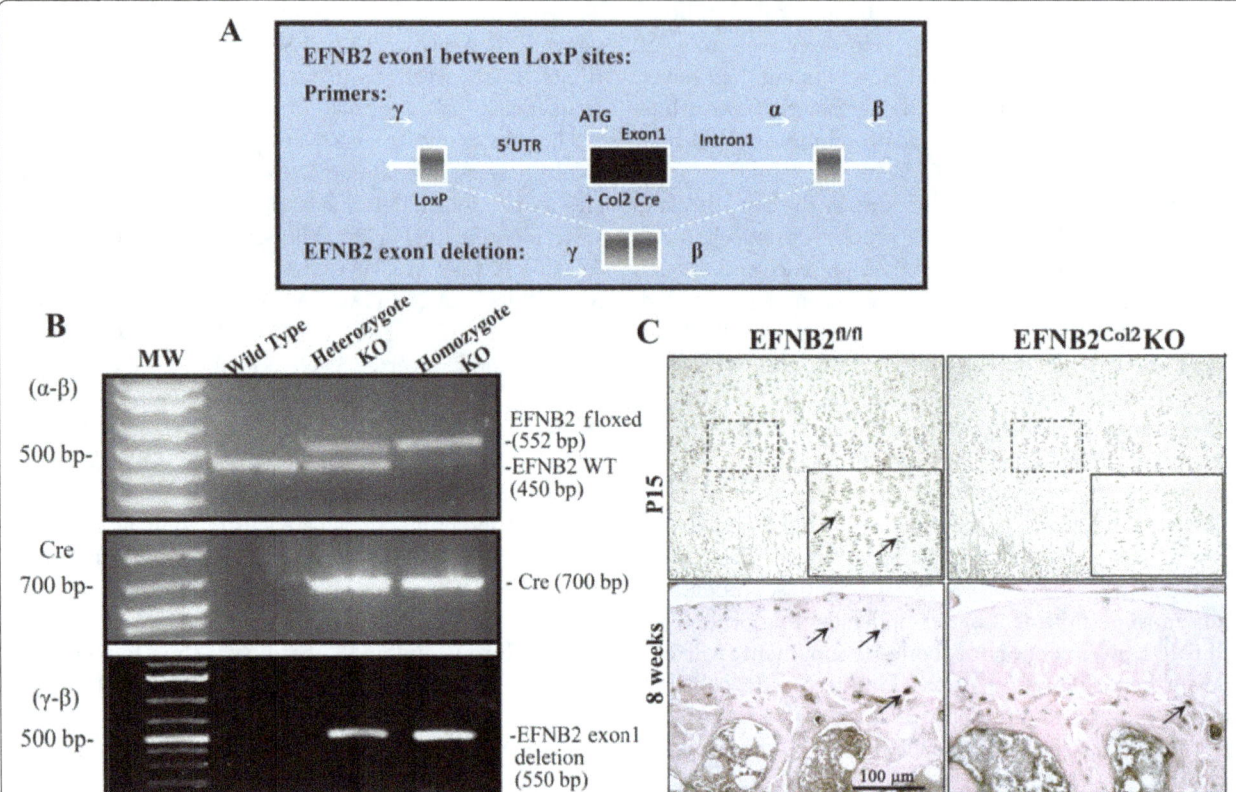

Fig. 1 Genetically modified mice harboring a cartilage-specific deletion of ephrin-B2 (*EFNB2*) were generated using the Cre Lox methodology. **a** Schematic representation of the EFNB2 knockout construct and primer design for the LoxP insertion in the EFNB2 gene (α-β) and EFNB2 exon 1 deletion (γ-β). **b** Representative genotyping that detects LoxP insertion in EFNB2 (552 base pairs (bp)), the presence of Cre transgene (700 bp) and EFNB2 exon 1 deletion (550 bp) in heterozygous (n = 8) and homozygous knockout (KO) (n = 8) mice at postnatal day zero (P0) (birth) and their absence in wild type (n = 8) mice assessed by PCR. *MW* molecular weight, *KO* knockout **c** Representative EFNB2 immunohistological staining of the tibial growth plate at P15 (n = 4) counterstained with methyl green, and of tibial cartilage and subchondral bone at 8 weeks old (n = 4) counterstained with hematoxylin and eosin. Immunohistological original magnification × 250 and insets × 400. *Dotted-line boxes* indicate the location of the insets; *scale bar* 100 μm; *arrows* indicate positive-stained cells

bones using digital calipers (model 2071 M; Mitutoyo Corporation, Kawasaki, Japan).

Micro-computed tomography (μCT)

The left femora of 8-week-old mice were dissected free of tissue, fixed as above and the distal metaphysis scanned with a SKYSCAN 1176 in vivo μCT instrument as described [15]. For the trabecular bone, 100 reconstructed grayscale images were selected from immediately below the tibial and femoral growth plate, and a 3D analysis was used to calculate morphometric parameters, including the bone volume (% bone volume/total volume), trabecular thickness (μm), trabecular number (l/mm) and trabecular separation (mm) at the same threshold with the 3D-Creator software supplied with the instrument.

Pelvic and hip acetabular evaluations

Mice at 8 weeks and 1 year old were evaluated for hip dysplasia from the acquired μCT images by measuring

the acetabular rim length (ARL, mm), the dorsal acetabular rim angle (DARA, angle degrees) and the acetabular angle (AA, angle degrees) [18]. Values were manually acquired on selected 2D μCT images by two independent observers who were blinded to group allocation. The ARL and the DARA of the right and left acetabula were measured and averaged.

Histological, histochemical and immunohistochemical analysis

The dissected right long bones were fixed in 4 % paraformaldehyde for 16 h at 4 °C, decalcified in RDO Rapid Decalcifier (Apex Engineering, Plainfield, IL, USA), and embedded in paraffin, as described [15]. Deparaffinized sections (5 μm) were stained with Safranin *O*/fast green (Sigma-Aldrich, Oakville, ON, Canada) and assessed by the BIOQUANT OSTEO II Image Analysis Software. Briefly, a region of 500 μm under the growth plate was selected and the total area was measured. In the same region, the mineralized cartilage matrix (in red) was selected by the color intensity, the area measured, and the ratio calculated.

Immunohistochemical analysis was performed on 5-μm paraffin sections, decalcified in 10 % ethylenediamine tetraacetic acid (EDTA) for 14 days at 4 °C. Briefly, sections were pretreated with 0.25 units/ml of protease-free chondroitinase ABC in phosphate-buffered saline (PBS) (Sigma-Aldrich, St. Louis, MO, USA) for 60 minutes at 37 °C. The specimens were incubated for 18 h at 4 °C with the following primary polyclonal antibodies; rabbit anti-EFNB2 (1:50 dilution; Santa Cruz Biotechnology, Dallas, TX, USA), rabbit anti-type II collagen (1:30 dilution; EMD Millipore, Billerica, MA, USA), mouse anti-proliferating cell nuclear antigen (PCNA) (1:500 dilution; Abcam, Cambridge, MA, USA), rabbit anti-vascular endothelial growth factor (VEGF) (1:1500 dilution; Abcam) and rabbit anti-type X collagen (1:100 dilution; provided by Dr E. Lee, Shriners Hospital for Children, McGill University Hospital Centre, Montreal, QC, Canada) [19]. Each slide was washed three times in PBS (pH 7.4) and incubated with a secondary biotinylated antibody (anti-mouse, or anti-rabbit when appropriate) (Vector Laboratories Inc., Burlingame, CA, USA), then processed using the Vectastain ABC kit (Vector Laboratories) following the manufacturer's instructions. The color was developed with 3,3'-diaminobenzidine (DAB) containing hydrogen peroxide, and slides were counterstained with methyl green.

Control procedures were performed according to the same experimental protocol as follows: 1) omission of the primary antibody and 2) substitution of the primary antibody with a nonspecific immunoglobulin from the same host as the primary antibody (Santa Cruz Biotechnology).

Tartrate resistant acid phosphatase (TRAP) detection was performed on paraffin sections, decalcified in 10 % EDTA for 14 days at 4 °C. Sections were stained for enzyme activity and processed as described [20] and counterstaining was performed with 0.4 % methyl green. Negative staining was performed without substrate and for all antibodies IgG controls displayed only background staining.

For the calcium deposition, freshly dissected left-side long bones were fixed as above and embedded in glycidyl methacrylate (GMA) plastic. Sections (2 μm) were stained using the von Kossa method with 5 % silver nitrate for 30 minutes under ultraviolet light, and with 0.2 % toluidine blue to determine trabecular bone thickness and bone volume. Histomorphometric data were obtained using BIOQUANT OSTEO II Image Analysis software.

To determine the number of TRAP-, VEGF- and type X collagen-positive cells the chondro-osseous junction area comprising the hypertrophic chondrocyte zone and the cartilage bone junction as the upper and lower limits

was evaluated. Hence, for type X collagen, the area analyzed comprised a box of 300×100 μm in the hypertrophic chondrocyte zone close to the chondro-osseous junction. The staining intensity of the total hypertrophic zone was assessed on one section/specimen using a Leitz Diaplan microscope (Leica Microsystems) connected to BIOQUANT OSTEO II Image Analysis software [15].

Knee and hip cartilage evaluation

At one year old, the knee and hip joints were evaluated. Sagittal sections (5 μm) from the mid-medial tibiofemoral joint were stained with Safranin O/fast green as described [15]. Cartilage was assessed using the Osteoarthritis Research Society International (OARSI) scoring system (knee) [21] and the modified Mankin system (hip) [22]. For the synovial membrane, histomorphometric quantitative analysis of the anterior synovial membrane thickness was performed as described [16]. Images were captured at $\times 63$ with a Leitz Diaplan microscope coupled to a personal computer, and histomorphometric data determined with BIOQUANT OSTEO II Image Analysis Software; data are expressed as μm. The anterior synovial membrane lining hyperplasia was graded on a scale of 0–2, where 0 = absence, 1 = hyperplasia of lining <50 % of the surface, and 2 = hyperplasia of lining >50 % of the surface, as described [23].

For both the cartilage and the synovial membrane, two independent observers graded the severity of the tissue, blinded to group allocation. Three sections were made from each block, each slide was examined, and the final score was a consensus between the two observations.

Tracing of the corticospinal tract
Surgical procedures and tracer injections

Surgical procedures and tracer injections were performed on 6-week-old EFNB2^{Col2}KO and control mice anesthetized with a mixture of ketamine (70 mg/kg IP, Ketalar; Pfizer, New York, NY, USA) and xylazine (3 mg/kg IP; Sigma-Aldrich). Mice were placed in a stereotaxic frame and transitioned to an inhalation anesthetic, isoflurane (approximately 2 %) in 100 % oxygen, delivered via a custom-made facial mask as described [24]. After the EFNB2^{Col2}KO and control mice were anesthetized, two small holes were made in the skull bone overlying the left primary motor cortex, based on stereotaxic coordinates (0.0, +1 mm anteroposterior, +1.5 mm mediolateral to the bregma). In each hole, 1 μl of the anterograde tracer biotinylated dextran amine (BDA; molecular weight (MW) 10,000, 5 % in saline solution; Invitrogen) was pressure injected with a Hamilton syringe and a microsyringe pump controller (Harvard Apparatus, Holliston, MA, USA). Tracer (1 μl) was injected in three boluses at different depths to create a column that labeled all layers of the gray matter. First, 500 nl was injected at a depth of 2,500 μm from the top of the skull. After a 2-minute rest period to favor the absorption of the tracer by the tissue, a second bolus of 300 nl was injected at 2,000 μm, again followed by a 2-minute rest period. A third bolus of 200 nl was injected at 1,500 μm, followed by a 5-minute rest period. Following injections into the two holes, mice received buprenorphine hydrochloride (0.05 mg/ml IP, Temgesic) and their recovery was monitored during a period of 2 h post surgery. They were then returned to their home cage and given access to food and water *ad libitum*. The mice were sacrificed 14 days after the injections of BDA. They were transcardially perfused with 0.1 M PBS, followed by 4 % paraformaldehyde in 0.1 M PBS. The cervical spinal cords were dissected and post fixed (20 % sucrose, 4 % paraformaldehyde solution in 0.1 M PBS for 2 h; 20 % sucrose, 2 % dimethyl sulfoxide (DMSO) in 0.1 M PBS for 24 h; and 20 % sucrose for 48 h or until the tissues sank). The cervical cord specimens (C4–C7) were quickly frozen at −55 °C with methyl butane, embedded with optimum cutting temperature compound (OCT, Tissue-Tek, Sakura Finetek USA Inc., Torrance, CA, USA) and frozen at −80 °C until sectioning. Transverse sections between C4 and C7 were cut with a cryostat (20 μm thickness). One out of three sections was stained for BDA and used to quantify the number of synaptic boutons.

Tissue processing

Tissue processing, in which the BDA staining was revealed, was carried out according to the protocol of Dancause et al. [25]. In brief, after sectioning, the tissues were rinsed in cold 0.05 M potassium phosphate buffer in saline solution (KPBS), treated with 0.4 % Triton X-100 in 0.05 M KPBS and rinsed again in 0.05 M KPBS. They were then incubated overnight in avidin-biotin (ABC) solution (two drops of solution A and B per 5 ml of 0.05 KPBS; Vectastain Elite ABC kit; Vector Laboratories, Burlingame, CA, USA). The following day, following four rinses with 0.1 M KPBS, the tissue was incubated in fresh 0.05 % DAB 0.015 % H_2O_2 in KPBS solution for 5–10 minutes. After three additional rinses in 0.1 M KPBS, the sections were mounted on subbed slides and dried overnight. DAB staining was intensified the following day. Sections were dehydrated in ascending alcohol solutions, transferred to xylene, rehydrated and incubated in a 1.42 % $AgNO_3$ solution for 1 h at 56 °C. They were then passed through H_2O (15 minutes), 0.2 % $HAuCl_4$ (10 minutes), 5 % $Na_2S_2O_3$ (5 minutes) and H_2O (15 minutes). Finally, they were dehydrated again followed by xylene and coverslipped the next day. Other sections were either Nissl stained with Cresyl violet to reveal spinal cord architecture (1/3) or kept for future staining (1/3).

Image capture and quantitative analysis of BDA

Image capture and quantitative analysis of BDA was performed as described [26]. In brief, the tissue was examined using a BX51 light microscope (Olympus, Tokyo, Japan). Photographs were digitally captured using an MBF CX9000 digital camera (MicroBrightField, Colchester, VT, USA) with a resolution of 1600 × 1200 active pixels and images imported to Adobe Photoshop CS5. A neuroanatomical reconstruction system, consisting of a computer-interfaced motorized stage mounted on a microscope and associated software (Neurolucida; MicroBrightField), was used to reconstruct sections stained for BDA and to quantify the number of labeled boutons at the C4–C7 levels. The most rostral section of the block to be reconstructed was randomly chosen. Then, one section out of every six BDA-stained sections was reconstructed up to a total of ten sections. A varicosity was considered to be a terminal bouton if it appeared as a small, darkly labeled sphere contacting a small fiber as described [26]. To quantify the number of labeled boutons within each hemisphere of the spinal cord, we examined the tissue using a grid pattern (100 × 100 μm) overlaid on the section image. If at least two synaptic boutons were located within a square of the grid, a marker was placed in the center of the square. Following inspection of the entire gray matter, the numbers of positive squares in each hemisphere were compared.

Statistical analysis

Values are expressed as mean ± standard error of the mean (SEM). Statistical analysis was performed using the Mann–Whitney U test (GraphPad Prism software, GraphPad, San Diego, CA, USA).

Results

Characterization of EFNB2^{Col2}KO cartilage conditional mice

The genotyping demonstrated the presence of the Cre transgene in P0 heterozygous and homozygous knockout mice and its absence in wild type mice (Fig. 1b). To confirm the cartilage specific deletion, immunohistochemical analysis using a specific EFNB2 antibody was performed on the tibiae at P15 and at 8 weeks old. EFNB2 was present in the cartilage of the control (EFNB2$^{fl/fl}$) and absent in the EFNB2^{Col2}KO (Fig. 1c). Of note, EFNB2 was present in the subchondral bone of both the EFNB2$^{fl/fl}$ and EFNB2^{Col2}KO mice (Fig. 1c).

Reduction in growth of EFNB2^{Col2}KO mice

In newborn litters EFNB2^{Col2}KO were smaller in size compared to control mice (Fig. 2a). The delayed pattern was observed in both genders but only data on male animals are presented in this article.

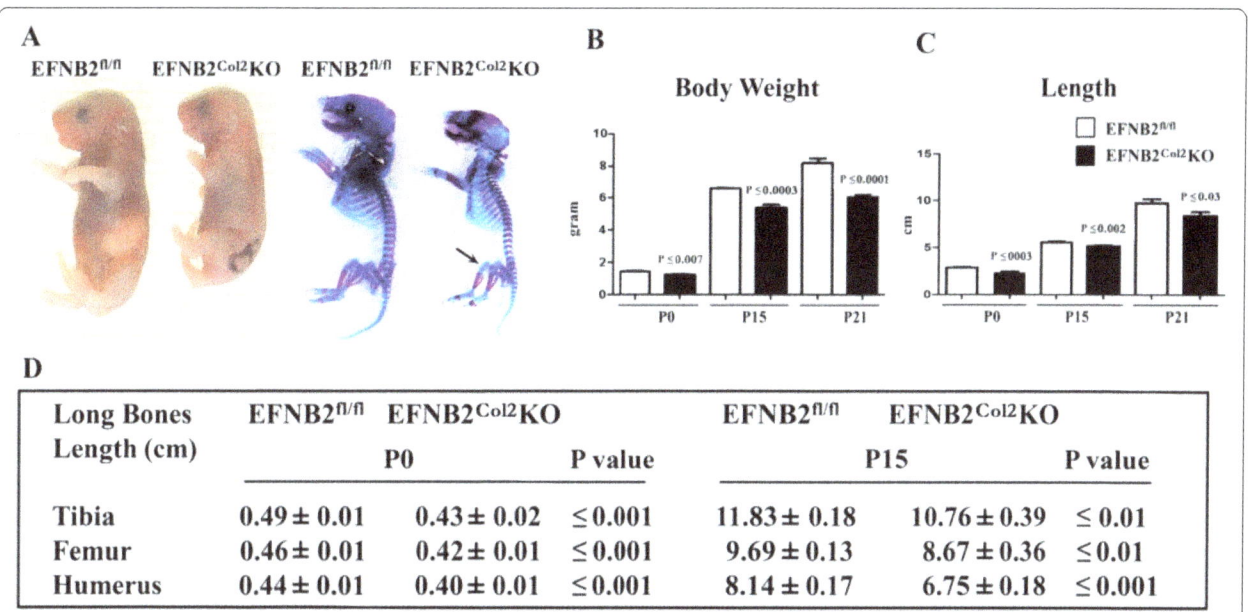

Fig. 2 Macroscopy and morphological assessments of male ephrin-B2 (*EFNB2*)$^{fl/fl}$ and EFNB2^{Col2}knockout (*KO*) cartilage conditional mice. **a** Representative mascroscopic and histochemical results of EFNB2$^{fl/fl}$ (n = 6) and EFNB2^{Col2}KO cartilage conditional (n = 6) mice at postnatal day zero (*P0*) (birth) showing that the latter displayed reduced growth and skeletal development. *Arrow* indicates thinner stained region in the EFNB2^{Col2}KO. Histograms show body weight (**b**) and length (**c**) of EFNB2$^{fl/fl}$ and EFNB2^{Col2}KO cartilage conditional mice at P0 (n = 8 and n = 9, respectively), P15 (n = 10 and n = 8) and P21 (n = 13 and n = 11). **d** Morphometric analysis of long bone length of EFNB2$^{fl/fl}$ and EFNB2^{Col2}KO cartilage conditional mice at P0 and P15 (n = 8–13). Data are expressed as mean ± standard error of the mean and *P* values were determined by Mann–Whitney *U* test

Skeletal staining confirmed the reduced growth in the homozygote EFNB2^{Col2}KO mice compared to controls at birth, and there was less skeletal staining in some regions of the limbs of mutant mice than in the control mice (Fig. 2a).

Morphometric analysis at P0, P15 and P21 showed that the EFNB2^{Col2}KO mice displayed a significant reduction in body weight and length (Fig. 2b, c) when compared with control mice. In addition, on measurement of individual long bones at P0 and P15 there was a significant reduction in the long bone length (tibia, femur and humerus) in the EFNB2^{Col2}KO mice (Fig. 2d). At P21, 8 weeks and 1 year, the EFNB2^{Col2}KO mice had significantly smaller tibiae ($P \leq 0.03$, $P \leq 0.01$, and $P \leq 0.02$, respectively) and femora ($P \leq 0.03$, $P \leq 0.03$, and $P \leq 0.04$) compared with their controls.

Impaired angiogenesis and delayed cartilage resorption in EFNB2^{Col2}KO mice

As bone length is determined in part by the activity of the growth plate during endochondral bone formation, we further examined the growth plate morphology in the EFNB2^{Col2}KO mice. At P0, EFNB2^{Col2}KO mice had abnormalities at the growth plates of appendicular bones (tibia, femur and humerus); there was a disorganized hypertrophic cartilage zone with no difference in the reserve or proliferating zones.

Type II collagen is the principal collagen laid down by proliferating, non-hypertrophic chondrocytes, whereas type X collagen production is restricted to hypertrophic cells in the epiphyseal cartilage. There were no differences in type II collagen (Fig. 3a, b) or the proliferation marker, PCNA (data not shown), implying that early stages of chondrocyte development were not affected by the lack of EFNB2. However, type X collagen immunostaining displayed disorganized hypertrophic chondrocyte columns (Fig. 3c-f) with increased staining ($P < 0.03$) accompanied by a decrease in mineralized cartilage matrix ($P < 0.007$) (Fig. 3g-j) at the chondro-osseous junction, which was also observed at P15 ($P < 0.03$). In addition, P15 EFNB2^{Col2}KO mice had a delay at the secondary center of ossification (Fig. 3k, l) and significantly decreased VEGF staining (Fig. 4a-c). The disturbed vascularization was associated with alterations in bone mineralization; the percentage of bone volume/tissue volume and the trabecular thickness were also significantly reduced in the EFNB2^{Col2}KO mice compared to controls (Fig. 4d-f).

The terminal stage of hypertrophic chondrocyte development is associated with invasion and resorption of the calcified cartilage core. Given the delay in calcification in the EFNB2^{Col2}KO mice, we further investigated whether the lack of EFNB2 disturbed the cartilage resorption process. The recruitment of and invasion by TRAP-positive cells was significantly

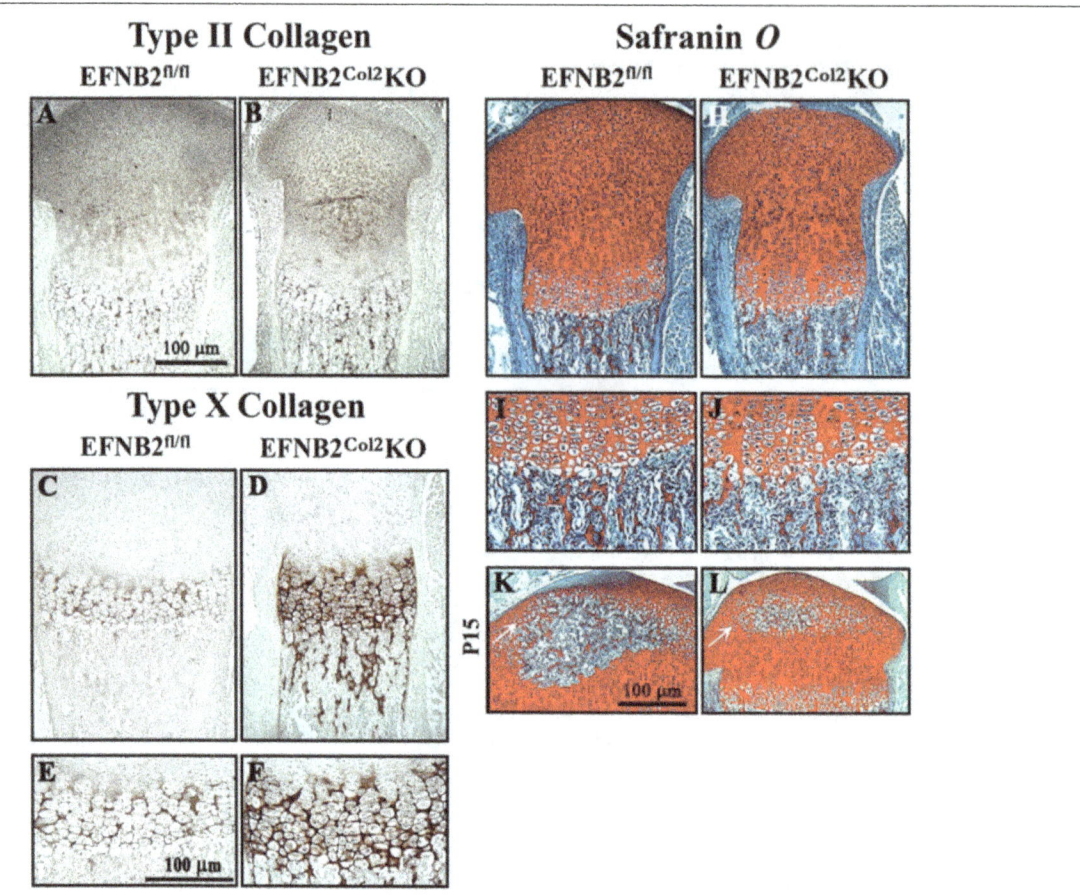

Fig. 3 Immunohistochemical localization of type II collagen, type X collagen and Safranin *O* in epiphyseal cartilage. Representative immunohistological sections of ephrin-B2 (*EFNB2*)$^{fl/fl}$ (n = 7) and EFNB2^{Col2}knockout (*KO*) cartilage conditional (n = 7) mice at postnatal day zero (P0) (birth) for type II collagen (**a-b**), type X collagen (**c-f**) and Safranin *O* (**g-l**) of the entire epiphyseal cartilage. **e, f** Higher magnification of **c** and **d**. **i, j** Higher magnification of **g** and **h**. The secondary center of ossification at P15 is indicated by *white arrows* (**k** and **l**). **a-f** Slides were counterstained with methyl green. Original magnification × 250 (**a-d, g, h, k, l**) and × 400 (**e, f, i, j**). *Scale bars* at 100 μm (**a, e, k**)

reduced in the EFNB2^{Col2}KO mice compared to controls (Fig. 4g-i).

Postnatal bone abnormalities in EFNB2^{Col2}KO mice

Macroscopic and radiographic assessments at P21 showed reduced body size of EFNB2^{Col2}KO mice (Fig. 5a). Although no bone deformities were found in the EFNB2^{Col2}KO mice, osteopenia was observed in the long bones (Fig. 5a). BMD analysis (Fig. 5b) showed that EFNB2^{Col2}KO mice had a significant reduction in the BMD of the whole body, femoral head, and lumbar vertebrae L4 and L5 at P21 and 8 weeks. At 1 year, although BMD values were lower for each of the bones studied, only for the femoral head BMD was statistically significant.

μCT of the femur and tibia in the 8-week-old EFNB2^{Col2}KO mice showed a statistically significant reduction in the mineralized tissue (about 35 %, as evaluated by the % bone volume/tissue volume) (Fig. 5c, d). Trabecular number and thickness in the proximal tibia were

also significantly decreased with an increase in trabecular separation compared to control (Fig. 5d). Similar differences were observed in the distal femur with the exception of trabecular number (Fig. 5c). Histological sections of the proximal tibia confirmed μCT data revealing thinner trabeculae and an increase in the trabecular separation (Fig. 5e). This decrease in mineralized tissue in the EFNB2^{Col2}KO could be the result of improper cartilage matrix degradation caused by EFNB2 deficiency in late hypertrophic chondrocytes.

Osteoarthritis (OA) phenotypic features in aged EFNB2^{Col2}KO mice

One-year-old EFNB2^{Col2}KO mice demonstrated OA phenotypic features associated with cartilage degeneration in both the knee and hip (Fig. 6). Radiologically, EFNB2^{Col2}KO mice exhibited a collapse of the joint with decreased joint space (Fig. 6a, b). Histological analysis of both the knee (medial tibia and condyle) and the proximal femoral condyle showed that EFNB2^{Col2}KO mice

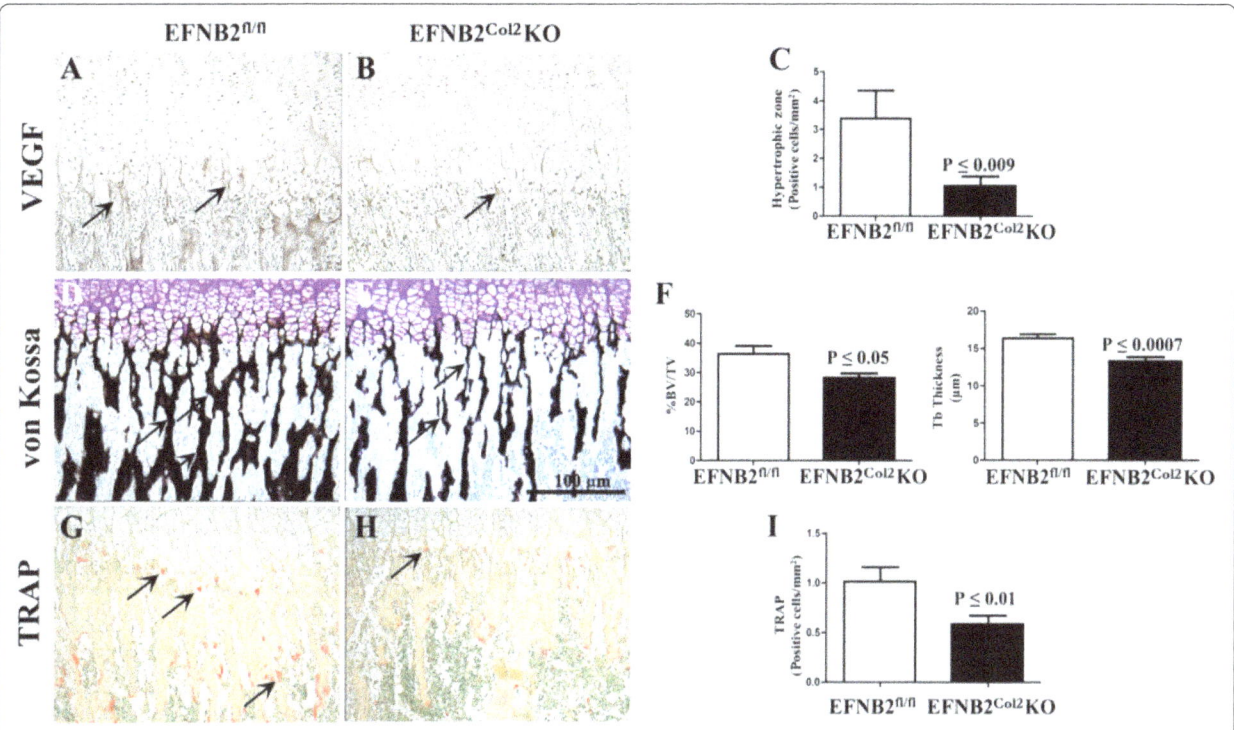

Fig. 4 Impaired vascularization of ephrin-B2 (*EFNB2*)^Col2^knockout (*KO*) cartilage conditional mice at postnatal day P15. Representative immunohistochemical and histochemical sections of proximal tibia, and histograms of EFNB2^fl/fl^ (n = 7) and EFNB2^Col2^KO cartilage conditional (n = 7) mice at P15 for vascular endothelial growth factor (*VEGF*) (**a-c**)), von Kossa (**d-f**) and tartrate resistant alkaline phosphatase (*TRAP*) (**g-i**). Sections were counterstained with methyl green. Original magnification × 400. **e** *Scale bar* at 100 μm. **f** *%BV/TV* % bone volume/tissue volume, *Tb Thickness* trabecular thickness. *Arrows* indicate positive staining (**a**, **b**, **g**, **h**) and trabecular thickness (**d**, **e**). Data are expressed as the mean ± standard error of the mean and *P* values were determined using the Mann–Whitney *U* test

had increased cartilage degradation with a loss of Safranin *O*, reduced cellularity and thinning of the cartilage (Fig. 6c-i). As synovial membrane also demonstrated alterations during the OA process, we further assessed the effects of cartilage-specific EFNB2 deletion on this tissue in 1-year-old mice. The synovial thickness was significantly greater in the knee in the EFNB2^Col2^KO mice (43.4 μm ± 5.6) than in the control mice (113.7 μm ± 27.2) (*P* ≤0.02) and in the hip (86.9 μm ± 5.9 compared to 143.3 μm ± 18.5, respectively) (*P* ≤0.03). There were no significant differences in the synovial lining cells between EFNB2^Col2^KO and the control mice.

Some EFNB2^Col2^KO mice exhibit a locomotor phenotype related to an abnormal corticospinal tract

A surprising feature of the EFNB2^Col2^KO mice was a locomotor phenotype observed in about 27 % of this mouse population, which appeared as soon as the mice started to walk at 2–3 weeks of age. It consisted of a lack of unilateral hip motor control yielding a simultaneous movement of the right and left limbs, resulting in a hopping gait (Fig. 7), unlike the alternate step gait displayed by control mice. Additional movie files show this in more detail (see Additional file 1 and Additional file 2).

The EFNB2^Col2^KO long bone developmental abnormalities could not account for the observed locomotor phenotype. However, the EFNB2^Col2^KO mice had a significantly (*P* ≤0.01) smaller pelvic bone at 8 weeks compared to controls, but not at 1 year (data not shown). We then further investigated the possibility of abnormal development of the hip joint. μCT of the EFNB2^Col2^KO proximal femoral head of the acetabular rim angle, acetabular angle and acetabular rim length of 8-week-old and 1-year-old mice did not differ from controls (Fig. 8), suggesting that the EFNB2^Col2^KO mice did not have any hip joint abnormalities that could explain the locomotor phenotype.

The above finding indicates that a cause other than the hip development is responsible for the EFNB2^Col2^KO locomotor phenotype. A search of the literature revealed that this locomotor phenotype resembles those reported for mice lacking the EFNB3 ligand or its receptor EphA4 [27–30]. This defect has been related to a critical role played by these factors in establishing corticospinal projection, in which the lack of unilateral control results from an embryonic midline abnormality involving the corticospinal tract [28, 29]. This points to the possibility that the EFNB2^Col2^KO mice might have had

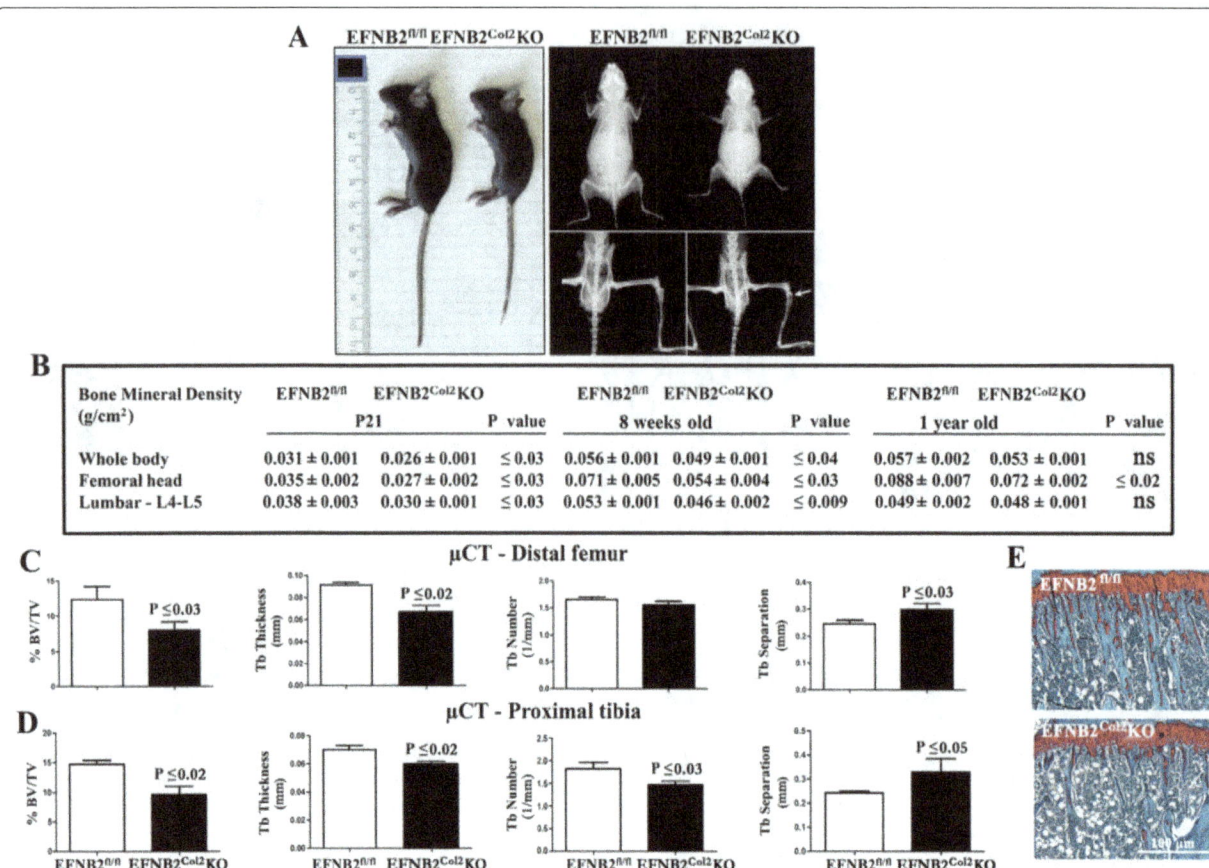

Fig. 5 Bone abnormalities of the ephrin-B2 (*EFNB2*)^Col2 knockout (*KO*) cartilage conditional mice. **a** Representative macroscopic and radiographic EFNB2^fl/fl (n = 6) and EFNB2^Col2KO cartilage conditional (n = 6) mice at postnatal day P21. In the radiographs, the lower portion of EFNB2^Col2KO cartilage conditional mice shows osteopenia (*arrow*) compared to EFNB2^fl/fl mice. **b** Bone mineral density measurements of EFNB2^fl/fl and EFNB2^Col2KO cartilage conditional mice at P21, 8 weeks and 1 year (n = 8–10 for each category). Micro-computed tomography (μCT) analysis of the distal femur (**c**) and proximal tibia (**d**) (n = 8) at 8 weeks. **e** Representative histological sections of the proximal tibia stained with Safranin *O*; original magnification × 400, *scale bar* at 100 μm. % *BV/TV*o % bone volume/tissue volume, *Tb* trabecular thickness. Data are expressed as mean ± standard error of the mean and the *P* values were determined by Mann–Whitney *U* test

abnormalities in the cortical tract even though the deletion was conditional to type II collagen.

We then looked at the corticospinal tract axons of the mice with the locomotor phenotype. To visualize the path taken by the corticospinal tract axons, we performed anterograde axon tracing experiments by injecting a tracer into one side of the motor cortex and observing the terminal projections in the spinal cord. Compared to the control mice, there was a dramatic difference in the path of EFNB2^Col2KO mouse corticospinal axons on entering the spinal dorsal gray matter. In the control mice, projections into the gray matter remained confined to the contralateral gray matter, never crossing the midline, as shown in cervical sections (Fig. 9a, c, d). In contrast, the corticospinal tract projections of EFNB2^Col2KO mice clearly crossed over the midline into the ipsilateral gray matter (Fig. 9b, e, f). Indeed, in the control mice, a high level of labeled fibers was visible in the hemisphere contralateral to the injection site, which

is close to the midline (Fig. 9a, c), whereas few labeled fibers were found in the ipsilateral hemisphere (Fig. 9d). In contrast, the EFNB2^Col2KO mice exhibited labeled fibers in both hemispheres (contralateral and ipsilateral) (Fig. 9b, e, f), which, compared to the control mice, were significantly fewer in the contralateral hemisphere but more numerous in the ipsilateral hemisphere (Fig. 9g). These neuroanatomical findings suggest that the locomotive phenotype was due to a neurological defect in corticospinal projections.

Discussion

In this study, we investigated the role of EFNB2 during endochondral bone development and its effect on adult articular cartilage integrity, by generating cartilage-specific EFNB2 KO mice. This model was chosen because global deletion of EFNB2 in mice leads to embryonic lethality [9, 10]. This study is the first to show that EFNB2 is essential for postnatal skeletal growth, as

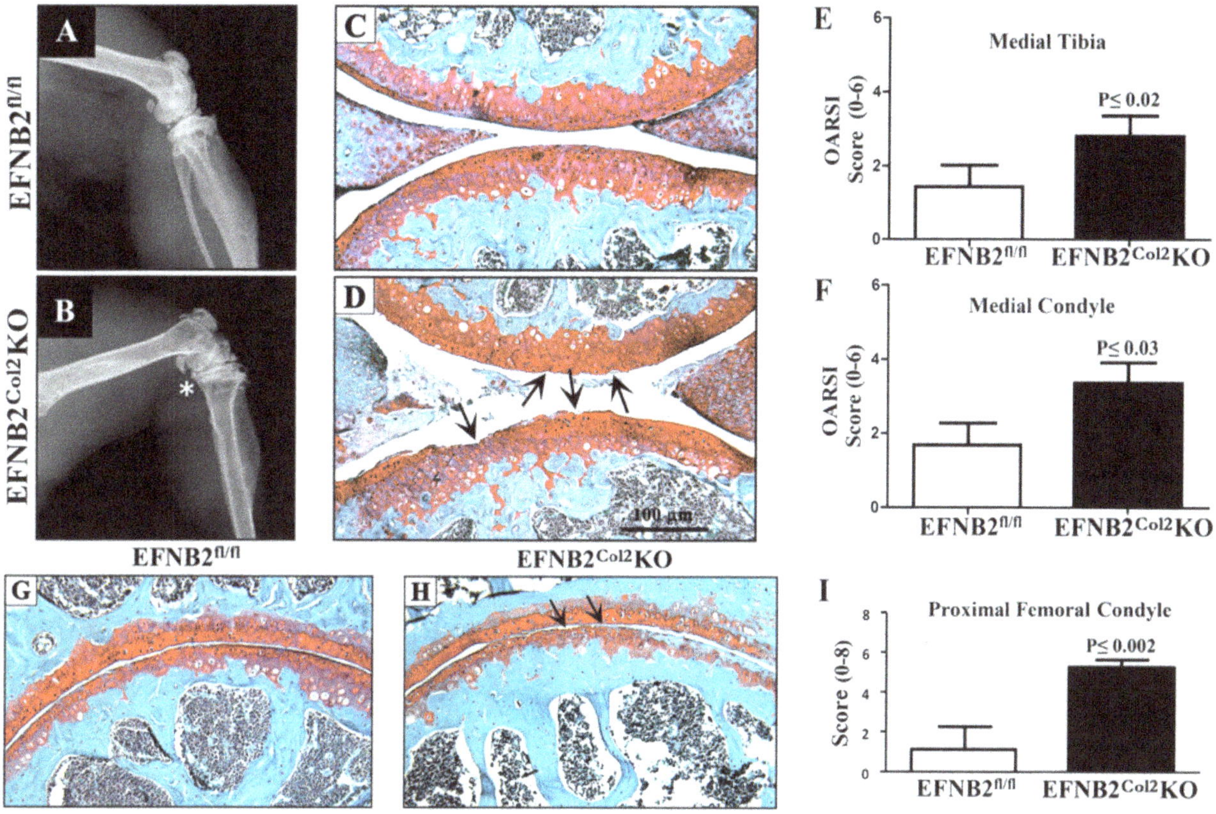

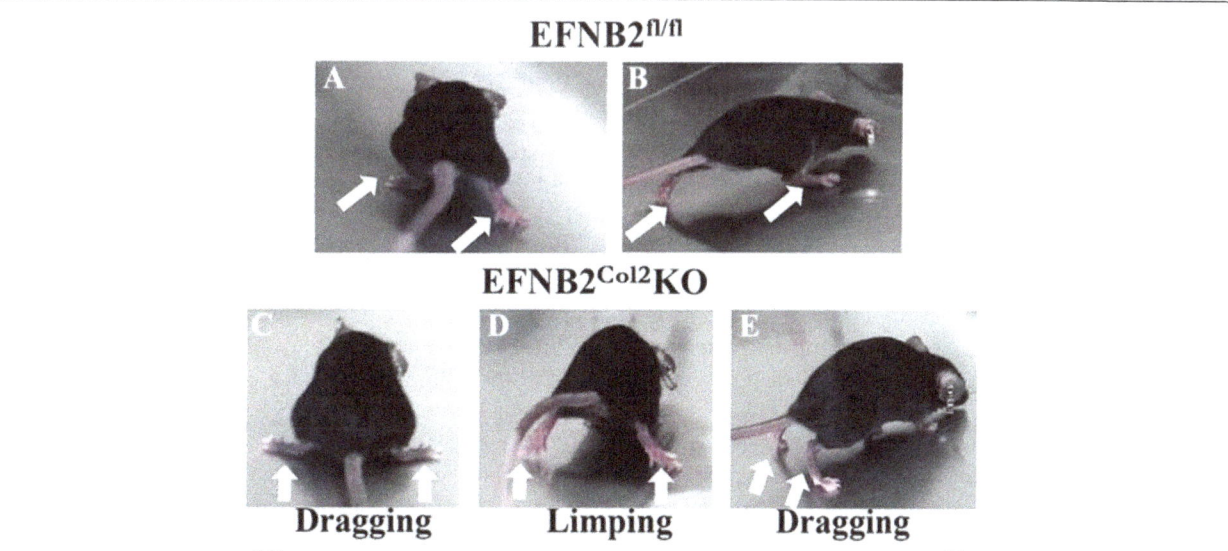

Fig. 6 Osteoarthritis features in ephrin-B2 (*EFNB2*)^Col2 knockout (*KO*) cartilage conditional mice at 1 year old. Representative radiographs (**a**, **b**) and histological sections (**c**, **d**) of the knee joint of EFNB2^fl/fl (n = 8) and EFNB2^Col2KO cartilage conditional (n = 8) mice stained with Safranin *O*/fast green. Histograms show Osteoarthritis Research Society International (*OARSI*) scoring of the medial tibia (**e**) and medial condyle (**f**). **g**, **h** Histological sections of the hip joint stained with Safranin *O*/fast green. **i** Hip scoring according to the modified Mankin system. *Decrease in the joint space (**b**). *Scale bar* at 100 μm (**d**). *Arrows* indicate cartilage degradation (**d**, **h**). Histological sections at original magnification × 100. Data are expressed as the mean ± standard error of the mean and *P* values were determined by Mann–Whitney *U* test

Fig. 7 Some ephrin-B2 (*EFNB2*)^Col2 knockout (*KO*) cartilage conditional mice exhibited a locomotor phenotype. EFNB2^fl/fl (**a**, **b**) and about 27 % of the EFNB2^Col2KO cartilage conditional mice (**c-e**) demonstrated a locomotor phenotype consisting of dragging and limping as soon as they started to walk. Additional movie files show the locomotor phenotype in more detail (see Additional file 1 (EFNB2^fl/fl) and Additional file 2 (EFNB2^Col2KO))

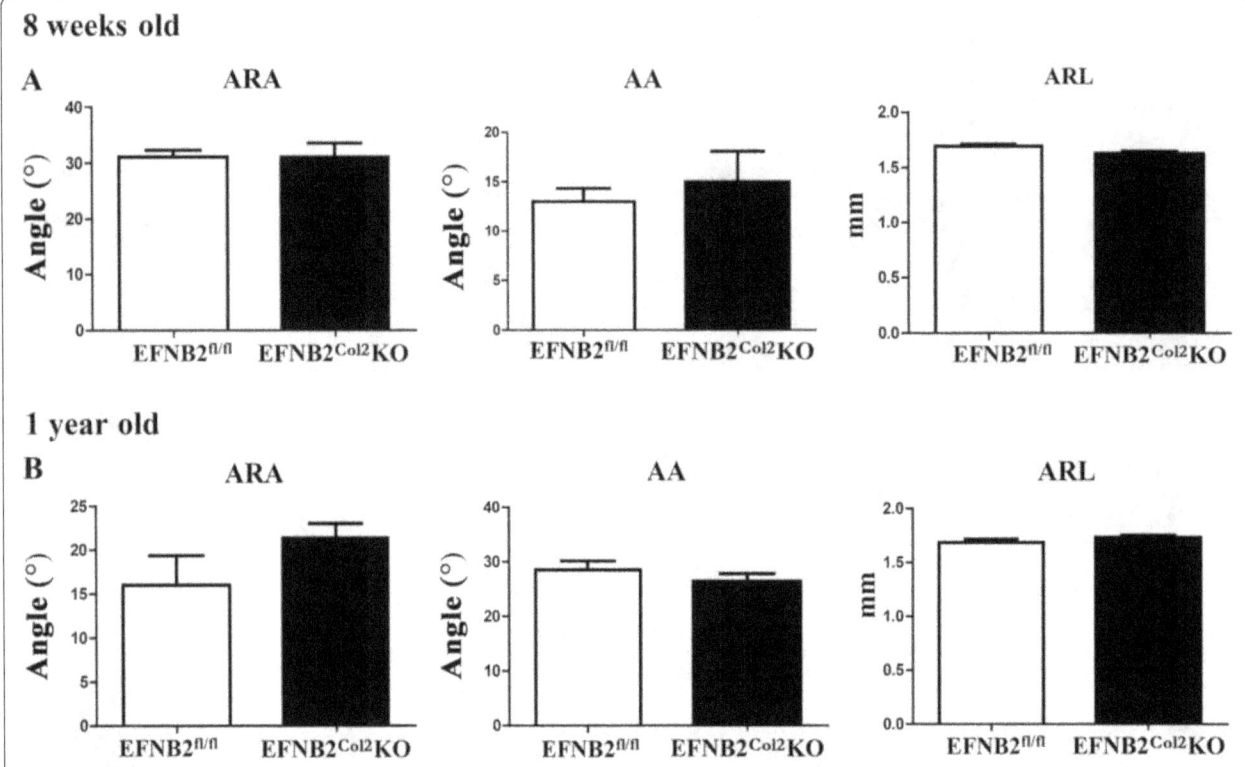

Fig. 8 Micro-computed tomography evaluations of the proximal femoral head of the acetabular rim angle, acetabular angle and acetabular rim length of the ephrin-B2 (*EFNB2*)^{Col2}knockout (*KO*) mice with a locomotor phenotype at both 8 weeks of age and 1 year. **a** Acetabular rim angle (*ARA*), acetabular angle (*AA*) and acetabular rim length (*ARL*) of EFNB2^{Col2}KO and EFNB2$^{fl/fl}$ (n = 5 and 4, respectively) at 8 weeks and **b** at 1 year (n = 5 for both groups). Data are expressed as the mean ± standard error of the mean and the *P* values were determined by Mann–Whitney *U* test

its absence in growth plates resulted in a delay of long bone growth including delayed primary and secondary centers of ossification, accompanied by increased mineralized cartilage, delayed vascular invasion, and a reduction in TRAP-positive cells, bone density and formation of bone trabeculae. Furthermore, the cartilage-specific ablation of EFNB2 also led to spontaneous features of OA associated with a decrease in joint space, cartilage degeneration and synovial membrane alterations in both knee and hip joints. Importantly, the latter was not related to the locomotor phenotype, as this was observed in only 27 % of EFNB2 KO mice, and all mice had the OA defects. Collectively, these data reinforce the hypothesis that EFNB2 plays an important role in cartilage growth and maintenance; its absence impairs endochondral ossification and cartilage development and predisposes the joint to degeneration resembling OA.

Endochondral bone formation and growth, during which the cartilage provides a template on which bone is laid down, are critically dependent on chondrocyte metabolism and this process involves highly organized cartilaginous growth plates [31–33]. Here, we demonstrated that the delayed ossification and growth plate alteration observed in the EFNB2^{Col2}KO mice appears not to be due to abnormal growth and differentiation of chondrocytes, as shown by the normal pattern of PCNA and type II collagen, markers of proliferation and chondrocyte differentiation [34]. Thus, EFNB2 seems to have no significant influence on either the influx of resting zone cells or on the mitogenic activity of proliferative cells in the growth plate. However, the increased type X collagen observed in the growth plates of EFNB2^{Col2}KO mice suggests an abnormal chondrocyte metabolism that could lead to shortening of the long bones, as this collagen facilitates endochondral ossification by regulating matrix mineralization and compartmentalizing matrix components [35, 36]. As our data showed that EFNB2 does not appear to be involved in the early stages of chondrocyte development, but affects the hypertrophic cells in the epiphyseal cartilage, it would be of interest to conduct a further study in which the loss of EFNB2 is specifically restricted to the hypertrophic chondrocytes of the growth plate cartilage, using the Col10a1 promoter.

A mechanistic explanation by which EFNB2 affects endochondral ossification could be as follows. At the chondro-ossesous junction in the growth plates, osteoclast activity follows vascular invasion and is required for the conversion of cartilage to bone. The communication

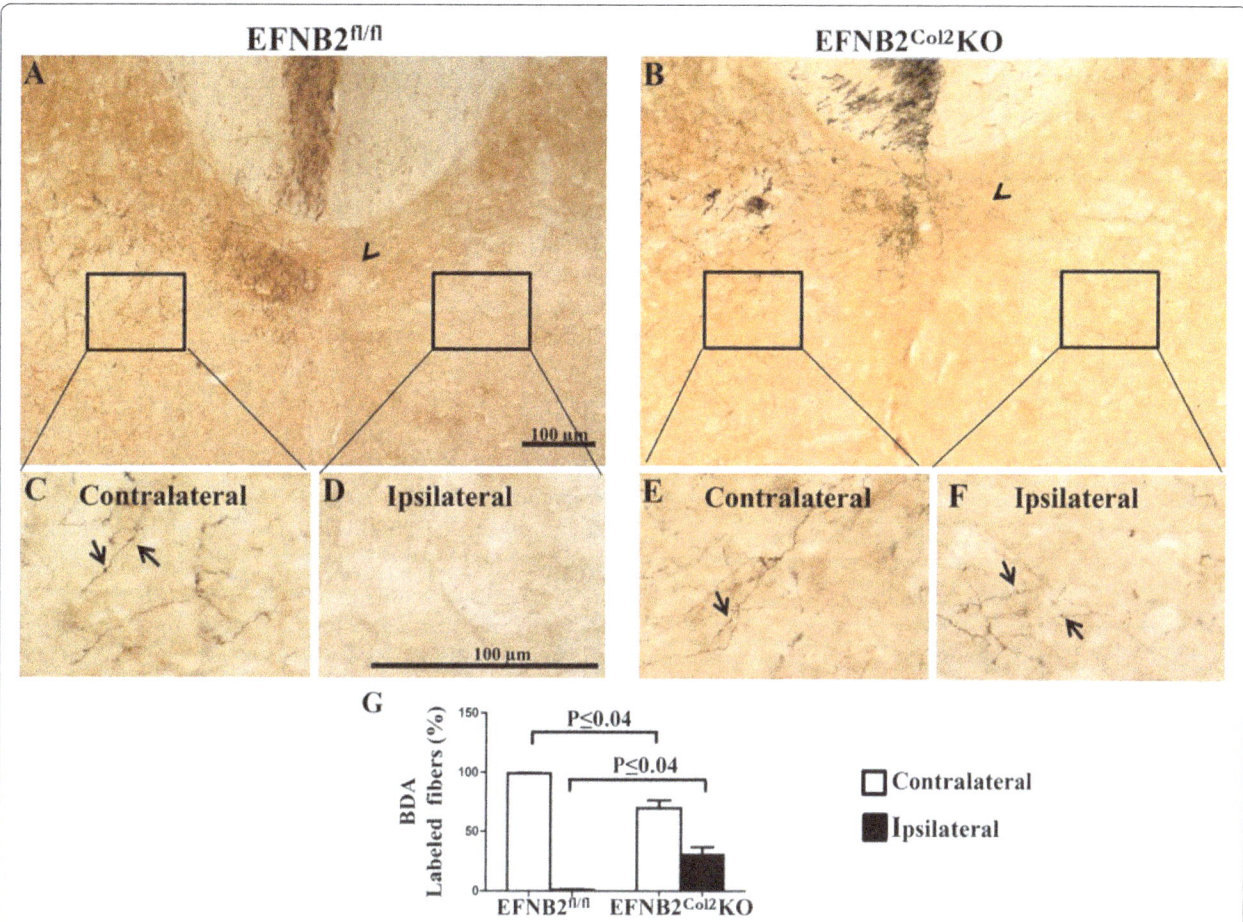

Fig. 9 Locomotor phenotype of some ephrin-B2 (*EFNB2*)^{Col2}knockout (*KO*) cartilage conditional mice is related to an abnormal corticospinal tract. **a-f** Brain tracing experiments to visualize the corticospinal path with biotinylated dextran amines (*BDA*) performed in 6-week-old EFNB2$^{fl/fl}$ (n = 2) and EFNB2^{Col2}KO cartilage conditional (n = 3) mice. Representative photomicrographs of the cervical spinal cord of EFNB2$^{fl/fl}$ (**a, c, d**) and EFNB2^{Col2}KO cartilage conditional mice (**b, e, f**) at the level of the fifth cervical vertebra. **g** Percentage of BDA-labeled fibers in the contralateral and ipsilateral hemispheres. *Arrowheads* indicate the injection site (**a, b**) and labeled fibers (**c-f**). *Scale bars* at 100 μm (**a, d**). Data are expressed as the mean ± standard error of the mean and the *P* values were determined by Mann–Whitney *U* test

between chondrocytes and adjacent osteoclasts is critical for this process. Although RANKL/RANK signaling has been implicated, additional studies have demonstrated that there is an alternative pathway in which the insulin-like growth factor (IGF)-1/IGF-1 receptor (IGF-1R) signaling, a system well known to play a fundamental role during endochondral bone formation [37–39], regulates EFNB2 and its specific receptor EphB4. Hence, IGF-1 signaling induces EFNB2/EphB4 expression in osteoblasts and chondrocytes and EFNB2 expression in osteoclasts. This upregulation of EFNB2/EphB4 mediates cell-cell communication necessary for IGF-1 stimulation of osteoblast, osteoclast and chondrocyte differentiation required for endochondral bone formation [40]. In addition, during the endochondral bone formation, VEGF, among other factors, directs adjacent inner perichondrial cells to become osteoblasts and form the bone collar [41]. Interestingly, Wang et al. [42] showed that IGF-1-increased EFNB2 production

stimulates VEGF expression and vascularization. Data from the present study demonstrate that in the absence of EFNB2, decreased VEGF is found in the hypertrophic zone of developing growth plate cartilage, reflecting, at least in part, reduced vascularization in this zone.

Vascularization of the un-mineralized transverse partition of cartilage columns is a critical step in endochondral bone formation; chondrocytes within cartilage terminally differentiate into hypertrophic chondrocytes, which produce VEGF to stimulate angiogenesis. Such an effect in EFNB2^{Col2}KO mice was not surprising, as EFNB2 has been found to be expressed by hypertrophic chondrocytes in the developing growth plate [43], to play a crucial role in VEGF-induced angiogenesis [44, 45], to act as a pro-angiogenic factor in postnatal neovascularization, and to be involved in the formation of the primary blood capillary [9, 10, 46–48].

Ossification begins with invasion of the calcified hypertrophic cartilage by capillaries, but the remodeling of bone matrix by osteoclasts is also of major importance, as it results in a cavity filled with vascular channels containing hematopoietic cells. The newly formed blood vessels bring in osteoclast-like cells, which resorb the mineralized cartilage [49]. The decreased number of TRAP-positive cells and increase in mineralized cartilage in EFNB2^{Col2}KO probably resulted from a delay in degradation of mineralized cartilage from the hypertrophic chondrocytes themselves [50] and chondroclasts and/or preosteclasts and osteoclasts, due to defective vascularization [43], culminating in altered bone growth. These findings suggest that EFNB2 acts on blood capillary invasion into hypertrophic chondrocytes, regulating angiogenesis at the chondro-osseous junction, thus facilitating endochondral bone development.

Endochondral ossification is a process that occurs from the embryonic stages through adulthood, permitting skeletal structures to be sustained during rapid bone growth. Our findings from imaging and bone densitometry showed that EFNB2^{Col2}KO mice at P21 and 8 weeks of age displayed reduced bone mass with lower mineral content and trabeculae formation, resulting from the altered endochondral ossification, which impacted the long-term long bone development. However, although 1-year-old EFNB2^{Col2}KO mice were smaller in size and length and had a significantly lower mineral content in the distal femur, other features such as pelvic size and whole body and vertebral mineral content did not differ from controls. An explanation for the latter observation could be that the independent, highly coordinated bone remodeling process [51, 52], which is responsible for removal and repair of damaged bone to maintain the integrity of the adult skeleton and mineral homeostasis, could have superseded the effect of the lack of EFNB2. Furthermore, several compensatory mechanisms that evolve during development could also compensate for the loss of EFNB2.

Importantly, cartilage-specific EFNB2 deletion also leads to spontaneous OA features, in which both cartilage and synovial membrane display alterations. However, the effect is not due to the abnormal gait of the cartilage-specific EFNB2^{Col2}KO mice, as only 27 % demonstrated the locomotor phenotype, and the OA features were present in all mutant mice. Data from this study, in which the lack of EFNB2 led to OA, concur with and substantiate findings demonstrating that the presence and role of this factor in human chondrocytes positively impact the abnormal metabolism of cartilage in OA [12]. Moreover, this study also concurs with in vivo overexpression of the EFNB2 specific receptor, EphB4, in articular tissue, also demonstrating a significant decrease in progression of OA [15]. All these data thus suggest EFNB2 as an attractive therapeutic target in OA. As a continuation of this study, it would be of interest to explore whether, using this EFNB2^{Col2}KO mouse model, surgically induced OA, such as the destabilization of the medial meniscus (DMM), would lead to development of more OA features.

Of the cartilage-specific EFNB2^{Col2}KO mice 27 % displayed a locomotor phenotype, which occurred as soon as they learned to walk at P15 and continued throughout their lifespan. One could question the low or incomplete penetrance of the locomotor phenotype. Most explanations of incomplete penetrance in genetically identical individuals assumed differences in gene expression or somatic genetic or epigenetic variations [53, 54]. Recently, an additional model of a fundamentally different mechanism was suggested, involving stochastic cell behavior in the colonization process during embryonic development, which results in variable success in colonization, hence allowing for incomplete penetrance [55]. All these may arise stochastically, but once present, they drive the phenotype so that some individuals are affected while others with the same primary disease-causing mutation are not.

We speculated that this locomotor phenotype was due to abnormalities in hip development. However, for mice with this phenotype, although pelvic bone and canal width were smaller at 8 weeks, no differences were observed at 1 year of age. Furthermore, there were no differences in the acetabular parameters, suggesting that it did not result from any developmental hip abnormality. Yet, the walking defect in these EFNB2^{Col2}KO mice resembled that which was previously demonstrated by two other members of the EFN family, specifically in mice lacking EFNB3 and its specific receptor EphA4 [28, 29]. For these EFN members, the defect was demonstrated to be related to a neurological defect occurring during the neurodevelopment in which there is a major disruption in the corticospinal tract, a pathway that sends messages from the brain to the moving limbs. How can this be related to our cartilage conditional KO model? The Col2a1 Cre promoter is reported to be expressed during early embryonic development (E9.5-11.5) on the notochord and developing brain [56] and at later stages in all cartilaginous tissues. As EFNB2 also plays an important role during neuronal development [57], in which it is found to guide boundary and synapse formation, cell migration and axon guidance, to name a few [4, 58–61], we therefore further explored the cause of the phenotype using a tracer of the corticospinal tract. The mice had an abnormal corticospinal projection pattern, with far more numerous ipsilateral projections in comparison to control mice. This finding is in line with reports on mice with EphA4 deletion [62] and EFNB3 deletion [29], which have similar behavioral defects. In brief, this pathway depends on the crossing of neurons from one side of the central nervous system to the other. The axons extending from neurons in the motor cortex of one hemisphere of the brain typically connect to targets on the opposite side of the spinal column. Therefore, the left side of the brain controls limb movement on the right side, and the right side of the brain controls limb movement on the left side. This result demonstrates the need for caution when the Col2a1 Cre promoter is used in transgenic mice. However, the vascular impairment, delayed mineralization and osteopenia displayed by the EFNB2^{Col2}KO mice are clearly independent of the neurological defect found in these mice. From the present data, it cannot yet be determined whether the spontaneous OA phenotype observed during aging is secondary to the observed developmental defects or whether it is caused by an independent role of EFNB2 in adult articular cartilage. An in vivo study with a specific inactivation of the EFNB2 gene in adult articular cartilage using an inducible Cre system could resolve this issue.

Conclusion

In summary, we showed for the first time that EFNB2 is required for normal endochondral ossification, cartilage/bone growth and development, and adult articular cartilage and synovial membrane preservation in vivo.

Competing interests

The authors declare that they have no competing interests.

Authors' contributions

GVF, JPP, and JMP conceived the study. GVF, BL, DH, AH, and ND were responsible for the data collection and analysis. GVF, BL, JW, AH, ND, HF, MK, JPP, and JMP interpreted the data. GVF, BL, JPP, and JMP undertook the literature search. GVF, AH, ND, and JMP generated the figures. GVF, BL, DH, JW, AH, ND, HF, MK, JPP, and JMP were involved in the drafting or critical revision of the manuscript and approved the final submitted version.

Acknowledgements

The authors wish to express their gratitude to Frédéric Paré, MSc and François Mineau, BSc for their expert technical support; François Depault, PhD for the initiation of the EFNB2^{Col2}KO cartilage-specific model; John S. Mort, PhD and Eunice Lee, PhD (Shriners Hospital for Children, McGill University Hospital Centre, Montreal, Quebec, Canada) for generously providing an antibody used in this project; and Virginia Wallis for her assistance with the manuscript preparation. We also wish to acknowledge the professionalism of the animal care technicians at the University of Montreal Hospital Research Centre (CRCHUM), and the excellent technical assistance of the Centre for Bone and Periodontal Research at McGill University. Dr. Valverde-Franco received postdoctoral bursaries from the Chair in Osteoarthritis of the University of Montreal and the MENTOR/Canadian Institutes of Health Research (CIHR) program.

Author details

[1]Osteoarthritis Research Unit, University of Montreal Hospital Research Centre (CRCHUM), 900 Saint-Denis, R11.412B, Montreal, QC H2X 0A9, Canada. [2]Faculty of Veterinary Medicine, Clinical Science, University of Montreal, Saint-Hyacinthe, QC, Canada. [3]Laboratory of Immunology, University of Montreal Hospital Research Centre (CRCHUM), Montreal, QC, Canada. [4]Neurosciences Department, Faculty of Medicine, University of Montreal, Montreal, QC, Canada. [5]Groupe de recherche sur le sytème nerveux central (GRSNC), Neurosciences Department, Faculty of Medicine, University of Montreal, Montreal, QC, Canada. [6]Division of Genetics and Development, Toronto Western Research Institute, University Health Network (UHN) and Department of Surgery, University of Toronto, Toronto, ON, Canada.

References

1. Hirai H, Maru Y, Hagiwara K, Nishida J, Takaku F. A novel putative tyrosine kinase receptor encoded by the eph gene. Science. 1987;238(4834):1717–20.
2. Committee EN. Unified nomenclature for Eph family receptors and their ligands, the ephrins. Eph Nomenclature Committee. Cell. 1997;90(3):403–4.
3. Wilkinson DG. Eph receptors and ephrins: regulators of guidance and assembly. Int Rev Cytol. 2000;196:177–244.
4. Flanagan JG, Vanderhaeghen P. The ephrins and Eph receptors in neural development. Annu Rev Neurosci. 1998;21:309–45.
5. Edwards CM, Mundy GR. Eph receptors and ephrin signaling pathways: a role in bone homeostasis. Int J Med Sci. 2008;5(5):263–72.
6. Davy A, Bush JO, Soriano P. Inhibition of gap junction communication at ectopic Eph/ephrin boundaries underlies craniofrontonasal syndrome. PLoS Biol. 2006;4(10):e315.
7. Zhao C, Irie N, Takada Y, Shimoda K, Miyamoto T, Nishiwaki T, et al. Bidirectional ephrinB2-EphB4 signaling controls bone homeostasis. Cell Metab. 2006;4(2):111–21.
8. Matsuo K, Otaki N. Bone cell interactions through Eph/ephrin: bone modeling, remodeling and associated diseases. Cell Adh Migr. 2012;6(2):148–56.
9. Wang HU, Chen ZF, Anderson DJ. Molecular distinction and angiogenic interaction between embryonic arteries and veins revealed by ephrin-B2 and its receptor Eph-B4. Cell. 1998;93(5):741–53.
10. Adams RH, Wilkinson GA, Weiss C, Diella F, Gale NW, Deutsch U, et al. Roles of ephrinB ligands and EphB receptors in cardiovascular development: demarcation of arterial/venous domains, vascular morphogenesis, and sprouting angiogenesis. Genes Dev. 1999;13(3):295–306.
11. Arthur A, Panagopoulos RA, Cooper L, Menicanin D, Parkinson IH, Codrington JD, et al. EphB4 enhances the process of endochondral ossification and inhibits remodeling during bone fracture repair. J Bone Miner Res. 2013;28(4):926–35.
12. Kwan Tat S, Pelletier JP, Amiable N, Boileau C, Lavigne M, Martel-Pelletier J. Treatment with ephrin B2 positively impacts the abnormal metabolism of human osteoarthritic chondrocytes. Arthritis Res Ther. 2009;11(4):R119.
13. Luo H, Charpentier T, Wang X, Qi S, Han B, Wu T, et al. Efnb1 and Efnb2 proteins regulate thymocyte development, peripheral T cell differentiation, and antiviral immune responses and are essential for interleukin-6 (IL-6) signaling. J Biol Chem. 2011;286(48):41135–52.
14. Monemdjou R, Vasheghani F, Fahmi H, Perez G, Blati M, Taniguchi N, et al. Association of cartilage-specific deletion of peroxisome proliferator-activated receptor gamma with abnormal endochondral ossification and impaired cartilage growth and development in a murine model. Arthritis Rheum. 2012;64(5):1551–61.
15. Valverde-Franco G, Pelletier JP, Fahmi H, Hum D, Matsuo K, Lussier B, et al. In vivo bone-specific EphB4 overexpression in mice protects both subchondral bone and cartilage during osteoarthritis. Arthritis Rheum. 2012;64(11):3614–25.
16. Valverde-Franco G, Hum D, Matsuo K, Lussier B, Pelletier JP, Fahmi H, et al. The in vivo effect of prophylactic subchondral bone protection of osteoarthritic synovial membrane in bone-specific Ephb4-overexpressing mice. Am J Pathol. 2015;185(2):335–46.
17. Wallin J, Wilting J, Koseki H, Fritsch R, Christ B, Balling R. The role of Pax-1 in axial skeleton development. Development. 1994;120(5):1109–21.
18. Dueland RT, Adams WM, Fialkowski JP, Patricelli AJ, Mathews KG, Nordheim EV. Effects of pubic symphysiodesis in dysplastic puppies. Vet Surg. 2001;30(3):201–17.
19. Lee ER, Lamplugh L, Kluczyk B, Leblond CP, Mort JS. Neoepitopes reveal the features of type II collagen cleavage and the identity of a collagenase involved in the transformation of the epiphyses anlagen in development. Dev Dyn. 2009;238(6):1547–63.
20. Valverde-Franco G, Liu H, Davidson D, Chai S, Valderrama-Carvajal H, Goltzman D, et al. Defective bone mineralization and osteopenia in young adult FGFR3-/- mice. Hum Mol Genet. 2004;13(3):271–84.

21. Glasson SS, Blanchet TJ, Morris EA. The surgical destabilization of the medial meniscus (DMM) model of osteoarthritis in the 129/SvEv mouse. Osteoarthritis Cartilage. 2007;15(9):1061–9.

22. Coles JM, Zhang L, Blum JJ, Warman ML, Jay GD, Guilak F, et al. Loss of cartilage structure, stiffness, and frictional properties in mice lacking PRG4. Arthritis Rheum. 2010;62(6):1666–74.

23. Morko J, Kiviranta R, Joronen K, Saamanen AM, Vuorio E, Salminen-Mankonen H. Spontaneous development of synovitis and cartilage degeneration in transgenic mice overexpressing cathepsin K. Arthritis Rheum. 2005;52(12):3713–7.

24. Dancause N, Barbay S, Frost SB, Plautz EJ, Popescu M, Dixon PM, et al. Topographically divergent and convergent connectivity between premotor and primary motor cortex. Cereb Cortex. 2006;16(8):1057–68.

25. Dancause N, Barbay S, Frost SB, Plautz EJ, Stowe AM, Friel KM, et al. Ipsilateral connections of the ventral premotor cortex in a new world primate. J Comp Neurol. 2006;495(4):374–90.

26. Dancause N, Barbay S, Frost SB, Plautz EJ, Chen D, Zoubina EV, et al. Extensive cortical rewiring after brain injury. J Neurosci. 2005;25(44):10167–79.

27. Coonan JR, Greferath U, Messenger J, Hartley L, Murphy M, Boyd AW, et al. Development and reorganization of corticospinal projections in EphA4 deficient mice. J Comp Neurol. 2001;436(2):248–62.

28. Dottori M, Hartley L, Galea M, Paxinos G, Polizzotto M, Kilpatrick T, et al. EphA4 (Sek1) receptor tyrosine kinase is required for the development of the corticospinal tract. Proc Natl Acad Sci U S A. 1998;95(22):13248–53.

29. Kullander K, Croll SD, Zimmer M, Pan L, McClain J, Hughes V, et al. Ephrin-B3 is the midline barrier that prevents corticospinal tract axons from recrossing, allowing for unilateral motor control. Genes Dev. 2001;15(7):877–88.

30. Yokoyama N, Romero MI, Cowan CA, Galvan P, Helmbacher F, Charnay P, et al. Forward signaling mediated by ephrin-B3 prevents contralateral corticospinal axons from recrossing the spinal cord midline. Neuron. 2001;29(1):85–97.

31. Cancedda R, Castagnola P, Cancedda FD, Dozin B, Quarto R. Developmental control of chondrogenesis and osteogenesis. Int J Dev Biol. 2000;44(6):707–14.

32. Dreier R. Hypertrophic differentiation of chondrocytes in osteoarthritis: the developmental aspect of degenerative joint disorders. Arthritis Res Ther. 2010;12(5):216.

33. Mackie EJ, Tatarczuch L, Mirams M. The skeleton: a multi-functional complex organ: the growth plate chondrocyte and endochondral ossification. J Endocrinol. 2011;211(2):109–21.

34. Mayne R. Collagen types and chondrogenesis. Ann NY Acad Sci. 1990;599:39–44.

35. Schmid TM, Linsenmayer TF. Immunohistochemical localization of short chain cartilage collagen (type X) in avian tissues. J Cell Biol. 1985;100(2):598–605.

36. Kwan KM, Pang MK, Zhou S, Cowan SK, Kong RY, Pfordte T, et al. Abnormal compartmentalization of cartilage matrix components in mice lacking collagen X: implications for function. J Cell Biol. 1997;136(2):459–71.

37. Liu J-P, Baker J, Perkins AS, Robertson EJ, Efstratiadis A. Mice carrying null mutations of the genes encoding insulin-like growth factor I (Igf-1) and type 1 IGF receptor (Igf1r). Cell. 1993;75:59–72.

38. Wang Y, Nishida S, Sakata T, Elalieh HZ, Chang W, Halloran BP, et al. Insulin-like growth factor-I is essential for embryonic bone development. Endocrinology. 2006;147(10):4753–61.

39. Wang Y, Cheng Z, Elalieh HZ, Nakamura E, Nguyen MT, Mackem S, et al. IGF-1R signaling in chondrocytes modulates growth plate development by interacting with the PTHrP/Ihh pathway. J Bone Miner Res. 2011;26(7):1437–46.

40. Wang Y, Menendez A, Fong C, ElAlieh HZ, Chang W, Bikle DD. Ephrin B2/EphB4 mediates the actions of IGF-I signaling in regulating endochondral bone formation. J Bone Miner Res. 2014;29(8):1900–13.

41. Kronenberg HM. Developmental regulation of the growth plate. Nature. 2003;423(6937):332–6.

42. Wang Y, Menendez A, Fong C, ElAlieh HZ, Kubota T, Long R, et al. IGF-I signaling in osterix-expressing cells regulates secondary ossification center formation, growth plate maturation, and metaphyseal formation during postnatal bone development. J Bone Miner Res. 2015;30(12):2239–48.

43. Gerber HP, Vu TH, Ryan AM, Kowalski J, Werb Z, Ferrara N. VEGF couples hypertrophic cartilage remodeling, ossification and angiogenesis during endochondral bone formation. Nat Med. 1999;5(6):623–8.

44. Sawamiphak S, Seidel S, Essmann CL, Wilkinson GA, Pitulescu ME, Acker T, et al. Ephrin-B2 regulates VEGFR2 function in developmental and tumour angiogenesis. Nature. 2010;465(7297):487–91.

45. Wang Y, Nakayama M, Pitulescu ME, Schmidt TS, Bochenek ML, Sakakibara A, et al. Ephrin-B2 controls VEGF-induced angiogenesis and lymphangiogenesis. Nature. 2010;465(7297):483–6.

46. Gerety SS, Wang HU, Chen ZF, Anderson DJ. Symmetrical mutant phenotypes of the receptor EphB4 and its specific transmembrane ligand ephrin-B2 in cardiovascular development. Mol Cell. 1999;4(3):403–14.

47. Maes C, Kobayashi T, Selig MK, Torrekens S, Roth SI, Mackem S, et al. Osteoblast precursors, but not mature osteoblasts, move into developing and fractured bones along with invading blood vessels. Dev Cell. 2010;19(2):329–44.

48. Bai J, Wang YJ, Liu L, Zhao YL. Ephrin B2 and EphB4 selectively mark arterial and venous vessels in cerebral arteriovenous malformation. J Int Med Res. 2014;42(2):405–15.

49. Nordahl J, Andersson G, Reinholt FP. Chondroclasts and osteoclasts in bones of young rats: comparison of ultrastructural and functional features. Calcif Tissue Int. 1998;63(5):401–8.

50. Blair HC, Zaidi M, Schlesinger PH. Mechanisms balancing skeletal matrix synthesis and degradation. Biochem J. 2002;364(Pt 2):329–41.

51. Raggatt LJ, Partridge NC. Cellular and molecular mechanisms of bone remodeling. J Biol Chem. 2010;285(33):25103–8.

52. Crockett JC, Rogers MJ, Coxon FP, Hocking LJ, Helfrich MH. Bone remodelling at a glance. J Cell Sci. 2011;124(Pt 7):991-8.

53. Gordon L, Joo JE, Powell JE, Ollikainen M, Novakovic B, Li X, et al. Neonatal DNA methylation profile in human twins is specified by a complex interplay between intrauterine environmental and genetic factors, subject to tissue-specific influence. Genome Res. 2012;22(8):1395–406.

54. Nadeau JH. Modifier genes and protective alleles in humans and mice. Curr Opin Genet Dev. 2003;13(3):290–5.

55. Binder BJ, Landman KA, Newgreen DF, Ross JV. Incomplete penetrance: The role of stochasticity in developmental cell colonization. J Theor Biol. 2015; 380:309–14.

56. Sakai K, Hiripi L, Glumoff V, Brandau O, Eerola R, Vuorio E, et al. Stage-and tissue-specific expression of a Col2a1-Cre fusion gene in transgenic mice. Matrix Biol. 2001;19(8):761–7.

57. Migani P, Bartlett C, Dunlop S, Beazley L, Rodger J. Ephrin-B2 immunoreactivity distribution in adult mouse brain. Brain Res. 2007;1182:60–72.

58. Holder N, Klein R. Eph receptors and ephrins: effectors of morphogenesis. Development. 1999;126(10):2033–44.

59. Klein R. Excitatory Eph receptors and adhesive ephrin ligands. Curr Opin Cell Biol. 2001;13(2):196–203.

60. Knoll B, Drescher U. Ephrin-As as receptors in topographic projections. Trends Neurosci. 2002;25(3):145–9.

61. Zhou R. The Eph family receptors and ligands. Pharmacol Ther. 1998;77(3):151–81.

62. Serradj N, Paixao S, Sobocki T, Feinberg M, Klein R, Kullander K, et al. EphA4-mediated ipsilateral corticospinal tract misprojections are necessary for bilateral voluntary movements but not bilateral stereotypic locomotion. J Neurosci. 2014;34(15):5211–21.

13

The autocrine role of proteoglycan-4 (PRG4) in modulating osteoarthritic synoviocyte proliferation and expression of matrix degrading enzymes

Ali Alquraini[1,6], Maha Jamal[1], Ling Zhang[2], Tannin Schmidt[3], Gregory D. Jay[2,4] and Khaled A. Elsaid[5*]

Abstract

Background: Lubricin/proteoglycan 4 (PRG4) is a mucinous glycoprotein secreted by synovial fibroblasts and superficial zone chondrocytes. Recently, we showed that recombinant human PRG4 (rhPRG4) is a putative ligand for CD44 receptor. rhPRG4-CD44 interaction inhibits cytokine-induced rheumatoid arthritis synoviocyte proliferation. The objective of this study is to decipher the autocrine function of PRG4 in regulating osteoarthritic synoviocyte proliferation and expression of catabolic and pro-inflammatory mediators under basal and interleukin-1 beta (IL-1β)-stimulated conditions.

Methods: Cytosolic and nuclear levels of nuclear factor kappa B (NFκB) p50 and p65 subunits in $Prg4^{+/+}$ and $Prg4^{-/-}$ synoviocytes were studied using western blot. Nuclear translocation of p50 and p65 proteins in osteoarthritis (OA) fibroblast-like synoviocytes (FLS) in response to IL-1β stimulation in the absence or presence of rhPRG4 was studied using DNA binding assays. OA synoviocyte (5000 cells per well) proliferation following IL-1β (20 ng/ml) treatment in the absence or presence of rhPRG4 (50–200 μg/ml) over 48 hours was determined using a colorimetric assay. Gene expression of matrix metalloproteinases (*MMPs*), tissue inhibitor of metallproteinases-1 (*TIMP-1*), *TIMP-2*, *IL-1β*, *IL-6*, *IL-8*, *TNF-α*, cycloxygenae-2 (*COX2*) and *PRG4* in unstimulated and IL-1β (1 ng/ml)-stimulated OA synoviocytes, in the presence or absence of rhPRG4 (100 and 200 μg/ml), was studied following incubation for 24 hours.

Results: $Prg4^{-/-}$ synoviocytes contained higher nuclear p50 and p65 levels compared to $Prg4^{+/+}$ synoviocytes ($p < 0.05$). rhPRG4 (100 μg/ml) reduced p50 and p65 nuclear levels in $Prg4^{+/+}$ and $Prg4^{-/-}$ synoviocytes ($p < 0.001$). Similarly, rhPRG4 (200 μg/ml) inhibited NFκB translocation and cell proliferation in OA synoviocytes in a CD44-dependent manner ($p < 0.001$) via inhibition of IκBα phosphorylation. IL-1β reduced *PRG4* expression in OA synoviocytes and rhPRG4 (100 μg/ml) treatment reversed this effect ($p < 0.001$). rhPRG4 (200 μg/ml) reduced basal gene expression of *MMP-1*, *MMP-3*, *MMP-13*, *IL-6*, *IL-8*, and *PRG4* in OA synoviocytes, while increasing *TIMP-2* and cycloxygenase-2 (*COX2*) expression ($p < 0.001$). rhPRG4 (200 μg/ml) reduced IL-1β induction of *MMP-1*, *MMP-3*, *MMP-9*, *MMP-13*, *IL-6*, *IL-8*, and *COX2* expression in a CD44-dependent manner ($p < 0.001$).

Conclusion: PRG4 plays an important anti-inflammatory role in regulating OA synoviocyte proliferation and reduces basal and IL-1β-stimulated expression of catabolic mediators. Exogenous rhPRG4 autoregulates native PRG4 expression in OA synoviocytes.

Keywords: Lubricin, Proteoglycan-4, CD44, Osteoarthritis, Fibroblast-like synoviocytes

---

* Correspondence: elsaid@chapman.edu
[5]Department of Biomedical and Pharmaceutical Sciences, Chapman University School of Pharmacy, Rinker Health Sciences Campus, 9401 Jeronimo Road, Irvine, CA 92618, USA
Full list of author information is available at the end of the article

Background

Lubricin/proteoglycan-4 (PRG4) is a glycoprotein secreted by synovial fibroblasts and superficial zone chondrocytes [1–3]. The importance of PRG4 to joint hemostasis is evidenced in the loss-of-function mutations in the *Prg4* gene in the autosomal recessive disease, camptodactylyl-arthropathy-coxa vara pericarditis (CACP) syndrome, characterized by juvenile-onset arthropathy [4, 5]. The joints of *Prg4* knockout (*Prg4$^{-/-}$*) mice display progressive synovial hyperplasia, cartilage surface fibrillations, and chondrocyte apoptosis, which may not be completely reversed by PRG4 re-expression [6–8]. Therapeutically, the recombinant and native forms of PRG4 have been shown to exhibit a disease-modifying effect in pre-clinical osteoarthritis (OA) models [9–14].

A biological role for recombinant human PRG4 (rhPRG4) was recently reported. rhPRG4 was shown to compete with hyaluronan for binding to the CD44 receptor resulting in downstream inhibition of nuclear factor kappa B (NFκB) nuclear translocation in synoviocytes from patients with rheumatoid arthritis (RA) [15]. Furthermore, rhPRG4 inhibits cytokine-induced proliferation of murine *Prg4$^{-/-}$* synovial fibroblasts and human synovial fibroblasts derived from patients with RA [15]. rhPRG4 has also been shown to interact with toll-like receptors 2 and 4 (TLR2 and TLR4) and may fulfill an anti-inflammatory role [15–17].

CD44 is a major cell surface receptor, with various isoforms generated by alternative splicing and glycosylations, which possesses the ability to bind different ligands and exert different biological functions in inflammation and cancer [18, 19]. Increased expression of CD44 was reported in experimental OA and in cartilage and synovia of patients with different severities of OA [20–23]. Given the emerging evidence on the role of PRG4 in regulating synoviocyte proliferation in response to inflammatory stimuli, we sought to decipher the autocrine role of PRG4 in regulating OA synoviocyte proliferation and expression of matrix metalloproteinases (MMPs), tissue inhibitors of matrix metalloproteinases (TIMPs), aggrecanase-1 (a disintegrin and metalloproteinase with thrombospondin motifs 4 (ADAMTS4)), aggrecanase-2 (ADAMTS5), and pro-inflammatory and chemotactic cytokines. Additionally, we studied the regulation of *PRG4* gene expression in OA fibroblast-like synoviocytes (FLS) in response to interleukin-1 beta (IL-1β) and rhPRG4 treatments. We hypothesized that PRG4 is an important autocrine modulator of synovial cells, mediated by its interaction with CD44.

Methods

NFκB p50 and p65 cytosolic and nuclear levels in *Prg4$^{+/+}$* and *Prg4$^{-/-}$* synoviocytes and impact of rhPRG4 treatment

Synovial tissues were harvested from *Prg4$^{+/+}$* and *Prg4$^{-/-}$* male mice 8–10 weeks old and synoviocytes were isolated as described [15]. *Prg4$^{+/+}$* and *Prg4$^{-/-}$* synoviocytes were cultured in T-25 flasks until confluence. *Prg4$^{+/+}$* and *Prg4$^{-/-}$* synoviocytes were treated with rhPRG4 (100 μg/ml) [24], CD44 monoclonal antibody (CD44 Ab) (1.25 μg/ml) (Abcam, USA) or a combination of rhPRG4 and CD44 Ab for 48 hours. Nuclear and cytosolic cell extractions were performed using NE-PER nuclear and cytoplasmic extraction reagents kit (Thermo Fisher Scientific, USA). A total of 20 μg of protein was loaded into the wells of 4–12% Bis-Tris gels (Thermo Fisher Scientific) followed by gel electrophoresis and western blotting. Membranes were blocked using 5% nonfat dry milk in PBS-T for 1 hour at room temperature. Subsequently, membranes were incubated with anti-NFκB p50 antibody (Santa Cruz Biotechnology, USA) (1:1000 dilution) or anti-NFκB p65 antibody (Abcam) (1:1000 dilution) overnight at 4 °C. Membranes were also incubated with anti-Lamin B1 antibody (Abcam) (nuclear loading control) or anti β-Actin antibody (Cell signaling Technologies, USA) (cytosolic loading control). After washing three times with PBS-T, membranes were incubated with IRDye 800CW goat anti-rabbit secondary antibody (1:10,000 dilution) (LI-COR, USA) at room temperature for 1 hour. After washing three times with PBS-T, membranes were imaged using Odyssey CLx imaging system (LI-COR). Densitometry analysis was performed using Image J software. Data are presented as the densitometry ratio of p50 or p65 and either Lamin B1 or β-Actin in the same sample. Data are presented as the average ± standard deviation of three independent experiments.

IL-1β induced NFκB p50 and p65 nuclear translocation in OA FLS, and IL-1β induced cell proliferation and impact of rhPRG4 treatment

OA FLS (Cell Applications, USA) were harvested from patients undergoing total knee replacement. Cells were used between the third and sixth passages in all experiments. OA FLS (300,000 cells per well) were stimulated with IL-1β (20 ng/ml; R&D Systems, USA) for 6 hours at 37 °C in the presence or absence of rhPRG4 (100 μg/ml), rhPRG4 (200 μg/ml), rhPRG4 (200 μg/ml) + CD44 Ab (2.5 μg/ml; Abcam) or CD44 Ab (2.5 μg/ml). Cells were harvested and nuclear extraction was performed using a commercially available kit (Thermo Fisher Scientific). Total protein was quantified, and 3 μg of nuclear extract from each experimental group was used. The p50 and p65 proteins were detected in the nuclear extract using NFκB DNA binding assay kits (Abcam). Data are presented as p50 or p65 nuclear levels normalized to untreated controls. Data are presented as the average ± the standard deviation of four independent experiments, each with duplicate wells per group.

OA FLS were seeded in T-25 flasks at 1,000,000 cells in DMEM + 10% FBS for 48 hours. The total volume was 4 ml. After 48 hours, medium was removed and re-placed with DMEM + 1% FBS. Cells were incubated for 6 hours in the absence or presence of rhPRG4 (100 and 200 μg/ml) and/or CD44 Ab (2.5 μg/ml; pre-treatment for 2 hours prior to rhPRG4 treatment) followed by treatment with IL-1β (1 ng/ml) for 30 minutes.

Subsequently, medium was removed and cells were rinsed twice with ice cold PBS (1 ml). Protein extraction reagent (M-PER, Thermo Fisher Scientific) supplemented with protease and phosphatase cocktail inhibitor (1:100 dilution; Thermo Fisher Scientific) and EDTA (1:100 dilution; Thermo Fisher Scientific) was added (300 μl per flask) and cells were collected. Protein samples (20 μg/ml; 40 μl per well) were loaded in 10% PAGE pre-cast gels (Bio-Rad, USA). Following gel electrophoresis and transfer, membranes were blocked using 5% bovine serum albumin (BSA) for 1 hour at room temperature. Membranes were probed for phosphorylated inhibitor kappa B alpha (p-IκBα) or total IκBα using commercially available rabbit antibodies (Abcam). Antibodies were diluted 1:1000 in 5% BSA and incubated with membranes overnight at 4 °C. After washing with Tris-buffered saline Tween 20 (TBS-T), membranes were incubated with horseradish peroxidase (HRP)-conjugated goat anti-rabbit (1:5000) for 1 hour at room temperature. Membranes were also probed for β-Actin using a commercially available β-Actin antibody (1: 10,000) (Abcam). Protein bands were developed using SuperSignal West Pico PLUS chemiluminescent substrate (Thermo Fisher Scientific) and visualized using C-Digit Target (LI-COR, USA).

OA FLS in 96-well plates (5000 cells per well) in DMEM supplemented with 1% FBS and 1 mM pyruvate were stimulated with IL-1β (20 ng/ml) for 48 hours at 37 °C in the absence or presence of rhPRG4 at a final concentration of 50, 100, or 200 μg/ml. The total volume in each well was 200 μl. Cell proliferation was determined using the Cell Titer 96 AQueous one solution cell proliferation assay (MTS; Promega, USA) and absorbance at 490 nm was measured. In a separate set of experiments, rhPRG4 (200 μg/ml) treatment was performed in the absence or presence of a CD44 Ab (2.5 μg/ml; Abcam) and cell proliferation was determined as described previously. Data are presented as fold of OA FLS proliferation normalized to untreated controls. Data are presented as the average ± standard deviation of four independent experiments, each with triplicate wells per group.

Modulation of PRG4 secretion by OA FLS and RA FLS and impact of rhPRG4 on PRG4 gene expression in unstimulated and IL-1β stimulated OA synoviocytes

OA FLS and RA FLS (Cell Applications) were grown in DMEM + 10% FBS and used between the third and sixth passages: 20,000 cells per well were plated in sterile 96-well plates and incubated at 37 °C for 48 hours to allow cell attachment. The total volume per well was 200 μl. The medium was changed to DMEM + 1% FBS and cells were treated with IL-1β (1 ng/ml), tumor necrosis factor alpha (TNF-α) (1 ng/ml; R&D Systems), or transforming growth factor beta (TGF-β) (1 ng/ml; R&D Systems) for 72 hours. Subsequently, medium supernatants were collected and PRG4 concentrations were determined using an inhibition ELISA as previously described [16]. PRG4 concentrations were normalized to cell density, determined colorimetrically using the Cell Titer 96 AQueous one solution cell proliferation assay (MTS; Promega) and the 490 nm absorbance was measured. Data are presented as media PRG4 content normalized to cell density. Data are presented as the average ± standard deviation of four independent experiments, each with duplicate wells per group.

OA FLS (250,000 cells per well) were treated with IL-1β (1 ng/ml) in the absence or presence of rhPRG4 (100 or 200 μg/ml) for 24 hours followed by RNA extraction using Triazol reagent (Thermo Fisher Scientific), and RNA concentrations were determined using a NanoDrop ND-2000 spectrophotometer (NanoDrop Technologies, USA). cDNA was synthesized using Transcriptor First Strand cDNA Synthesis Kit (Roche, USA). Quantitative PCR (qPCR) was performed on Applied Biosystems StepOnePlus Real-Time PCR System (Thermo Fisher Scientific) using TaqMan Fast Advanced Master Mix (Life Technologies, USA). The cycle threshold (Ct) value of PRG4 (Hs00981633_m1; Thermo Fisher Scientific) was normalized to the Ct value of GAPDH (Hs02758991_g1; Thermo Fisher Scientific) in the same sample, and the relative expression was calculated using the $2^{-\Delta\Delta Ct}$ method [25]. In another set of experiments, rhPRG4 (100 and 200 μg/ml) was incubated with OA FLS for 24 hours followed by RNA isolation, cDNA synthesis, and PRG4 qPCR as described above. Data are presented as fold PRG4 gene expression compared to untreated control. Data are presented as the average plus on minus standard deviation of four independent experiments with duplicate wells per treatment.

Modulation of IL-1β-induced OA FLS proliferation by OA SF and the role of synovial fluid PRG4

Synovial fluid (SF) samples were collected from patients with OA (n = 5) (Articular Engineering, USA) following knee replacement surgery [16]. Four of the OA patients were female and the median age of the group was 65 years. OA SF was pooled from the five patients. PRG4 immunoprecipitation was conducted as described previously [16]. PRG4 depletion was confirmed by assaying pooled OA SF for PRG4 levels using an inhibition ELISA as previously described [16].

IL-1β-induced OA FLS proliferation was conducted as described previously in the absence or presence of pooled OA SF or PRG4-immunoprecipitated OA SF at 20 μl or 40 μl per well (corresponding to 10% or 20% dilution). Cell proliferation was determined using the Cell Titer 96 AQueous one solution cell proliferation assay (MTS; Promega) and the 490 nm absorbance was measured. Data are presented as fold OA FLS proliferation compared to untreated controls. Data are presented as the average ± standard deviation of four independent experiments, each with duplicate wells per treatment.

PRG4 knockdown in OA FLS and proliferation of PRG4-silenced OA FLS

OA FLS (250,000 cells per well) were treated with a pre-validated PRG4 small interfering RNA (siRNA) (Thermo Fisher Scientific) (25 pmol per well) or a non-targeted negative control (NC) siRNA (25pmoles) (Thermo Fisher Scientific) for 48 hours. Transfection was performed using Lipofectamine RNAiMAX (Thermo Fisher Scientific) per manufacturer's recommendations. To confirm PRG4 knockdown, PRG4 gene expression was determined in PRG4 siRNA and NC siRNA-treated OA FLS as described previously and compared to PRG4 gene expression in untreated control OA FLS. IL-1β stimulation of OA FLS proliferation in control, NC siRNA, and PRG4 siRNA-treated cells was performed as described previously. IL-1β stimulation was performed for 24 hours and cell proliferation was measured as described previously. OA FLS proliferation of the different experimental groups was normalized to untreated control cells. Data are presented as the average ± standard deviation of three independent experiments with duplicate wells per treatment.

Impact of rhPRG4 treatment on target gene expression in unstimulated and IL-1β-stimulated OA FLS

OA FLS (250,000 cells per well) were treated with rhPRG4 (100 and 200 μg/ml) for 24 hours followed by RNA isolation, cDNA synthesis and qPCR was performed as described previously. Target genes included MMP-1 (Hs00899658_m1), MMP-2 (Hs00234422_m1), MMP-3 (Hs00968305_m1), MMP-9 (Hs00234579_m1), MMP-13 (Hs00233992_m1), TIMP-1 (Hs00171558_m1), TIMP-2 (Hs00234278_m1), ADAMTS4 (Hs00192708_m1), ADAMTS5 (Hs00199841_m1), IL-1β (Hs00174097_m1), IL-6 (Hs00985639_m1), IL-8 (Hs00174103_m1), TNF-α (Hs00174128_m1), and cycloxygenase-2 (COX2) (HS0 0153133_m1). All primers and probes are commercially available (Thermo Fisher Scientific). The Ct values of target genes were calculated and normalized to the Ct value of GAPDH in the same sample and relative gene expression was calculated as described previously. Data are presented as fold expression of target genes in rhPRG4-treated OA FLS compared to expression in

untreated control OA FLS. Data are presented as the average ± standard error of the mean (SEM) of four independent experiments.

OA FLS (250,000 cells per well) were treated with IL-1β (1 ng/ml) in the absence or presence of rhPRG4 (100 and 200 μg/ml) for 24 hours followed by RNA isolation, cDNA synthesis, and qPCR as described previously. Target genes included MMP-1, MMP-2, MMP-3, MMP-9, MMP-13, TIMP-1, TIMP-2, ADAMTS4, ADAMTS5, IL-1β, IL-6, IL-8, TNF-α and COX2. The Ct values of target genes were calculated and normalized to the Ct value of GAPDH in the same sample, and relative gene expression was calculated as described previously. Data are presented as fold expression of target genes in the IL-1β group, IL-1β + rhPRG4 (100 μg/ml) or IL-1β + rhPRG4 (200 μg/ml)-treated OA FLS groups, compared to expression in the control group. Data are presented as the average ± SEM of four independent experiments.

In another set of experiments, CD44 neutralization was achieved by pre-incubating OA FLS (250,000 cells per well) with CD44 Ab (2.5 μg/ml; Abcam) for 2 hours followed by treating OA FLS with IL-1β + rhPRG4 (200 μg/ml) for 24 hours followed by RNA isolation, cDNA, and qPCR as described previously. Data are presented as the average ± SEM of four independent experiments.

Statistical analyses

The nuclear NFκB p50 and p65 protein levels in OA FLS treatments were normalized to untreated control levels. The average of the absorbance values in untreated control cells across the four independent experiments was used to normalize absorbance values in the different experimental groups across the four independent experiments. A similar approach was used to present OA FLS proliferation. Statistical analyses of gene expression data was performed using ΔCt values (C_t target gene-C_t GAPDH) for each gene of interest in each experimental group and data were graphically presented as fold expression relative to untreated controls using the $2^{-\Delta\Delta Ct}$ method. Continuous variables were initially tested for normality and equal variances. Variables that satisfied both assumptions were tested for statistical significance using Student's t test or analysis of variance (ANOVA) with Tukey's post-hoc test for comparisons of two groups and more than two groups, respectively. Variables that did not satisfy the normality assumption were tested using the Mann-Whitney U test or ANOVA on the ranks. The level of statistical significance was set at α = 0.05.

Results

Cytosolic and nuclear NFκB p50 and p65 proteins in Prg4$^{+/+}$ and Prg4$^{-/-}$ synoviocytes and impact of rhPRG4 treatment

Cytosolic and nuclear p50 in rhPRG4 and CD44 antibody (Ab)-treated and untreated synoviocytes is shown in Fig. 1. A representative blot of p50 protein, cytosolic and nuclear loading controls is shown in Fig. 1a. We have observed stronger p50 bands in the cytosolic and nuclear fractions of $Prg4^{-/-}$ synoviocytes compared to $Prg4^{+/+}$ cells. Consistently, rhPRG4 treatment reduced cytosolic and nuclear p50 levels in both $Prg4^{+/+}$ and $Prg4^{-/-}$ synoviocytes. Semi-quantitative analysis of normalized cytosolic and nuclear p50 band intensities from the different experimental groups is presented in Fig. 1b and c. Cytosolic and nuclear p50 subunit levels were significantly higher in $Prg4^{-/-}$ synoviocytes compared to $Prg4^{+/+}$ synoviocytes ($p < 0.05$). There was no significant difference in cytosolic and nuclear levels of p50 between untreated control and CD44 Ab-treated $Prg4^{+/+}$ synoviocytes or $Prg4^{-/-}$ synoviocytes. rhPRG4 treatment significantly reduced cytosolic and nuclear p50 levels compared to untreated control $Prg4^{+/+}$ and $Prg4^{-/-}$

synoviocytes ($p < 0.001$). A trend towards an increase in cytosolic and nuclear p50 levels in the CD44 Ab + rhPRG4 group compared to the rhPRG4 alone group was observed although it was not statistically significant ($p > 0.05$).

Cytosolic and nuclear p65 protein in rhPRG4 and CD44 Ab-treated and untreated synoviocytes is shown in Fig. 2. p65 protein was detectable in the cytosolic and nuclear fractions in $Prg4^{+/+}$ and $Prg4^{-/-}$ synoviocytes (Fig. 2a). rhPRG4 treatment consistently reduced p65 staining intensity in the cytosolic and nuclear fractions in both genotypes. Semi-quantitative analysis of normalized cytosolic and nuclear p50 band intensities from the different experimental groups is presented in Fig. 2b and c. Nuclear p65 subunit levels were significantly higher in $Prg4^{-/-}$ synoviocytes compared to $Prg4^{+/+}$ synoviocytes ($p < 0.01$). CD44 Ab-treated $Prg4^{-/-}$ synoviocytes had significantly higher nuclear p65 levels compared to untreated

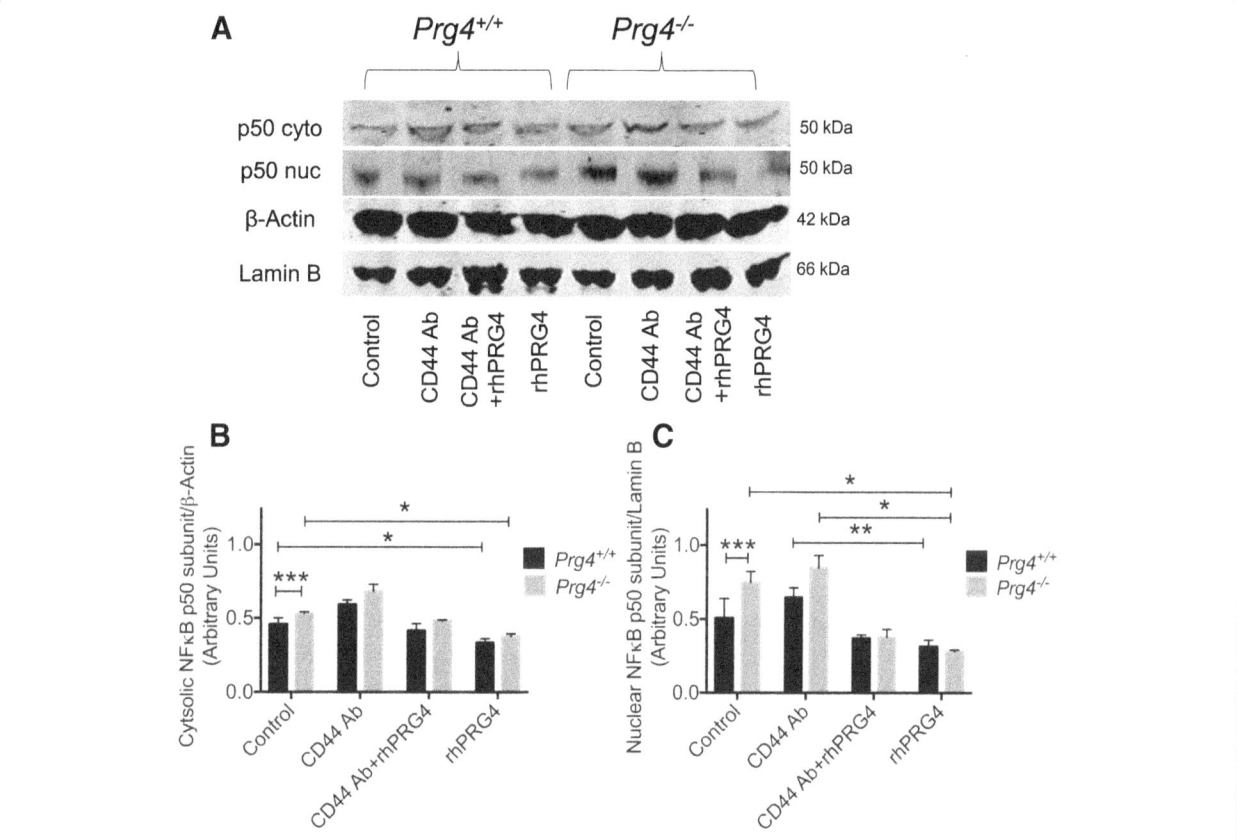

Fig. 1 The impact of recombinant human proteoglycan 4 (*rhPRG4*) treatment on cytosolic and nuclear levels of nuclear factor kappa B (*NFκB*) p50 subunit in $Prg4^{+/+}$ and $Prg4^{-/-}$ synoviocytes; *$p < 0.001$, **$p < 0.01$, ***$p < 0.05$. **a** Representative western blot showing cytosolic and nuclear p50 protein in $Prg4^{+/+}$ and $Prg4^{-/-}$ synoviocytes in control, CD44 antibody (*CD44 Ab*)-treated, CD44 Ab + rhPRG4-treated and rhPRG4-treated cells. Lamin B1 was used as a nuclear loading control and β-Actin was used as a cytosolic loading control. **b** Semi-quantitative densitometry analysis of normalized cytosolic p50 protein in untreated and rhPRG4-treated $Prg4^{+/+}$ and $Prg4^{-/-}$ synoviocytes. $Prg4^{-/-}$ synoviocytes had higher cytosolic p50 compared to $Prg4^{+/+}$ synoviocytes. rhPRG4 (100 μg/ml) reduced cytosolic p50 levels in $Prg4^{+/+}$ and $Prg4^{-/-}$ synoviocytes. Co-incubation with CD44 Ab (1.25 μg/ml) did not alter the effect of rhPRG4. Data are presented as mean ± standard deviation of three independent experiments. **c** Semi-quantitative densitometry analysis of normalized nuclear p50 protein in untreated and rhPRG4-treated $Prg4^{+/+}$ and $Prg4^{-/-}$ synoviocytes. $Prg4^{-/-}$ synoviocytes had higher nuclear p50 compared to $Prg4^{+/+}$ synoviocytes. rhPRG4 (100 μg/ml) reduced nuclear p50 levels in $Prg4^{+/+}$ and $Prg4^{-/-}$ synoviocytes. Co-incubation with CD44 Ab (1.25 μg/ml) did not alter the effect of rhPRG4. Data are presented as mean ± standard deviation of three independent experiments

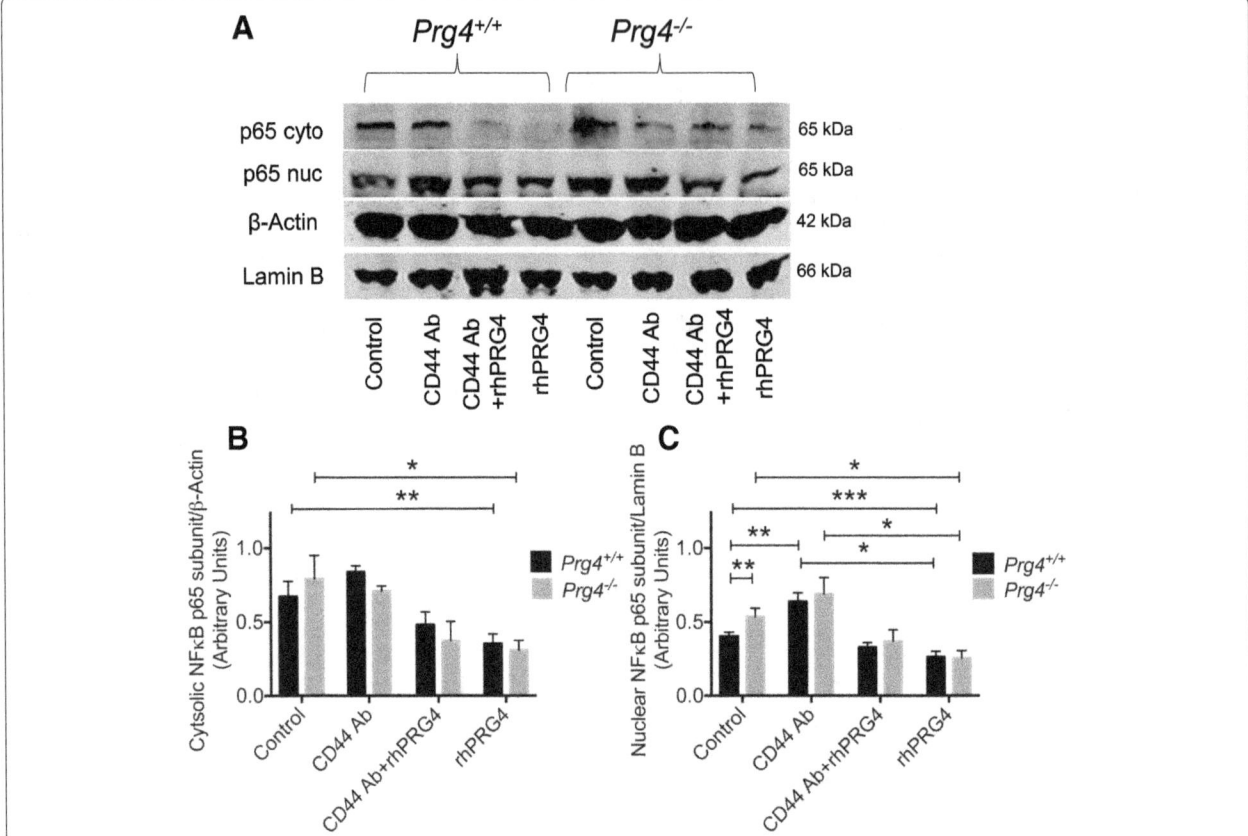

Fig. 2 The impact of recombinant human proteoglycan 4 (*rhPRG4*) treatment on cytosolic and nuclear levels of nuclear factor kappa B (*NFκB*) p65 subunit in *Prg4$^{+/+}$* and *Prg4$^{-/-}$* synoviocytes; *$p < 0.001$, **$p < 0.01$, ***$p < 0.05$. **a** Representative western blot showing cytosolic and nuclear p65 protein in *Prg4$^{+/+}$* and *Prg4$^{-/-}$* synoviocytes in control, CD44 antibody (*CD44 Ab*)-treated, CD44 Ab + rhPRG-treated, and rhPRG4-treated cells. Lamin B1 was used as a nuclear loading control and β-Actin was used as a cytosolic loading control. **b** Semi-quantitative densitometry analysis of normalized cytosolic p65 protein in untreated and rhPRG4-treated *Prg4$^{+/+}$* and *Prg4$^{-/-}$* synoviocytes. rhPRG4 (100 µg/ml) reduced cytosolic p65 levels in *Prg4$^{+/+}$* and *Prg4$^{-/-}$* synoviocytes. Co-incubation with CD44 Ab (1.25 µg/ml) did not alter the effect of rhPRG4. Data are presented as mean ± standard deviation of three independent experiments. **c** Semi-quantitative densitometry analysis of normalized nuclear p65 protein in untreated and rhPRG4-treated *Prg4$^{+/+}$* and *Prg4$^{-/-}$* synoviocytes. *Prg4$^{-/-}$* synoviocytes had higher nuclear p65 compared to *Prg4$^{+/+}$* synoviocytes. rhPRG4 (100 µg/ml) reduced nuclear p65 levels in *Prg4$^{+/+}$* and *Prg4$^{-/-}$* synoviocytes. Co-incubation with CD44 Ab (1.25 µg/ml) did not alter the effect of rhPRG4. Data are presented as mean ± standard deviation of three independent experiments

controls ($p < 0.01$). rhPRG4 treatment significantly reduced cytosolic and nuclear p65 levels compared to untreated control *Prg4$^{+/+}$* and *Prg4$^{-/-}$* synoviocytes ($p < 0.001$). Similarly, a trend towards an increase in cytosolic and nuclear p65 levels in the CD44 Ab + rhPRG4 group compared to the rhPRG4 alone group was observed although it was not statistically significant ($p > 0.05$).

rhPRG4 inhibited IL-1β-stimulated NFκB p50 and p65 nuclear translocation in OA FLS mediated by inhibition of IκBα phosphorylation in a CD44-dependent manner

IL-1β treatment significantly increased NFκB p50 and p65 nuclear levels in OA FLS compared to untreated OA FLS ($p < 0.001$) (Fig. 3a and b). rhPRG4 (100 µg/ml) treatment significantly reduced IL-1β-induced p50 and p65 nuclear translocation ($p < 0.01$). Similarly, rhPRG4 (200 µg/ml) treatment significantly reduced IL-1β

induced p50 and p65 nuclear translocation ($p < 0.001$). There was no significant difference in the p50 and p65 nuclear level in the IL-1β + CD44 Ab group and the IL-1β group. NFκB p50 and p65 nuclear levels in the IL-1β + rhPRG4 (200 µg/ml) + CD44 Ab group were significantly higher than corresponding levels in the IL-1β + rhPRG4 (200 µg/ml) group ($p < 0.001$) and were not significantly different from nuclear levels in the IL-1β + CD44 Ab group. The ability of rhPRG4 to lower NFκB nuclear levels was inhibited by co-incubation with CD44 Ab, which showed no difference from the IL-1β group.

A representative p-IκBα western blot in control and IL-1β-treated OA FLS in the presence or absence of rhPRG4 with or without CD44 Ab co-treatment is shown in Fig. 3c. IL-1β treatment increased p-IκBα levels compared to untreated control. rhPRG4 (200 µg/ml) treatment reduced IκBα phosphorylation compared to IL-1β alone. This effect

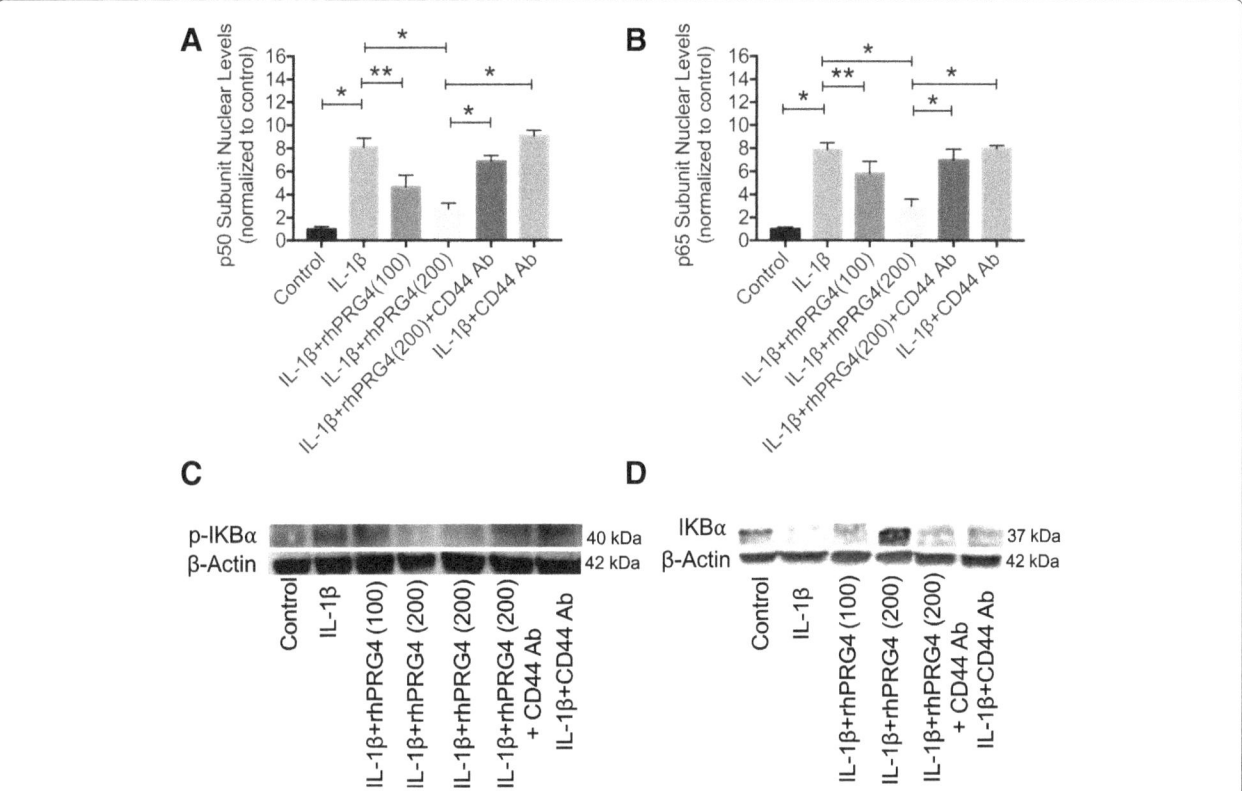

Fig. 3 The impact of recombinant human proteoglycan 4 (*rhPRG4*) treatment on interleukin-1 beta (*IL-1β*)-induced nuclear factor kappa b (*NFκB*) p50 and p65 nuclear translocation, inhibitor kappa B alpha (*IκBα*) phosphorylation and degradation. Data are presented as mean ± standard deviation of four independent experiments; *p < 0.001, **p < 0.01. **a** Impact of rhPRG4 treatment on IL-1β-induced p50 protein nuclear translocation in ostoarthritis fibroblast-like synoviocytes (OA FLS). IL1β treatment induced p50 protein nuclear translocation. rhPRG4 treatment (100 μg/ml and 200 μg/ml) inhibited IL-1β-induced p50 protein nuclear translocation. Co-incubation with a CD44 neutralizing monoclonal antibody (CD44 Ab) abolished the effect of rhPRG4 treatment. CD44 Ab treatment alone did not alter p50 nuclear translocation. **b** Impact of rhPRG4 treatment on IL-1β-induced p65 protein nuclear translocation in OA FLS. IL1β treatment induced p65 protein nuclear translocation. rhPRG4 treatment (100 μg/ml and 200 μg/ml) inhibited IL-1β-induced p65 protein nuclear translocation. Co-incubation with a CD44 neutralizing monoclonal antibody (CD44 Ab) abolished the effect of rhPRG4 treatment. CD44 Ab treatment alone did not alter p65 nuclear translocation. **c** Representative western blot of cytosolic phosphorylated inhibitor kappa B alpha (*p-IκBα*) in untreated and IL-1β-treated OA synoviocytes in the absence or presence of rhPRG4 and/or CD44 Ab. rhPRG4 (200 μg/ml) reduced p-IκBα levels in a CD44-dependent manner. **d** Representative western blot of cytosolic total inhibitor kappa B alpha (*IκBα*) in untreated and IL-1β-treated OA synoviocytes in the absence or presence of rhPRG4 and/or CD44 Ab. rhPRG4 (200 μg/ml) increased IκBα levels in a CD44-dependent manner

was reversed by a CD44 Ab. We did not observe a difference in p-IκBα level between the IL-1β group and the IL-1β + CD44 Ab group. A representative total IκBα western blot in control and IL-1β-treated OA FLS in the presence or absence of rhPRG4 with or without CD44 Ab co-treatment is shown in Fig. 3d. IL-1β treatment reduced total IκBα. Total IκBα was higher with IL-1β + rhPRG4 (200 μg/ml) compared to IL-1β alone. Co-incubation with a CD44 Ab abolished the effect of rhPRG4 on total IκBα following IL-1β stimulation. We did not observe a difference in total IκBα content between the IL-1β group and the IL-1β + CD44 Ab group.

rhPRG4 inhibited IL-1β-stimulated proliferation in OA FLS in a CD44-dependent manner

IL-1β induced OA FLS proliferation over 48 hours (p < 0.001) (Fig. 4a). rhPRG4 (50 μg/ml) treatment did not reduce IL-1β-induced OA FLS proliferation. In contrast, rhPRG4 (100 and 200 μg/ml) treatments significantly reduced IL-1β-induced OA FLS proliferation (p < 0.01; p < 0.001). CD44 Ab and rhPRG4 co-treatment resulted in significantly greater OA FLS proliferation compared to rhPRG4 treatment (p < 0.01) and was not significantly different from OA FLS proliferation in the IL1β alone group. Finally, there was no significant difference in OA FLS proliferation between the IL-1β + CD44 Ab group and the IL-1β group.

Modulation of PRG4 production in OA FLS and RA FLS and effect of rhPRG4

Basal PRG4 production in OA FLS was significantly higher than PRG4 production by RA FLS (p < 0.001) (Fig. 4b). IL-1β and TNF-α reduced PRG4 production by OA FLS compared to control untreated cells (p < 0.001).

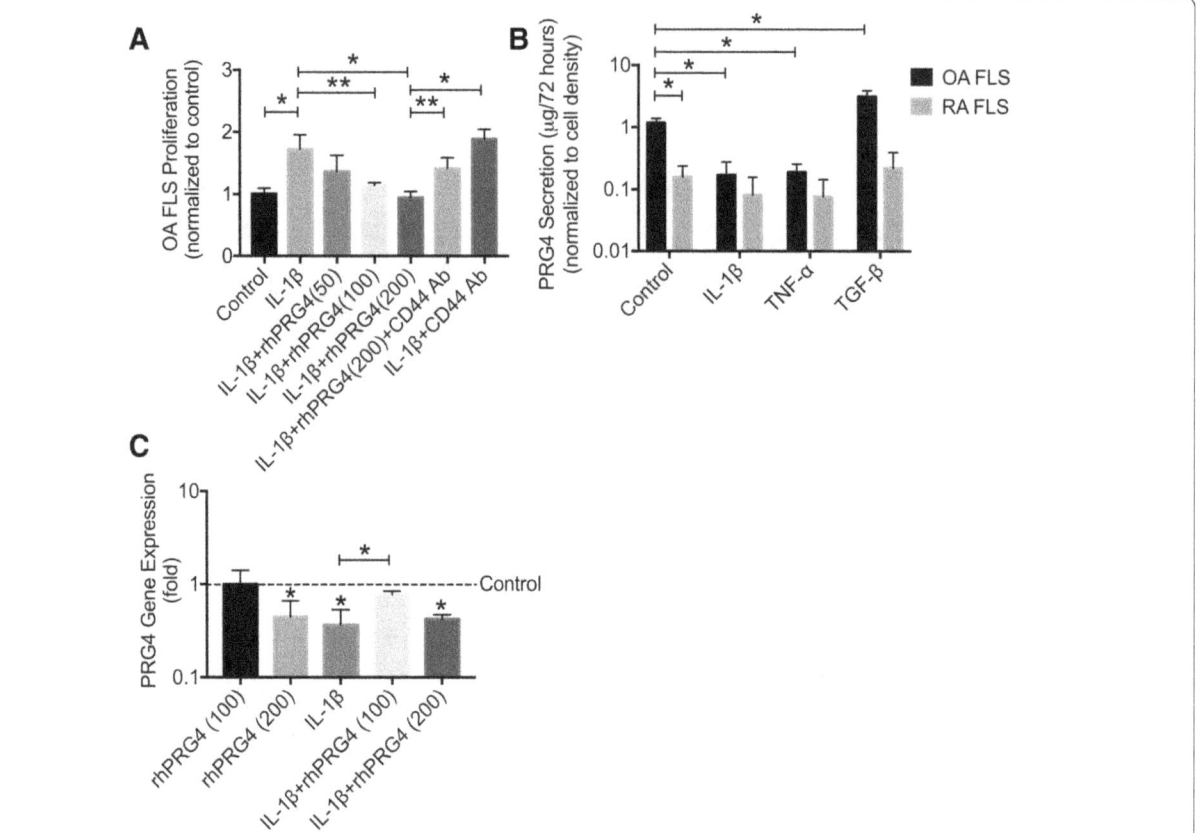

Fig. 4 The impact of recombinant human proteoglycan 4 (*rhPRG4*) treatment on interleukin-1 beta (*IL-1β*)-induced osteoarthritis fibroblast-like synoviocytes (*OA FLS*) proliferation and regulation of proteoglycan-4 (*PRG4*) gene expression and production. Data are presented as the average ± standard deviation of four independent experiments; *$p < 0.001$, **$p < 0.05$. **a** Impact of rhPRG4 treatment (50, 100, and 200 μg/ml) on IL-1β-induced proliferation of OA FLS over 48 hours. IL-1β induced OA FLS proliferation. rhPRG4 (100 and 200 μg/ml) reduced IL-1β-induced OA FLS proliferation. Co-treatment with a CD44 neutralizing monoclonal antibody (*CD44 Ab*) abolished the effect of rhPRG4 treatment. CD44 Ab treatment alone did not alter IL-1β-induced OA FLS proliferation. **b** Regulation of PRG4 production by cytokines in OA FLS and rheumatoid arthritis FLS (RA FLS). OA FLS produces significantly higher PRG4 protein compared to RA FLS. IL-1β and TNF-α reduce PRG4 production by OA FLS while transforming growth factor beta (*TGF-β*) increases PRG4 production by OA FLS. IL-1β, TNF-α, and TGF-β did not alter PRG4 production by RA FLS. **c** IL-1β downregulated *PRG4* gene expression in OA FLS. *PRG4* expression in the IL-1 β + rhPRG4(100 μg/ml) group was higher than *PRG4* expression in the IL-1β alone group and was not different from *PRG4* expression in control cells. *PRG4* expression in the IL-1β + rhPRG4(200 μg/ml) group was lower than *PRG4* expression in the control and in the IL-1β + rhPRG4(100 μg/ml) group. rhPRG4 (200 μg/ml) treatment reduced basal *PRG4* gene expression in OA FLS compared to control. Data are presented as fold change compared to untreated control OA FLS

TGF-β enhanced PRG4 production by OA FLS compared to control untreated cells ($p < 0.001$). IL-1β, TNF-α, and TGF-β did not significantly alter PRG4 production by RA FLS compared to untreated cells.

rhPRG4 (100 μg/ml) treatment did not alter basal *PRG4* gene expression in OA FLS (Fig. 4c). In contrast, rhPRG4 (200 μg/ml) significantly reduced *PRG4* gene expression in OA FLS ($p < 0.001$). IL-1β reduced *PRG4* gene expression in OA FLS ($p < 0.001$). *PRG4* expression in the IL-1β + rhPRG4 (100 μg/ml) group was significantly higher than *PRG4* expression in IL-1β alone ($p < 0.001$) and the IL-1β + rhPRG4 (200 μg/ml) group ($p < 0.01$). Alternatively, there was no significant difference in *PRG4* gene expression between the IL1β group and the IL1β + rhPRG4 (200 μg/ml) group. Finally, *PRG4* gene expression in the IL-1β + rhPRG4 (200 μg/ml) treatment

was significantly lower than PRG4 expression in untreated control OA FLS ($p < 0.001$).

SF PRG4 depletion and PRG4 downregulation promotes OA FLS proliferation

Mean PRG4 concentration in OA SF after PRG4 immunoprecipitation was 25.11 ± 3.18 μg/ml, compared to 280.43 ± 14.76 μg/ml in OA SF with no PRG4 immunoprecipitation. OA SF treatment at 10% dilution did not significantly alter IL-1β-induced OA FLS proliferation (Fig. 5a). PRG4-deficient OA SF (10% dilution) significantly increased IL-1β-induced OA FLS proliferation compared to OA SF (10% dilution) ($p < 0.001$) or no SF treatment ($p < 0.01$). OA SF (20% dilution) significantly reduced IL-1β-induced OA FLS proliferation ($p < 0.01$) (Fig. 5b). PRG4-deficient OA SF (20% dilution)

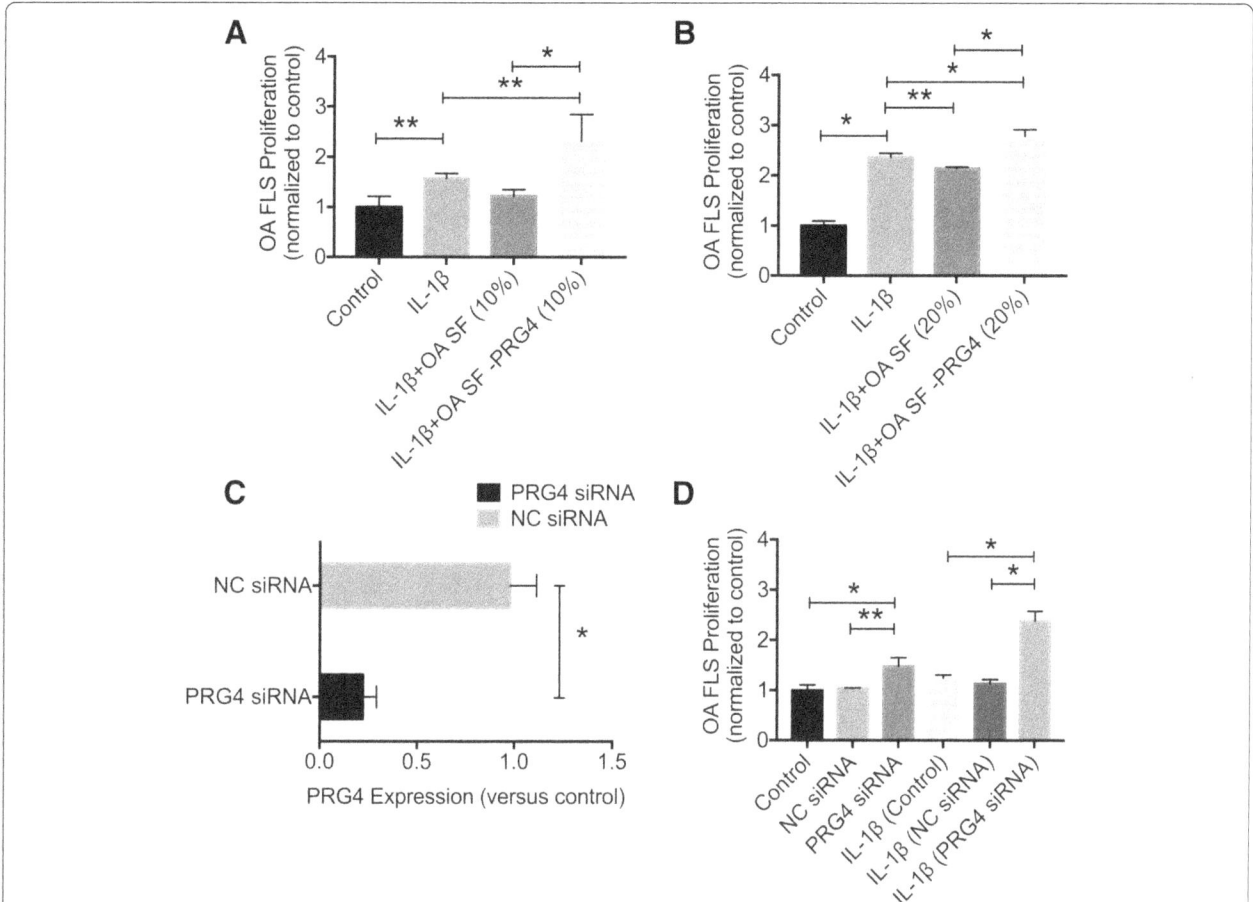

Fig. 5 The role of proteoglycan 4 (*PRG4*) resident in synovial fluids from patients with osteoarthritis (*OA*) and produced by OA fibroblast-like synoviocytes (*OA FLS*) in modulating interleukin-1 beta (*IL-1β*)-induced OA FLS proliferation. Data are presented as mean ± standard deviation of at least three independent experiments. OA FLS proliferation of the different experimental groups was normalized to untreated control cells; *p < 0.001, **p < 0.05. **a** Impact of synovial fluid PRG4 depletion on cellular proliferation in an in vitro model of IL-1β-induced OA FLS proliferation over 48 hours. IL-1β induced OA FLS proliferation and OA SF (10%) did not alter the effect of IL-1β on OA FLS. PRG4-depleted OA SF (*OA SF – PRG4*) enhanced the proliferative effect of IL-1β on OA FLS. **b** Impact of synovial fluid PRG4 depletion on cellular proliferation in an in vitro model of IL-1β-induced OA FLS proliferation over 48 hours. IL-1β induced OA FLS proliferation and OA SF (20%) significantly reduced IL-1β-induced OA FLS proliferation. PRG4 depletion reversed the effect of OA SF and enhanced the proliferative effect of IL-1β on OA FLS. **c** *PRG4* gene knockdown in OA FLS using PRG4 small interfering RNA (*siRNA*). Treatment with a non-targeting negative control (*NC*) siRNA over a 48-hour period did not alter PRG4 gene expression. PRG4 siRNA treatment reduced endogenous PRG4 expression in OA FLS. Data are normalized to PRG4 expression in untreated control OA FLS. **d** Impact of PRG4 knockdown on OA FLS proliferation under unstimulated and IL-1β stimulated conditions. PRG4 knockdown enhanced OA FLS proliferation under basal conditions compared to NC treatment over 24 hours. PRG4 knockdown enhanced IL-1β-induced OA FLS proliferation compared to NC treatment over 24 hours

significantly increased IL-1β induced OA FLS proliferation compared to OA SF (20% dilution) or no SF treatment ($p < 0.001$). NC siRNA treatment did not significantly alter *PRG4* gene expression in OA FLS compared to untreated OA FLS (Fig. 5c). In contrast, PRG4 siRNA treatment resulted in a significant reduction in *PRG4* gene expression, approximating an 80% reduction ($p < 0.001$) compared to untreated or NC siRNA-treated OA FLS. PRG4 siRNA-treated OA FLS displayed significantly higher basal cell proliferation compared to NC siRNA-treated OA FLS ($p < 0.01$) or untreated OA FLS ($p < 0.001$) over 24 hours (Fig. 5d). Similarly, and following IL-1β stimulation, PRG4 siRNA-treated OA FLS had significantly higher proliferation

compared to NC siRNA-treated OA FLS or non-silenced control OA FLS over 24 hours ($p < 0.001$).

Expression of OA-associated catabolic enzymes is affected by rhPRG4 in unstimulated and IL-1β-stimulated OA FLS

rhPRG4 (100 µg/ml) did not significantly alter basal expression of MMP-1, MMP-2, MMP-3, MMP-9, MMP-13, TIMP-1, TIMP-2, ADAMTS4, or ADAMTS5 (Fig. 6a). rhPRG4 (200 µg/ml) significantly reduced basal expression of MMP-1, MMP-3, and MMP-13 ($p < 0.001$). The magnitude of reduction in gene expression was approximately 45% for MMP-1 compared with 58% for MMP-3 and 62% for MMP-13. rhPRG4 (200 µg/ml) significantly increased basal expression of TIMP-2 ($p <$

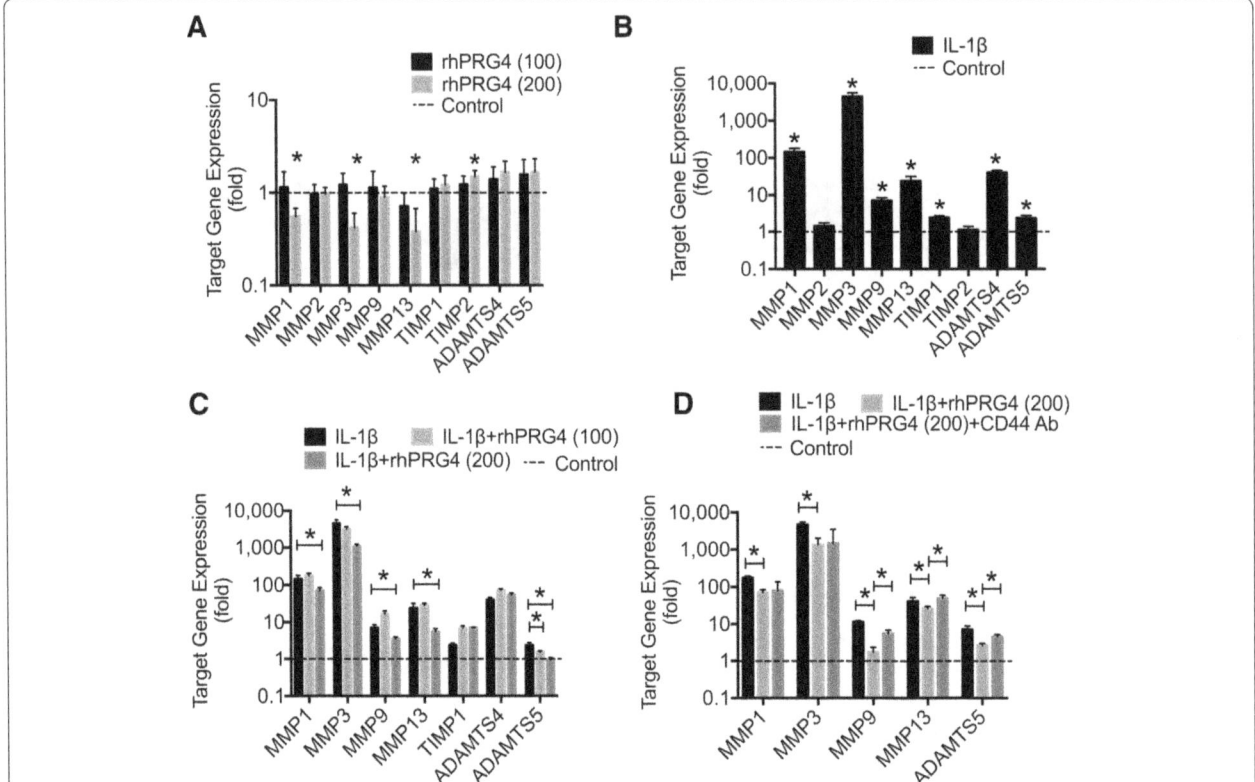

Fig. 6 The impact of recombinant human proteoglycan-4 (*rhPRG4*) treatment on basal and IL-1β-induced gene expression of matrix metalloproteinases (*MMPs*), aggrecanases 1 and 2 (*ADAMTS4* and *ADAMTS5*), and tissue inhibitor of metalloproteinases (*TIMPs*) in OA fibroblast-like synoviocytes (*OA FLS*). Data are presented as the average ± standard error of the mean (SEM) of four independent experiments. Data are represented as fold change compared to untreated control OA FLS; *$p < 0.001$. **a** Effect of rhPRG4 treatment on basal gene expression in OA FLS. rhPRG4 (200 μg/ml) reduced expression of *MMP1*, *MMP3*, and *MMP13*. rhPRG4 (200 μg/ml) increased expression of *TIMP-2*. **b** Impact of IL-1β treatment on catabolic enzyme gene expression in OA FLS. IL-1β induced *MMP1*, *MMP3*, *MMP9*, *MMP13*, *TIMP-1*, *ADAMTS4*, and *ADAMTS5* gene expression. **c** Impact of rhPRG4 treatment in IL-1β-stimulated OA FLS. rhPRG4 (200 μg/ml) treatment reduced *MMP1*, MMP3, *MMP9*, *MMP13* and *ADAMTS5* gene expression in IL-1β-stimulated OA FLS. **d** Role of CD44 in modulating the effect of rhPRG4 on *MMP1*, *MMP3*, *MMP9*, *MMP-13*, and *ADAMTS5* expression in IL-1β-stimulated OA FLS. CD44 neutralization using a CD44 monoclonal antibody (*CD44 Ab*) significantly inhibited the effect of rhPRG4 treatment on *MMP9*, *MMP13*, and *ADAMTS5* expression

0.001) (~50% increase) and did not alter the expression of MMP-2, TIMP-1, ADAMTS4, or ADAMTS5.

IL-1β significantly induced *MMP-1*, *MMP-3*, *MMP-9*, *MMP-13*, *ADAMTS4*, and *ADAMTS5* gene expression in OA FLS ($p < 0.001$) (Fig. 6b). rhPRG4 (100 μg/ml) treatment significantly reduced ADAMTS5 expression in IL-1β-stimulated OA FLS ($p < 0.001$) (~35% reduction) (Fig. 6c). rhPRG4 (200 μg/ml) treatment significantly reduced *MMP-1*, *MMP-3*, *MMP-9*, *MMP-13*, and *ADAMTS5* expression in IL-1β-stimulated OA FLS ($p < 0.001$). The magnitude of reduction in gene expression was approximately 51% for *MMP-1* compared with 76% for *MMP-3*, 49% for *MMP-9*, 77% for *MMP-13*, and 60% for *ADAMTS5*. rhPRG4 (100 or 200 μg/ml) treatment did not alter *ADAMTS4* expression. Expression of *MMP-9*, *MMP-13* and *ADAMTS5* genes was significantly higher in the IL-1β + rhPRG4 + CD44 Ab group compared to the IL-1β + rhPRG4 group ($p < 0.001$) (Fig. 6d). In contrast, there was no significant difference in fold expression of MMP-1 or MMP-3 between the IL-

1β + rhPRG4 + CD44 Ab group and the IL-1β + rhPRG4 group. Additionally, there was no significant difference in fold expression of *MMP-1*, *MMP-3* or *MMP-13* between the IL-1β + rhPRG4 + CD44 Ab group and the IL-1β group.

Expression of OA-associated inflammatory cytokines and mediators is affected by rhPRG4 in unstimulated and IL-1β-stimulated OA FLS

rhPRG4 (100 μg/ml) did not significantly alter basal expression of *IL-1β*, *IL-6*, *IL-8*, *TNF-α*, and significantly increased basal *COX2* gene expression ($p < 0.001$) (~96% increase) (Fig. 7a). rhPRG4 (200 μg/ml) significantly reduced basal expression of *IL-1β*, *IL-6* and *IL-8* ($p < 0.001$) (~37%, 59%, and 73% decrease) and significantly increased basal expression of *COX2* (~61% increase) ($p < 0.001$). rhPRG4 (100 or 200 μg/ml) did not alter basal expression of TNF-α.

IL-1β significantly induced *IL-1β*, *IL-6*, *IL-8*, *TNF-α*, and *COX2* gene expression ($p < 0.001$) (Fig. 7b). There

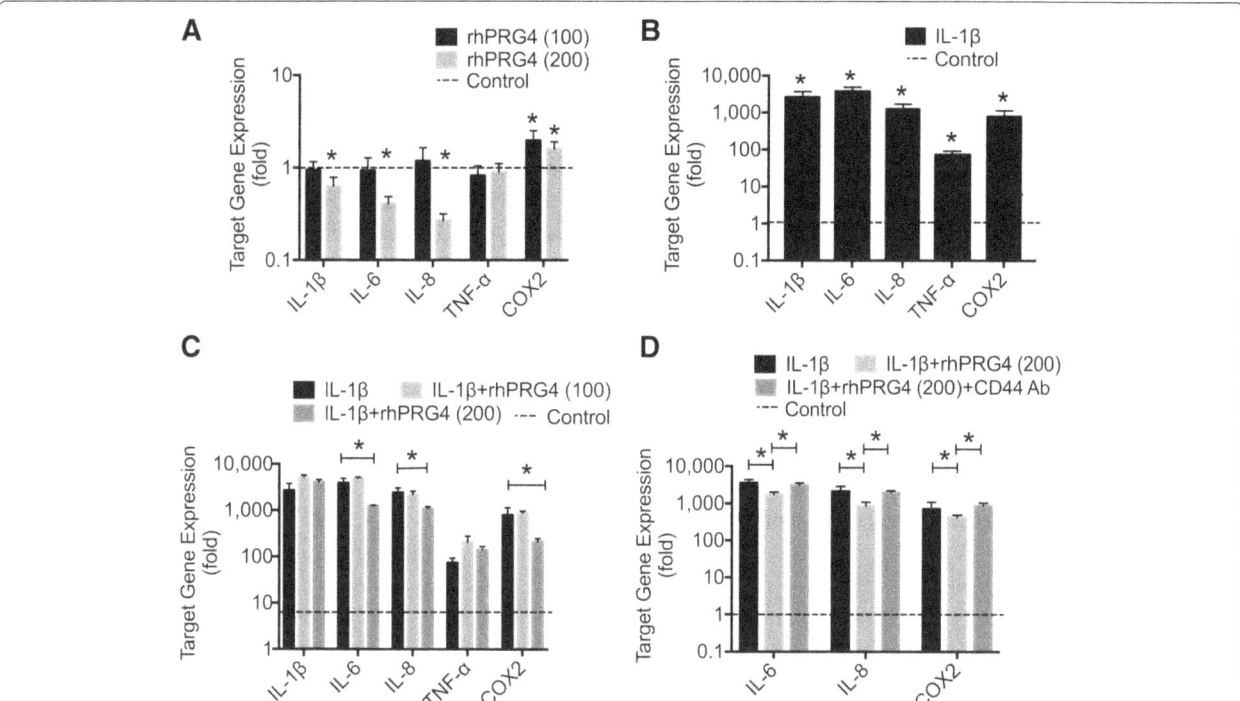

Fig. 7 The impact of recombinant human proteoglycan-4 (*rhPRG4*) treatment on basal and IL-1β-induced gene expression of *IL-1β, IL-6, IL-8, TNF-α,* and cyclooxygenase-2 (*COX2*) in osteoarthritis fibroblast-like synoviocytes (OA FLS). Data are presented as the average ± standard error of the mean of four independent experiments. Data are presented as fold change compared to untreated control OA FLS; *p < 0.001. **a** Effect of rhPRG4 treatment on basal gene expression in OA FLS. rhPRG4 (100 μg/ml and 200 μg/ml) increased basal *COX2* expression. rhPRG4 (200 μg/ml) reduced basal *IL-1β, IL-6,* and *IL-8* expression. **b** Impact of IL-1β treatment on pro-inflammatory cytokines and mediators of gene expression in OA FLS. IL-1β induced *IL-1β, IL-6, IL-8, TNF-α,* and *COX2* gene expression. **c** Impact of rhPRG4 treatment in IL-1β-stimulated OA FLS. rhPRG4 (200 μg/ml) treatment reduced *IL-1β, IL-6, IL-8, TNF-α,* and *COX2* gene expression in IL-1β-stimulated OA FLS. **d** Role of CD44 in modulating the effect of rhPRG4 on *IL-6, IL-8,* and *COX2* expression in IL-1β-stimulated OA FLS. CD44 neutralization using a CD44 monoclonal antibody (*CD44 Ab*) significantly inhibited the effect of rhPRG4 treatment on *IL-6, IL-8,* and *COX2* expression

was no significant difference in *IL-1β, IL-6, IL-8, TNF-α,* or *COX2* gene expression between the IL-1β + rhPRG4 (100 μg/ml) group and the IL-1β group (Fig. 7c). rhPRG4 (200 μg/ml) treatment significantly reduced *IL-6, IL-8,* and *COX2* gene expression in IL-1β-stimulated OA FLS (*p* < 0.001). The magnitude of reduction in gene expression was approximately 67% for *IL-6* compared with 55% for *IL-8* and 73% for *COX2*. Expression of *IL-6, IL-8* and *COX-2* genes was significantly higher in the IL-1β + rhPRG4 + CD44 Ab group compared to the IL-1β + rhPRG4 group (*p* < 0.001) (Fig. 7d). Finally, there was no significant difference in fold expression of *IL-6, IL-8,* or *COX-2* between the IL-1β + rhPRG4 + CD44 Ab group and the IL-1β group.

Discussion

In this work, we have shown that nuclear levels of NFκB p50 and p65 in *Prg4*$^{-/-}$ synoviocytes were higher compared to *Prg4*$^{+/+}$ synoviocytes. Additionally, *Prg4*$^{+/+}$ and *Prg4*$^{-/-}$ synoviocytes had similar levels of p65 subunits in the cytosol while the latter had elevated cytosolic p50 subunit levels. Enhanced nuclear localization of NFκB in

Prg4$^{-/-}$ synoviocytes may explain their pro-inflammatory and proliferative capacity under unstimulated conditions and in response to inflammatory stimuli compared to their wildtype counterparts [15]. rhPRG4 inhibited NFκB p50 and p65 nuclear translocation in *Prg4*$^{-/-}$ synoviocytes and *Prg4*$^{+/+}$ synoviocytes. Interestingly, rhPRG4 treatment reduced cytosolic levels of p50 and p65 proteins in *Prg4*$^{+/+}$ and *Prg4*$^{-/-}$ synoviocytes. This is a unique biological effect of rhPRG4 and may indicate that rhPRG4 functions to reduce the total cellular pool of NFκB, accounting for its anti-proliferative and anti-inflammatory activities. The observed effect of rhPRG4 in relation to nuclear NFκB translocation in murine synoviocytes may not be entirely due to its binding to CD44 receptor as neutralization of CD44 did not completely abolish the effect of rhPRG4.

OA synovitis is characterized by synovial hyperplasia with an increased number of synovial lining cells, neovascularization and inflammatory cell infiltration [26–31]. Patients with OA display a heterogeneous array of synovial pathologic changes and the severity of OA synovitis is correlated with pain and disease progression

[32–35]. OA synoviocytes proliferate in response to IL-1 as shown by us and others [36]. As expected, the degree of OA synoviocyte proliferation in our experiment was markedly reduced compared to RA synoviocyte proliferation under similar conditions [15, 36]. rhPRG4 dose-dependently reduced IL-1-induced OA synovial fibroblast proliferation, mediated by inhibition of NFκB p50 and p65 nuclear translocation, in a CD44-dependent manner. The biological effect of rhPRG4 is mediated by its ability to inhibit IκBα phosphorylation subsequent to IL-1 receptor stimulation. IκBα binds to NFκB subunits causing their cytoplasmic retention [37]. Phosphorylation of IκBα results in proteasome-mediated degradation [37]. rhPRG4 prevents IκBα degradation in a CD44-dependent manner; this is consistent with its ability to inhibit IL-1-induced NFκB nuclear translocation. This observation extends the efficacy of rhPRG4 as a biologic agent that inhibits synoviocyte proliferation in RA and OA, and establishes a role for CD44 in modulating OA synoviocyte proliferation [38]. The role of PRG4 in modulating OA synoviocyte proliferation is further highlighted by the ability of PRG4 in SF to reduce OA synoviocyte proliferation. Depleting PRG4 in OA SF enhanced the proliferative effect of IL-1 on OA synoviocytes. PRG4 acts in an autocrine manner to inhibit OA synoviocyte proliferation. This effect is manifested by the enhanced basal and IL-1-induced OA synoviocyte proliferation in response to PRG4 knockdown. This autocrine role for PRG4 validates the synovial hyperplasia observed in $Prg4^{-/-}$ mice and the partial regression of synovial hyperplasia upon Prg4 re-expression [5, 8].

PRG4 expression by articular chondrocytes and synovial fibroblasts is modulated by mechanical and biological stimuli. Shear upregulates *PRG4* gene expression in articular cartilage [39, 40] and intermittent hydrostatic pressure application enhances PRG4 expression in isolated rat mandibular fibroblasts [41]. Cartilage biosynthesis of PRG4 is reduced as a result of IL-1β and TNF-α exposure but is increased with TGF-β [42–44]. In synoviocytes, *PRG4* expression is reduced by IL-1β and is increased by TGF-β and TGF-β-linked PRG4 accumulation is counterbalanced by IL-1β [42, 45]. In our study, IL-1β and TNF-α reduced PRG4 production in OA synoviocytes but did not reduce PRG4 production in RA synoviocytes. Correspondingly, TGF-β enhanced PRG4 production in OA synoviocytes but did not enhance it in RA synoviocytes. These differences in synoviocyte production of PRG4 extends to basal conditions where OA synoviocytes produced PRG4 to a greater extent compared to RA synoviocytes. While the underlying mechanism of differential production of PRG4 by synoviocytes from different disease origins remains to be elucidated, these phenotypic differences may contribute to the enhanced proliferation and migration seen in RA synoviocytes compared to OA synoviocytes [36].

rhPRG4 exhibited a bimodal concentration-dependent response related to its ability to modulate PRG4 expression in IL-1β-stimulated OA synoviocytes. While rhPRG4 at a low concentration restored *PRG4* expression in OA synoviocytes following IL-1β challenge, rhPRG4 at a higher concentration did not antagonize IL-1β downregulation of PRG4 in OA synoviocytes. Moreover, exogenous PRG4 appeared to directly regulate *PRG4* production by OA synoviocytes. At a low concentration, rhPRG4 treatment did not change basal expression of *PRG4* in OA synoviocytes. Alternatively, exogenous PRG4 exhibited negative feedback on *PRG4* expression in OA synoviocytes as rhPRG4 treatment downregulated basal *PRG4* expression in OA synoviocytes. Our observations extend the understanding of how endogenous PRG4 expression is modulated by exogenous PRG4 in articular cartilage and in in vivo models of posttraumatic arthritis [14, 46].

Synoviocytes play an important role in driving OA pathogenesis. OA synoviocytes express a wide-range of matrix-degrading catabolic enzymes and cytokines. In our study, and in response to IL-1β stimulation, OA synoviocytes induced the expression of *MMP-1*, *MMP-3*, *MMP-9*, *MMP-13*, *TIMP-1*, *aggrecanase-1*, *aggrecanase-2*, *IL-1β*, *TNF-α*, *IL-6*, *IL-8*, and *COX2*. Our results are in agreement with previous studies that reported on the effect of IL-1β on OA synoviocytes [47, 48]. rhPRG4 dose-dependently reduced the expression of *MMP-1*, *MMP-3*, *MMP-9*, *MMP-13*, *aggrecanase-2*, *IL-6*, *IL-8*, and *COX2* in IL-1β-stimulated OA synoviocytes. This anti-inflammatory effect of rhPRG4 was partially mediated by the CD44 receptor, as blocking this receptor abolished the effect of rhPRG4 on *MMP-9*, *MMP-13*, *aggrecanase-2*, *IL-6*, *IL-8*, and *COX2* expression.

rhPRG4 dose-dependently downregulated basal expression of OA-associated enzymes and cytokines. Specifically, rhPRG4 downregulated the expression of *MMP-1*, *MMP-3*, *MMP-9*, and *MMP-13*, which are involved in synovial fibroblast proliferation and migration [49, 50] and cartilage destruction. Interestingly, rhPRG4 reduced the expression of *COX2* in IL-1β-stimulated OA synoviocytes, whereas rhPRG4 marginally increased the expression of COX2 in unstimulated OA synoviocytes. The significance of this observation in the overall biological effect of rhPRG4 remains to be elucidated.

In summary, we herein report on the biological effect of PRG4 on fibroblast-like synoviocytes derived from patients with OA. To our knowledge, this is the first report that delineates the biological role of PRG4 in regulating OA synoviocyte function. Our study adds to existing literature that describes a non-mechanical cartilage-protective effect of PRG4 through upregulation of hypoxia-inducible factor (HIF3α) [51]. An interesting finding in our work is the role of CD44 in modulating the biological activity of rhPRG4 in synoviocytes from different origins. While rhPRG4 functioned to reduce basal NFκB nuclear levels in murine synoviocytes, this effect did not appear to be mediated by the CD44 receptor. Furthermore, rhPRG4 had equal efficacy in $Prg4^{-/-}$ synoviocytes and $Prg4^{+/+}$ synoviocytes, despite the fact that $Prg4^{-/-}$ synoviocytes display enhanced CD44 protein expression compared to $Prg4^{+/+}$ synoviocytes [15]. The CD44-dependent activity of rhPRG4 is clearly evident in OA FLS following stimulation with IL-1. In this setting, rhPRG4 inhibited IL-1-induced NFκB activation and downstream expression of catabolic enzymes and inflammatory cytokines in a CD44-dependent manner.

Our findings may be limited by the small number of OA SF aspirates included in the study. Additionally, we have not studied the biological effect of rhPRG4 on FLS from patients with varying degrees of synovitis. A third limitation of our study is that we cannot exclude the possibility that other SF proteins were co-precipitated in the PRG4 immunoprecipitation experiments.

Conclusion

PRG4 is a glycoprotein secreted by synovial fibroblasts that regulates basal and IL-1-induced expression of matrix metalloproteinases that are involved in synovial proliferation and cartilage destruction. The full-length recombinant form of PRG4 inhibits proliferation of synovial fibroblasts through a mechanism that involves the CD44 receptor. Additionally, depletion of native PRG4 in OA SF stimulates synoviocyte proliferation.

Abbreviations

Ab: Antibody; ADAMTS: A disintegrin and metalloproteinase with thrombospondin motifs; ANOVA: Analysis of variance; BSA: Bovine serum albumin; COX2: Cycloxygenase-2; Ct: Cycle threshold; DMEM: Dulbecco's modified Eagle's medium; ELISA: Enzyme-linked immunosorbent assay; FBS: Fetal bovine serum; FLS: Fibroblast-like synoviocytes; GAPDH: Glyceraldehyde-3-phosphate dehydrogenase; IL-1β: Interleukin-1 beta; MMP: Matrix metalloproteinase; NC: Negative control; NFκB: Nuclear factor kappa B; OA: Osteoarthritis; PBS: Phosphate-buffered saline; p-IκBα: Phosphorylated inhibitor kappa B alpha; PRG4: Proteoglycan-4; qPCR: Quantitative PCR; RA: Rheumatoid arthritis; rhPRG4: Recombinant human PRG4; SF: Synovial fluid; siRNA: Small interfering RNA; TBS-T: Tris-buffered saline Tween 20; TGF-β: Transforming growth factor beta; TIMP: Tissue inhibitor of metalloproteinases; TNFα: Tumor necrosis factor alpha

Acknowledgements
Not applicable.

Funding
This work is supported by R01AR067748 to KE and GJ.

Authors' contributions
Authors AA, MJ, and LZ carried out the experiments and participated in the analysis of data. Author TS participated in study design and critical interpretation of results. Authors GJ and KE conceived the study and participated in data analysis and interpretation. All authors have participated in drafting and critical evaluation of the manuscript. All authors have read and approved the final version of the manuscript.

Authors' information
Ali Alquraini, MSc: Ph.D. candidate, MCPHS University, Boston, MA, USA. Maha Jamal, MSc: Ph.D. student, Chapman University, Irvine, CA, USA. Ling Zhang, MD: Senior Research Assistant, Rhode Island Hospital, Providence, RI, USA. Tannin Schmidt, Ph.D.: Associate Professor of Bioengineering, University of Calgary, Canada. Gregory D. Jay, MD, Ph.D.: Professor, Emergency Medicine, Rhode Island Hospital, Providence, RI, USA. Khaled A. Elsaid, Pharm.D, Ph.D.: Associate Professor of Biomedical and Pharmaceutical Sciences, Chapman University, Irvine, CA, USA.

Competing interests
Authors AA, MJ, and LZ have nothing to disclose. Author GJ holds patents on rhPRG4 and holds equity in Lubris LLC, MA, USA. Author TS holds patents on rhPRG4, is a paid consultant for Lubris LLC, MA, USA, and holds equity in Lubris LLC, MA, USA. Author KE holds patents on rhPRG4. All authors have no non-financial competing interests related to this manuscript.

Consent for publication
Not applicable.

Ethical approval and consent to participate
OA and RA synoviocytes were obtained from a commercial source (Cell Applications Inc.). Harvest of synoviocytes was performed following appropriate Institutional Review Board (IRB) approvals from partner sites with informed written consent from the donor. OA SF specimens were acquired from Articular Engineering, IL, USA, following knee replacement surgery or from donors within 24 hours of death, collected with partner site IRB approval with informed written consent from the donor or nearest relative. Harvest of synovial tissues from $Prg4^{-/-}$ and $Prg4^{+/+}$ mice was approved by the IACUC Committee at Rhode Island Hospital, Providence, RI, USA. This study was approved by the IRB at the MCPHS University. The biological samples (cells and SF) were obtained from a commercial source and patients were de-identified. The authors did not seek patients' consent to study these biological samples.

Author details
[1]Department of Pharmaceutical Sciences, MCPHS University, Boston, MA, USA. [2]Department of Emergency Medicine, Rhode Island Hospital, Providence, RI, USA. [3]Faculty of Kinesiology and Schulich School of Engineering, University of Calgary, Calgary, AB, Canada. [4]Department of Biomedical Engineering, Brown University, Providence, RI, USA. [5]Department of Biomedical and Pharmaceutical Sciences, Chapman University School of Pharmacy, Rinker Health Sciences Campus, 9401 Jeronimo Road, Irvine, CA 92618, USA. [6]School of Pharmacy, Albaha University, Albaha, Saudi Arabia.

References
1. Jay GD, Britt DE, Cha CJ. Lubricin is a product of megakaryocyte stimulating factor gene expression by human synovial fibroblasts. J Rheumatol. 2000; 27(3):594–600.
2. Jay GD, Tantravahi U, Britt DE, Barrach HJ, Cha CJ. Homology of lubricin and superficial zone protein (SZP): products of megakaryocyte stimulating factor (MSF) gene expression by human synovial fibroblasts and articular chondrocytes localized to chromosome 1q25. J Orthop Res. 2001;19(4):677–87.
3. Flannery CR, Hughes CE, Schumacher BL, Tudor D, Aydelotte MB, et al. Articular cartilage superficial zone protein (SZP) is homologous to megakaryocyte stimulating factor precursor and is a multifunctional proteoglycan with potential growth-promoting cytoprotective, and lubricating properties in cartilage metabolism. Biochem Biophys Res Commun. 1999;254(3):535–41.
4. Rhee DK, Marcelino J, Baker M, Gong Y, Smits P, et al. The secreted glycoprotein lubricin protects cartilage surfaces and inhibits synovial cell overgrowth. J Clin Invest. 2005;115(3):622–31.

5. Rhee DK, Marcelino J, Al-Mayouf S, Schelling DK, Bartels CF, et al. Consequences of disease-causing mutations on lubricin protein synthesis, secretion, and post-translational processing. J Biol Chem. 2005;280(35): 31325–32.

6. Jay GD, Torres JR, Rhee DK, Helminen HJ, Hytinnen MM, et al. Association between friction and wear in diarthrodial joint lacking lubricin. Arthritis Rheum. 2007;56(11):3662–9.

7. Waller KA, Zhang LX, Elsaid KA, Fleming BC, Warman ML, et al. Role of lubricin and boundary lubrication in the prevention of chondrocyte apoptosis. Proc Natl Acad Sci U S A. 2013;110(15):5852–7.

8. Hill A, Walker KA, Allen JM, Smits P, Zhang LX, et al. Lubricin restoration in a mouse model of congenital deficiency. Arthritis Rheumatol. 2015;67(11): 3070–81.

9. Jay GD, Fleming BC, Watkins BA, McHugh KA, Anderson SC, et al. Prevention of cartilage degeneration and restoration of chondroprotection by lubricin tribosupplementation in the rat following anterior cruciate ligament transection. Arthritis Rheum. 2010;62(8):2382–91.

10. Teeple E, Elsaid KA, Jay GD, Zhang L, Badger GJ, et al. Effects of supplemental intra-articular lubricin and hyaluronic acid on the progression of posttraumatic arthritis in the anterior cruciate ligament-deficient rat knee. Am J Sports Med. 2011;39(1):164–72.

11. Jay GD, Elsaid KA, Kelly KA, Anderson SC, Zhang L, et al. Prevention of cartilage degeneration and gait asymmetry by lubricin tribosupplementation in the rat following anterior cruciate ligament transection. Arthritis Rheum. 2012;64(4):1162–71.

12. Elsaid KA, Zhang L, Waller K, Tofte J, Teeple E, et al. The impact of forced joint exercise on lubricin biosynthesis from articular cartilage following ACL transection and intra-articular lubricin's effect in exercised joints following ACL transection. Osteoarthr Cartil. 2012;20:940–8.

13. Cui Z, Xu C, Li X, Song J, Yu B. Treatment with recombinant lubricin attenuates osteoarthritis by positive feedback loop between articular cartilage and subchondral bone in ovariectomized rats. Bone. 2015;74:37–47.

14. Elsaid KA, Zhang L, Shaman Z, Patel C, Schmidt TA, et al. The impact of early intra-articular administration of interleukin-1 receptor antagonist on lubricin metabolism and cartilage degeneration in an anterior cruciate ligament transection model. Osteoarthr Cartil. 2015;23:114–21.

15. Al-Sharif A, Jamal M, Zhang L, Larson K, Schmidt TA, et al. Lubricin/proteoglycan 4 binidng to CD44 receptor: a mechanism of lubricin's suppression of proinflammatory cytokine induced synoviocyte proliferation. Arthritis Rheumatol. 2015;67(6):1503–13.

16. Alquraini A, Garguilo S, D'Souza G, Zhang LX, Schmidt TA, et al. The interaction of lubricin/proteoglycan-4 (PRG4) with toll-like receptors 2 and 4: an anti-inflammatory role of PRG4 in synovial fluid. Arthritis Res Ther. 2015;17:353.

17. Iqbal SM, Leonard C, Regmi SC, De Rantere D, Tailor P, et al. Lubricin/proteoglycan 4 binds to and regulates the activity of toll-like receptors in vitro. Sci Rep. 2016;6:18910.

18. Cutly M, Nguyen HA, Underhill CB. The hyaluronan receptor (CD44) participates in the uptake and degradation of hyaluronan. J Cell Biol. 1992; 116(4):1055–62.

19. Underhill C. CD44: the hyaluronan receptor. J Cell Sci. 1992;103(Pt 2):293–8.

20. Tibesku CO, Szuwart T, Ocken SA, Skwara A, Fuchs S. Expression of the matrix receptor CD44v5 on chondrocytes changes with osteoarthritis: an experimental investigation in the rabbit. Ann Rheum Dis. 2006;65(1):105–8.

21. Fuchs S, Dankbar B, Wildenau G, Goetz W, Lohmann CH, et al. Expression of the CD44 variant isoform 5 in the human osteoarthritic knee joint: correlation with radiological, histomorphological, and biochemical parameters. J Orthop Res. 2004;22(4):774–80.

22. Zhang FJ, Luo W, Gao SG, Su DZ, Li YS, et al. Expression of CD44 in articular cartilage is associated with disease severity in knee osteoarthritis. Mod Rheumatol. 2013;23(6):1186–91.

23. Fuhrmann IK, Steinhagen J, Ruther W, Schumacher U. Comparative immunohistochemical evaluation of the zonal distribution of extracellular matrix and inflammation markers in human meniscus in osteoarthritis and rheumatoid arthritis. Acta Histochem. 2015;117:243–54.

24. Samson ML, Morrison S, Masala N, Sullivan BD, Sullivan DA, et al. Characterization of full-length recombinant human proteoglycan 4 as an ocular surface boundary lubricant. Exp Eye Res. 2014;127C:14–9.

25. Livak KJ, Schmittgen TD. Analysis of relative gene expression data using real-time quantitative PCR and the 2(-Delta Delta C(T)) method. Methods. 2001;25:402–8.

26. Wenham CY, Congahan PG. The role of synovitis in osteoarthritis. Ther Adv Musculoskelet Dis. 2010;2:349–59.

27. Loeuille D, Chary-Valckenaere I, Champigneulle J, Rat AC, Toussaint F, et al. Macroscopic and microscopic features of synovial membrane inflammation in the osteoarthritic knee: correlating magnetic resonance imaging findings with disease severity. Arthritis Rheum. 2005;52(11):3492–501.

28. Loeuille D, Rat AC, Goebel JC, Champigneulle J, Blum A, et al. Magnetic resonance imaging in osteoarthritis: which method best reflects synovial membrane inflammation? Correlations with clinical, macroscopic and microscopic features. Osteoarthr Cartil. 2009;17:1186–92.

29. Scanzello CR, McKeon B, Swaim BH, Dicarlo E, Asomugha EU, et al. Synovial inflammation in patients undergoing arthroscopic meniscectomy: molecular characterization and relationship to symptoms. Arthritis Rheum. 2011;63: 391–400.

30. Saito I, Koshino T, Nakashima K, Uesugi M, Saito T. Increased cellular infiltrate in inflammatory synovia of osteoarthritic knees. Osteoarthr Cartil. 2002;10:156–62.

31. Bondeson J, Wainwright SD, Lauder S, Amos N, Hughes CE. The role of synovial macrophages and macrophage-produced cytokines in driving aggrecanases, matrix metalloproteinases, and other destructive and inflammatory responses in osteoarthritis. Arthritis Res Ther. 2006;8:R187.

32. Hill CL, Hunter DJ, Niu J, Clancy M, Guermazi A, et al. Synovitis detected on magnetic resonance imaging and its relation to pain and cartilage loss in knee osteoarthritis. Ann Rheum Dis. 2007;66:1599–603.

33. Torres L, Dunlop DD, Peterfy C, Guermazi A, Prasad P, et al. The relationship between specific tissue lesions and pain severity in persons with knee osteoarthritis. Osteoarthr Cartil. 2006;14:1033–40.

34. Ishijima M, Watari T, Naito K, Kaneko H, Futami I, et al. Relationships between biomarkers of cartilage, bone, synovial metabolism and knee pain provide insights into the origins of pain in early knee osteoarthritis. Arthritis Res Ther. 2011;13:R22.

35. Roemer FW, Guermazi A, Felson DT, Niu J, Nevitt MC, et al. Presence of MRI-detected joint effusion and synovitis increases the risk of cartilage loss in knees without osteoarthritis at 30-month follow-up: the MOST study. Ann Rheum Dis. 2011;70:1804–9.

36. Inoue H, Takamori M, Nagata N, Nishikawa T, Oda H, et al. An investigation of cell proliferation and soluble mediators induced by interleukin-1 beta I human synovial fibroblasts: comparative response in osteoarthritis and rheumatoid arthritis. Inflamm Res. 2001;50:65–72.

37. Karin M. How NF-κB is activated: the role of the IκB kinase (IKK) complex. Oncogene. 1999;18:6867–74.

38. Brun P, Zavan B, Vindigni V, Schiavinato A, Pozzuoli A, et al. In vitro response of osteoarthritic chondrocytes and fibroblast-like synoviocytes to a 500-730 kDa hyalruonan amide derivative. J Biomed Mater Res B Appl Biomater. 2010;100:2073–81.

39. Nugent GE, Aneloski NM, Schmidt TA, Schumacher BL, Voegtline MS, et al. Dynamic shear stimulation of bovine cartilage biosynthesis of proteoglycan 4. Arthritis Rheum. 2006;54:1888–96.

40. Ogawa H, Kozhemyakina E, Hung HH, Grodzinsky AJ, Lassar AB. Mechanical motion promotes expression of Prg4 in articular cartilage via multiple CREB-dependent, fluid flow shear stress-induced signaling pathways. Genes Dev. 2014;28:127–39.

41. Xu T, Wu MJ, Feng JY, Lin XP, Gu ZY. Combination of intermittent hydrostatic pressure linking TGF-β1, TNF-α on modulation of proteoglycan 4 metabolism in rat temporomandibular synovial fibroblasts. Oral Surg Oral Pathol Oral Radiol. 2012;114:183–92.

42. Jones AR, Flannery CR. Bioregulation of lubricin expression by growth factors and cytokines. Eur Cell Mater. 2007;13:40–5.

43. Schmidt TA, Gastelum NS, Han EH, Nugent-Derfus GE, Schumacher BL, et al. Differential regulation of proteoglycan 4 metabolism in cartilage by IL-1 alpha, IGF-1, and TGF-beta 1. Osteoarthr Cartil. 2008;16(1):90–7.

44. McNary SM, Athanasiou KA, Reddi AH. Transforming growth factor-β induced superficial zone protein accumulation in the surface zone of articular cartilage is dependent on the cytoskeleton. Tissue Eng Part A. 2014; 20(5-6):921–9.

45. Blewis ME, Lao BJ, Schmuacher BL, Bugbee WD, Sah RL, et al. Interactive cytokine regulation of synoviocyte lubricant secretion. Tissue Eng Part A. 2010;16(4):1329–37.

46. Larson KM, Zhang L, Elsaid KA, Schmidt TA, Fleming BC, et al. Reduction of friction by recombinant human proteoglycan 4 in IL-1α stimulated bovine cartilage explants. J Orthop Res. 2016;35(3):580–9. doi:10.1002/jor.23367.

47. Wang CT, Lin YT, Chiang BL, Lin YH, Hou SM. High molecular weight hyaluronic acid down-regulates the gene expression of osteoarthritis-associated cytokines and enzymes in fibroblast-like synoviocytes from patients with early osteoarthritis. Osteoarthr Cartil. 2006;14:1237–47.
48. Fernandes JC, Martel-Pelletier J, Pelletier JP. The role of cytokines in osteoarthritis pathophysiology. Bioreheology. 2002;39:237–46.
49. Bartok N, Firestein GS. Fibroblast-like synoviocytes: key effector cells in rheumatoid arthritis. Immunol Rev. 2010;233:233–55.
50. Xue M, McKElvey K, Shen K, Minhas N, March L, et al. Endogenous MMP-9 and not MMP-2 promotes rheumatoid synovial fibroblast survival, inflammation and cartilage destruction. Rheumatology. 2014;53:2270–9.
51. Ruan M, Erez A, Guse K, Dawson B, Bertin T, et al. Proteoglycan 4 expression protects against the development of osteoarthritis. Sci Transl Med. 2013; 5(176):176ra34.

14

Transient receptor potential ankyrin 1 (TRPA1) is functionally expressed in primary human osteoarthritic chondrocytes

Elina Nummenmaa[1] [iD], Mari Hämäläinen[1], Lauri J. Moilanen[1], Erja-Leena Paukkeri[1], Riina M. Nieminen[1], Teemu Moilanen[1,2], Katriina Vuolteenaho[1] and Eeva Moilanen[1*]

Abstract

Background: Transient receptor potential ankyrin 1 (TRPA1) is a membrane-associated cation channel, widely expressed in neuronal cells and involved in nociception and neurogenic inflammation. We showed recently that TRPA1 mediates cartilage degradation and joint pain in the MIA-model of osteoarthritis (OA) suggesting a hitherto unknown role for TRPA1 in OA. Therefore, we aimed to investigate whether TRPA1 is expressed and functional in human OA chondrocytes.

Methods: Expression of TRPA1 in primary human OA chondrocytes was assessed by qRT-PCR and Western blot. The functionality of the TRPA1 channel was assessed by Ca^{2+}-influx measurements. Production of MMP-1, MMP-3, MMP-13, IL-6, and PGE_2 subsequent to TRPA1 activation was measured by immunoassay.

Results: We show here for the first time that TRPA1 is expressed in primary human OA chondrocytes and its expression is increased following stimulation with inflammatory factors IL-1β, IL-17, LPS, and resistin. Further, the TRPA1 channel was found to be functional, as stimulation with the TRPA1 agonist AITC caused an increase in Ca^{2+} influx, which was attenuated by the TRPA1 antagonist HC-030031. Genetic depletion and pharmacological inhibition of TRPA1 downregulated the production of MMP-1, MMP-3, MMP-13, IL-6, and PGE_2 in osteoarthritic chondrocytes and murine cartilage, respectively.

Conclusions: The TRPA1 cation channel was found to be functionally expressed in primary human OA chondrocytes, which is an original finding. The presence and inflammatory and catabolic effects of TRPA1 in human OA chondrocytes propose a highly intriguing role for TRPA1 as a pathogenic factor and drug target in OA.

Keywords: Osteoarthritis, Chondrocyte, TRPA1, Inflammation, Matrix metalloproteinase

Background

Transient receptor potential ankyrin 1 (TRPA1) is a membrane-associated cation channel which mediates pain and hyperalgesia [1, 2] and functions as a chemosensor of noxious compounds [3–5]. TRPA1 was first discovered in 1999 [6] and has since then been found to be widely expressed in afferent sensory neurons, especially in Aδ and C fibers of nociceptors [7, 8]. In addition to pain, TRPA1 also has a role in mediating neurogenic inflammation [9, 10]. More recently, TRPA1 has been found to be expressed also in some nonneuronal cells such as keratinocytes [11] and synoviocytes [12] but the functional roles of nonneuronal expression remain to be studied.

TRPA1 is activated by numerous exogenous pungent compounds such as allyl isothiocyanate (AITC) from mustard oil [5], acrolein from exhaust fumes and tobacco smoke [9], and allicin from garlic [3]. Interestingly, TRPA1 is also activated and sensitized by agents formed endogenously in inflammatory reactions, such as nitric oxide [13], hydrogen peroxide [14] and nitro-oleic acid [15]. The activation of TRPA1 causes an influx of cation ions, particularly Ca^{2+}, into the activated cells [16] and this elevation of intracellular Ca^{2+} has been

* Correspondence: eeva.moilanen@uta.fi
[1]The Immunopharmacology Research Group, University of Tampere School of Medicine and Tampere University Hospital, Tampere, Finland
Full list of author information is available at the end of the article

shown to trigger an action potential in neuronal cells [16, 17]. Interestingly, among the many regulatory effects of the alterations of intracellular Ca^{2+} concentration, its increase has also been shown to affect the gene expression of inflammatory mediators [18–20].

Recent evidence suggests TRPA1 to have a role in inflammation through exogenous activation by TRPA1 agonists and also through endogenous mechanisms. TRPA1 has been shown to mediate carrageenan-induced inflammatory edema [21], tumor necrosis factor (TNF)-triggered hyperalgesia [22], airway hyperreactivity and inflammation [23, 24], and to relate to acute gouty arthritis [25, 26]. Very recently we found that TRPA1 has a role in mediating acute inflammation, cartilage destruction, and joint pain in monosodium iodoacetate (MIA)-induced inflammation and osteoarthritis in the mouse [27].

Osteoarthritis (OA) is the most common cause of musculoskeletal disability and pain worldwide and its prevalence is constantly increasing as the population ages. OA is a degenerative disease of the joints, which is characterized by inflammation and hypoxia within the joint, leading to cartilage degradation, joint deformity, disability, and pain [28, 29]. OA-related cartilage degradation is caused by a growing imbalance between the production of catabolic, anabolic, and inflammatory mediators within the joint driven by the increased expression of matrix-degrading metalloproteinases and proinflammatory mediators such as interleukin (IL)-6 and prostaglandin E_2 (PGE_2) [28].

TRPA1 has not previously been investigated in chondrocytes. However, factors involved in hypoxia and inflammation, such as hydrogen peroxide (H_2O_2), nitric oxide (NO), and IL-6 have been shown to upregulate the expression or activation of TRPA1 in some other cells [12–14]. Furthermore, the activation of TRPA1 has been reported to enhance the production of inflammatory factors [12, 21, 26, 30]. Since there is a hypoxic and inflammatory state in OA joints [28, 31], and TRPA1 has been shown to be involved in the mediation of acute inflammation and cartilage degradation in MIA-induced osteoarthritis [27], we hypothesized that TRPA1 is expressed in the chondrocytes in osteoarthritic joints, where its activation could play a vital part in the inflammation and pathogenesis of OA. In the present study, we tested that hypothesis by measuring the expression and function of TRPA1 in primary human OA chondrocytes.

Methods
Cell culture
Primary chondrocyte cultures were carried out as previously described [32]. Leftover pieces of OA cartilage from knee joint replacement surgery were used under full patient consent. The patients in this study fulfilled the American College of Rheumatology classification criteria for OA [33] and the study was approved by the Ethics Committee of Tampere University Hospital, Tampere, Finland (reference number R09116), and carried out in accordance with the Declaration of Helsinki. The procedures to isolate and culture the primary chondrocytes are described in the supplementary data (Additional file 1). During experiments the cells were treated with IL-1β (R&D Systems Europe Ltd, Abingdon, UK), IL-17 (R&D Systems Europe Ltd.), lipopolysaccharide (LPS) (Millipore Sigma, St. Louis, MO, USA), resistin (BioVision Inc., Milpitas, CA, USA), the TRPA1 antagonist HC-030031 (Millipore Sigma) or with combinations of these compounds as indicated.

Immortalized human T/C28a2 chondrocytes [34] were cultured as described in the supplementary data (Additional file 1). During the experiments T/C28a2 chondrocytes were treated with IL-1β (R&D Systems Europe Ltd), IL-17 (R&D Systems Europe Ltd.), LPS (Millipore Sigma), HC-030031 (Millipore Sigma) or with combinations of these compounds as indicated.

HEK 293 human embryonic kidney cells (American Type Culture Collection, Manassas, VA, USA) were cultured as described in the supplementary data (Additional file 1). The cells were transfected using 0.42 mg/cm^2 of human TRPA1 plasmid DNA (pCMV6-XL4 by Origene, Rockville, MD, USA) with lipofectamine 2000 (Invitrogen, Life Technologies, Carlsbad, CA, USA) according to the manufacturer's instructions.

Animals
Wild-type (WT) and TRPA1 knockout (KO) male B6;129P-Trpa1(tm1Kykw)/J mice (Charles River Laboratories, Sulzfeld, Germany) aged 19–22 days were used in mouse cartilage culture experiments. Mice were housed under standard conditions (12–12 h light–dark cycle, 22 ± 1 °C) with food and water provided ad libitum. Animal experiments were carried out in accordance with the legislation for the protection of animals used for scientific purposes (Directive 2010/63/EU) and the experiments were approved by The National Animal Experiment Board (reference number UTA 845/712-86). Animals were sacrificed by carbon monoxide followed by cranial dislocation.

Mouse cartilage culture
After mice were euthanized, full-thickness articular cartilage from femoral heads were removed and cultured as described in the supplementary data (Additional file 1). The cartilage pieces were exposed to IL-1β (R&D Systems Europe Ltd.) or its vehicle for 42 h and thereafter culture media were collected and matrix metalloproteinase (MMP)-3, IL-6, and PGE_2 concentrations were measured by immunoassay.

Western blot measurements

After the cell culture experiments, total protein was extracted, and TRPA1 was immunoprecipitated and analyzed with Western blot as described in the supplementary data (Additional file 1). TRPA1 antibody NB110-40763 (Novus Biologicals, LCC, Littleton, CO, USA) was used as the primary antibody and goat anti-rabbit HRP-conjugate (sc-2004, Santa Cruz Biotechnology, Inc., Dallas, TX, USA) as the secondary antibody in the Western blot analysis.

Immunoassay

Concentrations of IL-6, MMP-1, MMP-3, MMP-13 and PGE_2 in medium samples were determined by enzyme-linked immunosorbent assay (ELISA) with commercial reagents (PGE_2: Cayman Chemical Co., Ann Arbor, MI, USA; human IL-6: eBioscience Inc. San Diego, CA, USA; MMP-1, MMP-3, MMP-13 and mouse IL-6: R&D Systems Europe Ltd).

RNA extraction and quantitative RT-PCR

At the indicated time points, total RNA was extracted and analyzed by quantitative reverse transcription polymerase chain reaction (qRT-PCR) for the expression of TRPA1 mRNA as described in the supplementary data (Additional file 1).

Ca^{2+}-influx measurements

TRPA1-mediated Ca^{2+} influx was measured in HEK293 cells [35] transfected with human TRPA1 plasmid, in human T/C28a2 chondrocytes, and in primary human OA chondrocytes as described previously [36]. Briefly, the cells were loaded with 4 μM fluo-3-acetoxymethyl ester (Fluo-3-AM, Millipore Sigma) and 0.08 % Pluronic F-127® (Millipore Sigma in Hanks' balanced salt solution (HBSS, Lonza, Verviers, Belgium) containing 1 mg/ml of bovine serum albumin, 2.5 mM probenecid and 25 mM HEPES pH 7.2 (all from Millipore Sigma) for 30 min at room temperature. The intracellular-free Ca^{2+} levels were assessed by Victor3 1420 multilabel counter (Perkin Elmer, Waltham, MA, USA) at excitation/emission wavelengths of 485/535 nm. In the experiments, the cells were first preincubated with the TRPA1 antagonist HC-030031 (100 μM, Millipore Sigma) or the vehicle for 30 min at +37 °C. Thereafter, the TRPA1 agonist allyl isothiocyanate (AITC, 50 μM, Millipore Sigma) was added and the measurements were continued for 30 s after which a robust Ca^{2+} influx was induced by application of the control ionophore compound ionomycin (1 μM, Millipore Sigma).

Statistical analysis

Data were analyzed using Graph-Pad InStat version 3.00 software (GraphPad Software, San Diego, CA, USA).

The results are presented as mean + standard error of the mean (SEM) unless otherwise indicated. Unpaired t test, paired t test, one-way analysis of variance (ANOVA) or repeated-measures ANOVA, followed by Dunnett's test were used in the statistical analysis. Differences were considered significant at $p < 0.05$, $p < 0.01$, and $p < 0.001$.

Results

TRPA1 is expressed in primary human OA chondrocytes and in immortalized human T/C28a2 chondrocyte cell line

Primary human OA chondrocytes and immortalized human T/C28a2 chondrocyte cell line expressed TRPA1. The expression was measured by quantitative RT-PCR on isolated total mRNA using a specific TaqMan assay. The proinflammatory cytokine IL-1β was found to increase TRPA1 expression in a time-dependent manner: in primary chondrocytes the expression of TRPA1 increased up to 48 hours and declined thereafter (Fig. 1a), whereas in the human T/C28a2 chondrocytes the expression maximum was at 6 hours (Fig. 1b). In addition, TRPA1 expression was also enhanced by inflammatory factors IL-17, LPS, and resistin (Fig. 2).

To verify the translation of TRPA1 mRNA into protein, we extracted total protein from primary human OA chondrocytes and human T/C28a2 chondrocytes and performed Western blot analysis. HEK293 cells transiently transfected with TRPA1 plasmid were used as positive control and the protein was detected with a specific human TRPA1 antibody. Remarkably, both cell types were found to express TRPA1 protein as seen in Fig. 3.

Human chondrocytes express a functional TRPA1 channel

To confirm that TRPA1 mRNA and the subsequent protein expressed by human chondrocytes produces a functional channel, Ca^{2+}-influx measurements were carried out. Primary human chondrocytes and T/C28a2 chondrocytes were cultured with IL-1β, which was found to stimulate TRPA1 expression, or with its vehicle for 24 h, and thereafter TRPA1 was activated with the TRPA1 agonist AITC. IL-1β stimulation resulted in an increased responsiveness to AITC as seen as an enhanced Ca^{2+} influx, and the selective TRPA1 antagonist HC-030031 was shown to prevent this effect (Fig. 4).

MMP, IL-6 and PGE_2 production is downregulated by genetic depletion and pharmacological inhibition of TRPA1

After finding that functional TRPA1 was indeed expressed in chondrocytes, we aimed to further examine the possible arthritogenic role of the TRPA1 channel. We investigated the effect of genetic depletion of TRPA1 on the production of OA-related factors MMP-3, IL-6, and PGE_2 by using articular cartilage samples from TRPA1-deficient (knockout, KO) and corresponding wild-type (WT) mice. IL-1β treatment increased MMP-

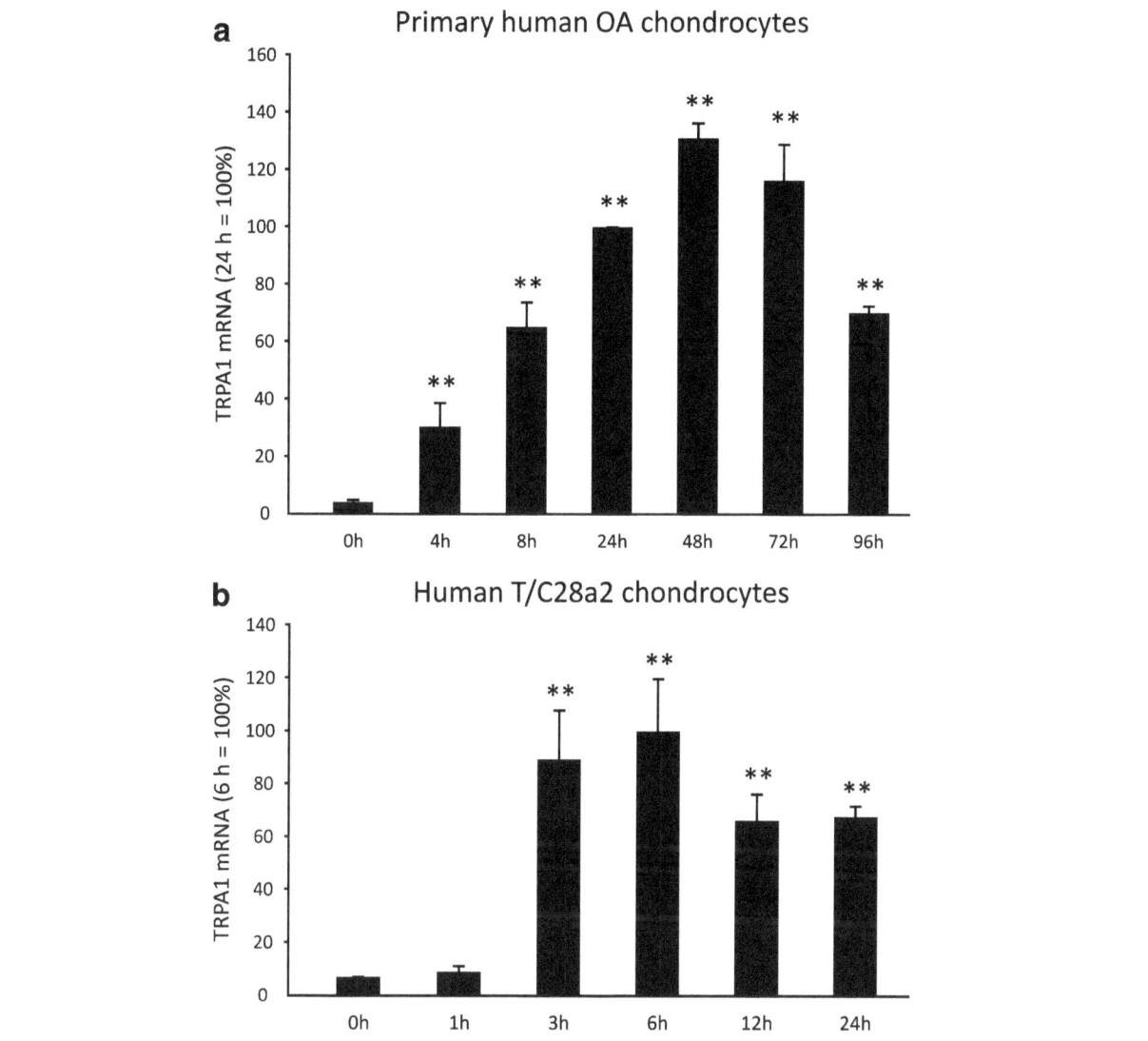

Fig. 1 Primary human OA chondrocytes (**a**) and human T/C28a2 chondrocyte cell line (**b**) express TRPA1 mRNA and its expression is enhanced by IL-1 in a time-dependent manner. Cultures of primary human OA chondrocytes (**a**) and human T/C28a2 chondrocytes (**b**) were stimulated with IL-1β (100 pg/ml) for 0–96 h and 0–24 h, respectively, and thereafter total RNA was extracted. TRPA1 mRNA levels were measured by qRT-PCR, and the results were normalized against GAPDH mRNA. The mRNA levels are expressed as arbitrary units with the levels measured at 24 h (**a**; primary OA chondrocytes) or 6 h (**b**; T/C28a2 chondrocytes) set as 100 %; and the values at the other time points are related to those values. Primary chondrocyte samples were obtained from three to five different donors and the experiments were carried out in duplicate. Human T/C28a2 chondrocyte experiments were carried out in quadruplicate. Results are expressed as mean + SEM. One-way ANOVA followed by Dunnett's post-test was used in the statistical analysis; **indicates $p < 0.01$ compared to the control (0 h) sample. *OA* osteoarthritis, *TRPA1* transient receptor potential ankyrin 1

3, IL-6, and PGE_2 production in cartilage as expected. Remarkably, this response was significantly attenuated in the cartilage from the TRPA1 KO mice as compared to the corresponding WT mice (Fig. 5). Further, we treated primary human chondrocytes with IL-1β alone and together with the selective TRPA1 antagonist HC-030031 for 24 h. Interestingly, the selective TRPA1 antagonist HC-030031 downregulated IL-1β-enhanced MMP-1, MMP-3, MMP-13, IL-6, and PGE_2 production by 25–45 % (Fig. 6), suggesting that TRPA1 plays a role in the

upregulation of these catabolic and inflammatory factors in OA cartilage.

Discussion

The findings of the present study suggest a hitherto unknown role for TRPA1 in the pathogenesis of OA. We have shown for the first time the expression of the TRPA1 channel in primary human OA chondrocytes and in the human T/C28a2 chondrocyte cell line. We showed the expression of TRPA1 mRNA and protein by

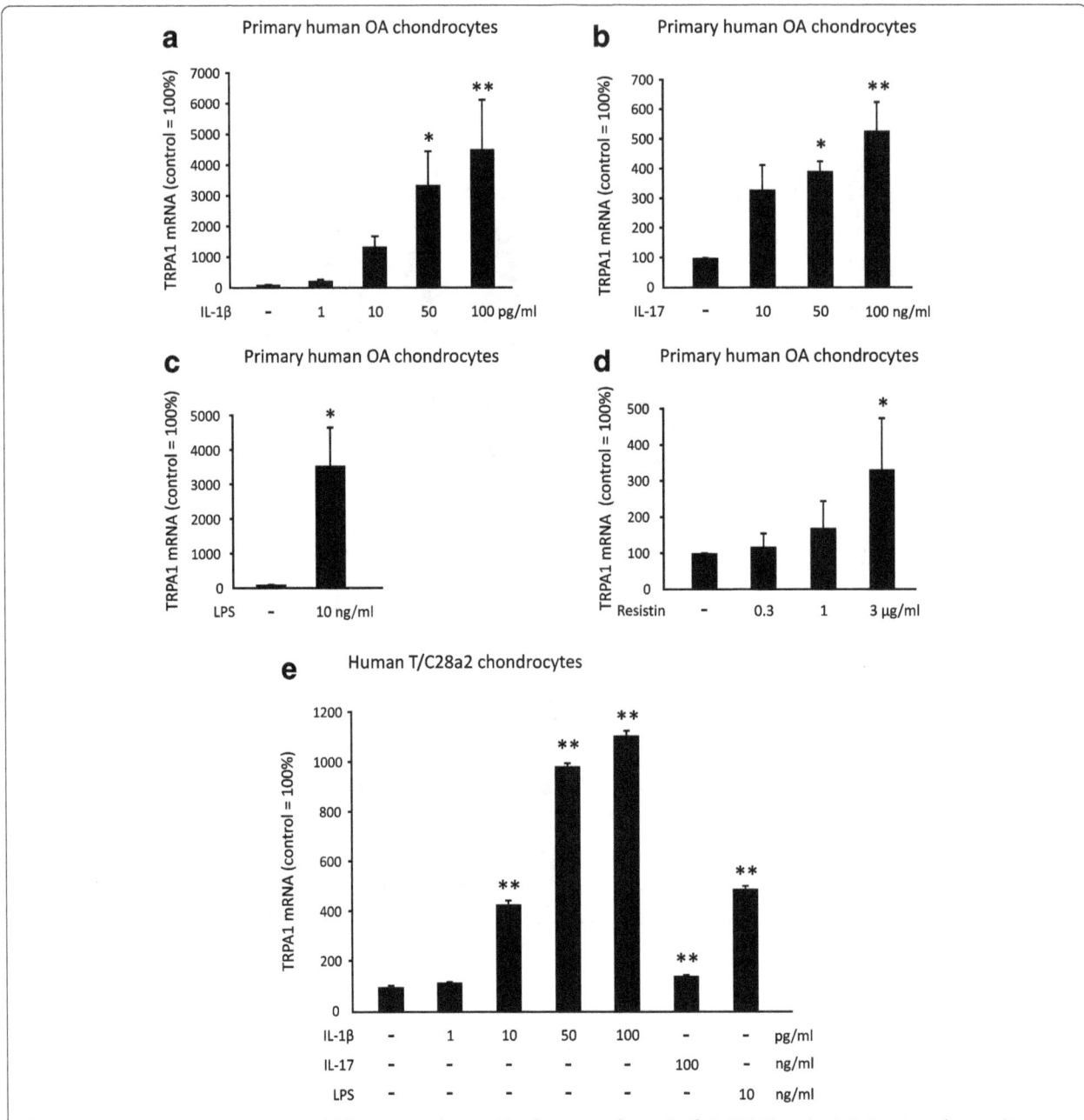

Fig. 2 TRPA1 mRNA expression is increased following stimulation with inflammatory factors IL-1β, IL-17, LPS, and resistin in primary human OA chondrocytes (**a-d**) and in human T/C28a2 chondrocyte cell line (**e**). Isolated primary human OA chondrocytes were stimulated with IL-1β (1–100 pg/ml) (**a**), IL-17 (10–100 ng/ml) (**b**), LPS (10 ng/ml) (**c**). and resistin (0.3–3 μg/ml) (**d**); and human T/C28a2 chondrocytes with IL-1β (1–100 pg/ml), IL-17 (100 ng/ml) and LPS (10 ng/ml) (**e**) for 24 h; and thereafter total RNA was extracted. TRPA1 mRNA levels were measured by qRT-PCR, and the results were normalized against GAPDH mRNA levels. The results are expressed as a percentage in comparison to untreated control samples, which was set as 100 %. Primary chondrocyte samples were obtained from four different donors and the experiments were performed in duplicate. Human T/C28a2 chondrocyte experiments were carried out in quadruplicate. Results are expressed as mean + SEM. Repeated measures ANOVA (**a**, **b**, **d**) and one-way ANOVA (**e**) followed by Dunnett's post-test or paired t test (**c**) was used in the statistical analysis; $^*p < 0.05$ and $^{**}p < 0.01$, compared to the untreated control samples. *IL* interleukin, *LPS* lipopolysaccharide, *OA* osteoarthritis, *TRPA1* transient receptor potential ankyrin 1

qRT-PCR and Western blot, respectively. We were also able to show that the expressed TRPA1 was functional, as evidenced by Ca^{2+}-influx measurements. Further, we found TRPA1 to have a role in mediating the production of OA-related factors MMP-1, MMP-3, MMP-13, IL-6,

and PGE$_2$ as evidenced by pharmacological inhibition and genetic depletion of TRPA1.

TRPA1 was first discovered in 1999 in fetal lung fibroblasts [6]. Since then it has been mainly studied in different afferent sensory neurons such as Aδ and C fibers of

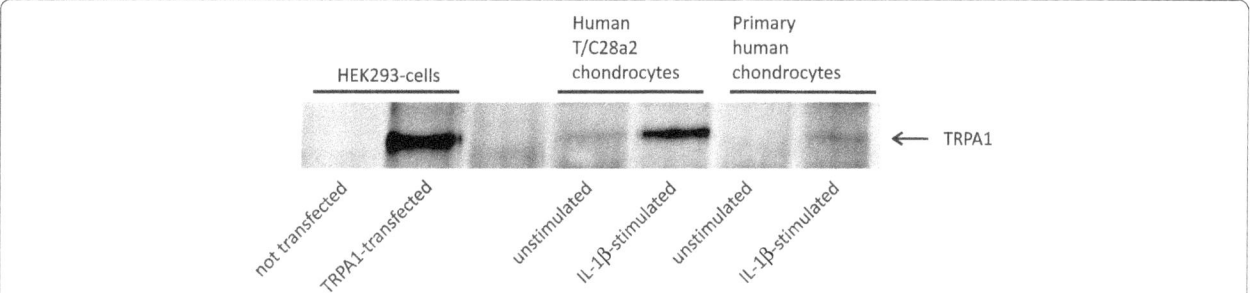

Fig. 3 TRPA1 protein is expressed in primary human OA chondrocytes and human T/C28a2 chondrocyte cell line. Chondrocyte cultures were stimulated with IL-1β (100 pg/ml) for 24 h. Extracted proteins were immunoprecipitated and TRPA1 was detected with Western blot analysis. HEK293 cells transiently transfected with human TRPA1 plasmid were used as a positive control. Representative blot of three independent experiments with similar results. *IL* interleukin, *TRPA1* transient receptor potential ankyrin 1

nociceptors [7, 8]. More recently, however, TRPA1 has also been found to be expressed in some nonneuronal cells such as keratinocytes [11, 37, 38], synoviocytes [12, 39] and airway epithelial and smooth muscle cells [30]. It is noteworthy, that not all of these studies have shown functionality of the TRPA1 ion channel and some have only reported the expression of TRPA1 at the mRNA level. In the present study, we have comprehensively shown the expression and activation of TRPA1 in human chondrocytes, to support the criteria set by Fernandes et al. [40]. We were able to show for the first time the expression of both TRPA1 mRNA and protein and the functionality of the TRPA1 channel in primary human OA chondrocytes and in human T/C28a2 chondrocyte cell line. This finding is particularly interesting as in OA joints there is a hypoxic [31] and inflammatory [28, 41] state and related factors, H_2O_2, NO, and IL-6, have previously been shown to upregulate the expression and activation of TRPA1 [12–14]. According to Hatano et al. [12] the human *TRPA1* promoter has at least six putative nuclear factor kappa B (NF-kB) binding sites and ten core hypoxia response elements (HREs), which are binding sites for hypoxia-inducible factor (HIF) transcription factors. HIFs are known to mediate adaptive responses to hypoxia as well as to be activated by inflammation [42, 43] and the binding of HIFs to consensus HREs on their target genes regulates gene transcription.

After discovering TRPA1 expression in chondrocytes, we aimed to investigate whether inflammatory factors/mechanisms related to the pathogenesis of OA [28, 29] regulate expression of TRPA1, which would indicate a role for TRPA1 as a mediator in OA. IL-1β is considered as a major player in OA associated with cartilage destruction. IL-1β is elevated in OA joints and it suppresses type II collagen and aggrecan expression, stimulates the release of MMP-1, MMP-3, and MMP-13, and induces the production of IL-6 and some other cytokines as well as PGE₂ [28]. In part IL-17 feeds forward

these mechanisms as it further induces IL-1β, TNF, and IL-6 production, upregulates NO and MMPs and downregulates proteoglycan levels related to the pathogenesis of OA [28]. Based on our results, IL-1β and IL-17 both also induce TPRA1 expression and intriguingly, some of the IL-1β-induced inflammatory and catabolic effects are partly mediated by TRPA1. In OA the innate immune system and in particular toll-like receptors (TLRs) activated by cartilage matrix degradation products, also play a significant part in disease progression. Chondrocytes express TLRs, which trigger major inflammatory pathways and are activated by bacterial lipopolysaccharide (LPS) and damage-associated molecular patterns [29], and also the adipocytokine resistin known to be expressed in OA joints [44] has been shown to transduce its effects through toll-like receptor 4 [45]. In the present study, we found that both LPS and resistin increased expression of TRPA1 in human chondrocytes, suggesting a TLR-mediated mechanism to enhance TRPA1 expression in OA cartilage. In support of the present results, Hatano et al. showed that TRPA1 gene expression was enhanced in synoviocytes by inflammatory factors TNF-α and IL-1 [12], and the present study together with that of Hatano et al. [12] suggests a previously unrecognized mechanism that links TRPA1 as an inducible factor to joint inflammation.

Activation of TRPA1 results in a substantial influx of Ca^{2+} into the stimulated cells [46]. Here we verified the functionality and activation of the TRPA1 channel in human chondrocytes by measuring Ca^{2+} influx using the TRPA1 agonist AITC as well as the TRPA1 antagonist HC-030031. As shown previously, elevated intracellular Ca^{2+} concentration may affect the expression of inflammatory genes both in a direct or indirect manner [20]. In the present study, we found that TRPA1 regulated the production of inflammatory and catabolic factors, namely MMP enzymes, IL-6, and PGE₂ in chondrocytes. IL-1-induced MMP-3, IL-6, and PGE₂ production in the cartilage from TRPA1-deficient mice was less than half

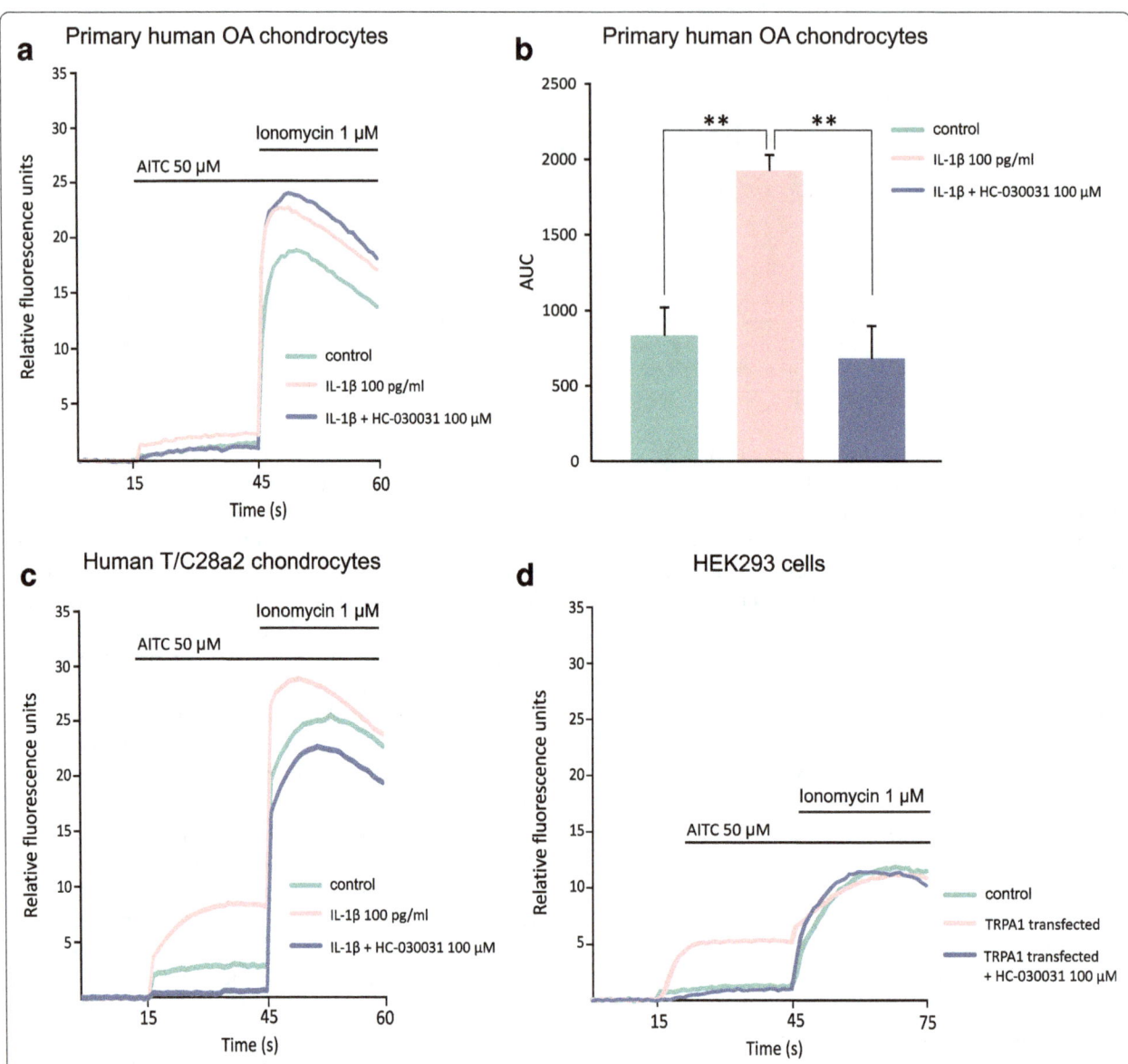

Fig. 4 The TRPA1 ion channel is functional in primary human OA chondrocytes (**a**, **b**) and human T/C28a2 chondrocyte cell line (**c**) as shown by TRPA1-mediated Ca^{2+} influx. Primary human chondrocytes (**a**, **b**) and human T/C28a2 chondrocytes (**c**) were cultured with or without (control) IL-1β (100 pg/ml) for 24 h. HEK293 cells transfected with plasmids encoding human TRPA1 were used as positive control cells (**d**). The cells were loaded with Fluo-3-AM and the TRPA1-mediated Ca^{2+} influx was measured by Victor3 multilabel counter at excitation/emission wavelengths of 485/535 nm at 1/s frequency. The cells were first preincubated with the TRPA1 antagonist HC-030031 (100 μM) or the vehicle for 30 min at +37 ° C. In the measurements, basal fluorescence was first recorded for 15 s and thereafter the selective TRPA1 agonist allyl isothiocyanate (AITC; 50 μM) was added and the measurement was continued for 30 s after which the control ionophore compound ionomycin (1 μM) was introduced to the cells. IL-1β stimulation resulted in an elevation in AITC-induced Ca^{2+} influx compared to unstimulated control cells, and it was attenuated by the selective TRPA1 antagonist HC-030031. The results were normalized against the background and expressed as mean of eight simultaneous measurements. Curves in *A*, *C* and *D* express results from one representative experiment. In (**b**) area under the curve (AUC) from 15 to 45 s was calculated from measurements of primary chondrocyte from four donors (each with eight repeats). Results are expressed as mean + SEM. Repeated measures ANOVA followed by Dunnett's post-test was used in the statistical analysis; $^{**}p < 0.01$ compared to the IL-1β-treated samples. *IL* interleukin, *OA* osteoarthritis, *TRPA1* transient receptor potential ankyrin 1

of that found in the cartilage from wild-type mice. Accordingly, the selective TRPA1 antagonist HC-030031 reduced IL-1-induced MMP-1, MMP-3, MMP-13, IL-6, and PGE_2 production by 25–45 % in primary human OA chondrocytes. In the latter experiment, the cells

were incubated in the presence of IL-1 and HC-030031 for 24 h; therefore the result may be an underestimate of the effect of total inhibition of TRPA1 in OA chondrocytes because HC-030031 is a reversible TRPA1 antagonist with a relatively short half-life [47]. These findings

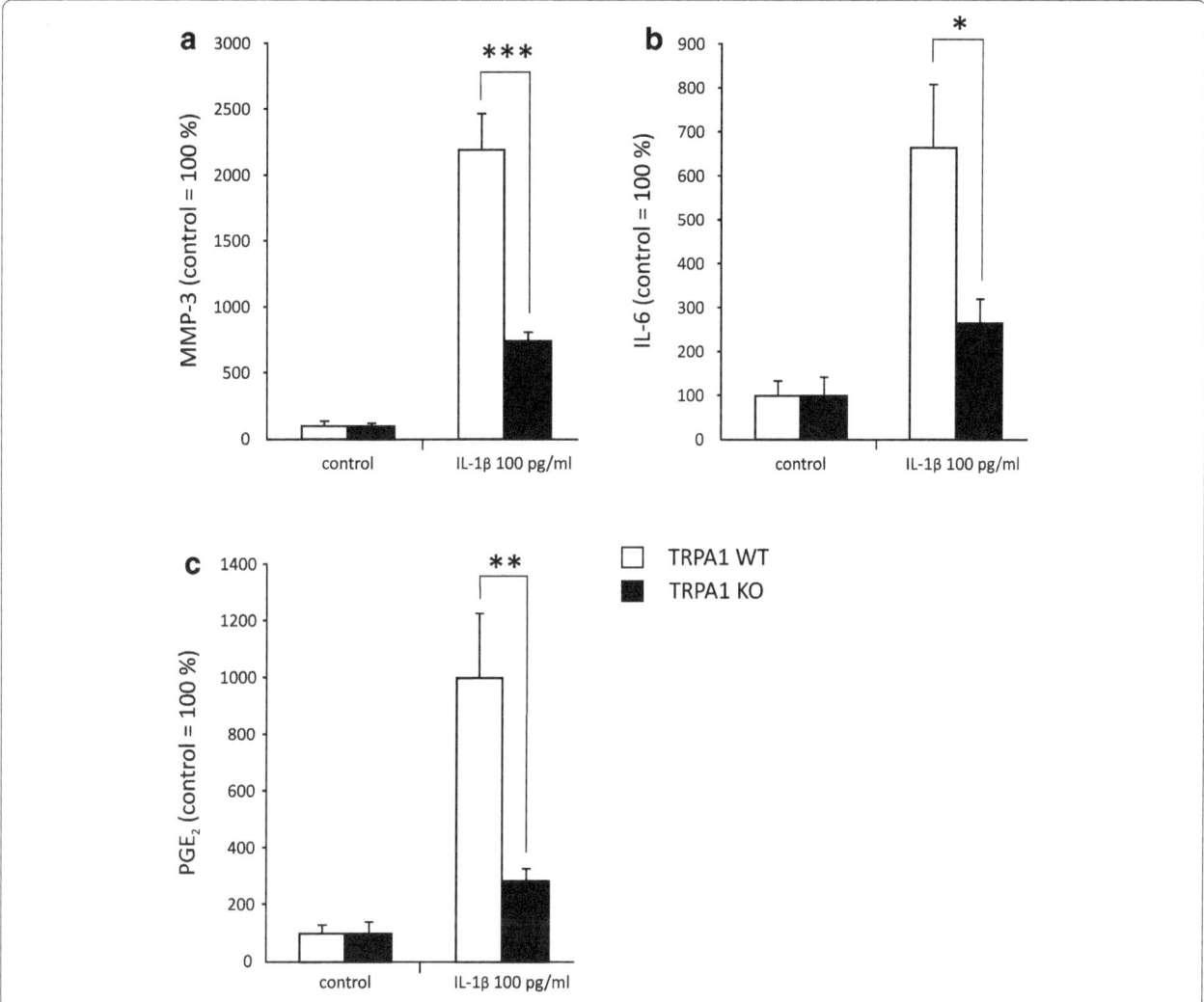

Fig. 5 IL-1β-induced production of MMP-3 (**a**), IL-6 (**b**), and PGE$_2$ (**c**) in the cartilage is attenuated by genetic depletion of TRPA1. Cartilage samples were obtained from TRPA1-deficient (knockout, KO) and corresponding wild-type (WT) mice. The samples were cultured with and without IL-1β (100 pg/ml) for 42 h and thereafter the culture medium was collected and analyzed for concentrations of MMP-3, IL-6, and PGE$_2$ by immunoassay. The results are expressed as mean + SEM, n = 6–9. Unpaired *t* test was used in the statistical analysis; $^*p < 0.05$, $^{**}p < 0.01$, and $^{***}p < 0.001$ compared to the WT mice. *IL* interleukin, *MMP* matrix metalloproteinase, *PGE$_2$* prostaglandin E$_2$, *TRPA1* transient receptor potential ankyrin 1

are supported by previous studies indicating that TRPA1 activation regulates the production of IL-1 in keratinocytes [38], IL-6 and IL-8 in synoviocytes [12], and PGE$_2$ along with leukotriene B$_4$ in fibroblasts and keratinocytes [48]. We have recently found that TRPA1 also regulates the expression of cyclooxygenase-2 (COX-2) [21, 27] and the production of monocyte chemotactic protein-1 (MCP-1), IL-6, IL-1β, myeloperoxidase (MPO), MIP-1α and MIP-2 in inflammatory conditions [26]. The detailed molecular mechanisms of this regulation remain, however, to be studied.

TRPA1 is shown to be involved in pain, hyperalgesia, and neurogenic inflammation [10, 16, 49, 50]. In OA-related pain, the role of TRPA1 has been investigated in studies by Moilanen et al. [27] McGaraughty et al. [51] and Okun et al. [52] using the MIA-model of OA. The two first-mentioned studies [27, 51] concluded TRPA1 to contribute

to joint pain in experimental OA. In addition, Moilanen et al. [27] reported that TRPA1-deficient mice developed less severe cartilage changes following MIA injections. Accordingly, we showed here that TRPA1 is functionally expressed in chondrocytes. We also examined the possible functions of the channel by treating primary chondrocyte cultures with IL-1β and the selective antagonist HC-030031 [2, 53, 54]. Our results suggest an inflammatory and catabolic role for TRPA1 in human chondrocytes, as we found inhibition of TRPA1 to suppress the production of OA-related factors MMP-1, MMP-3, MMP-13, IL-6, and PGE$_2$. These results were supported by experiments with cartilage from WT and TRPA1-deficient mice: following stimulation with IL-1β MMP-3, IL-6, and PGE$_2$ production was lower in the cartilage from TRPA1-deficient mice than from WT animals. These results together suggest that TRPA1-activating

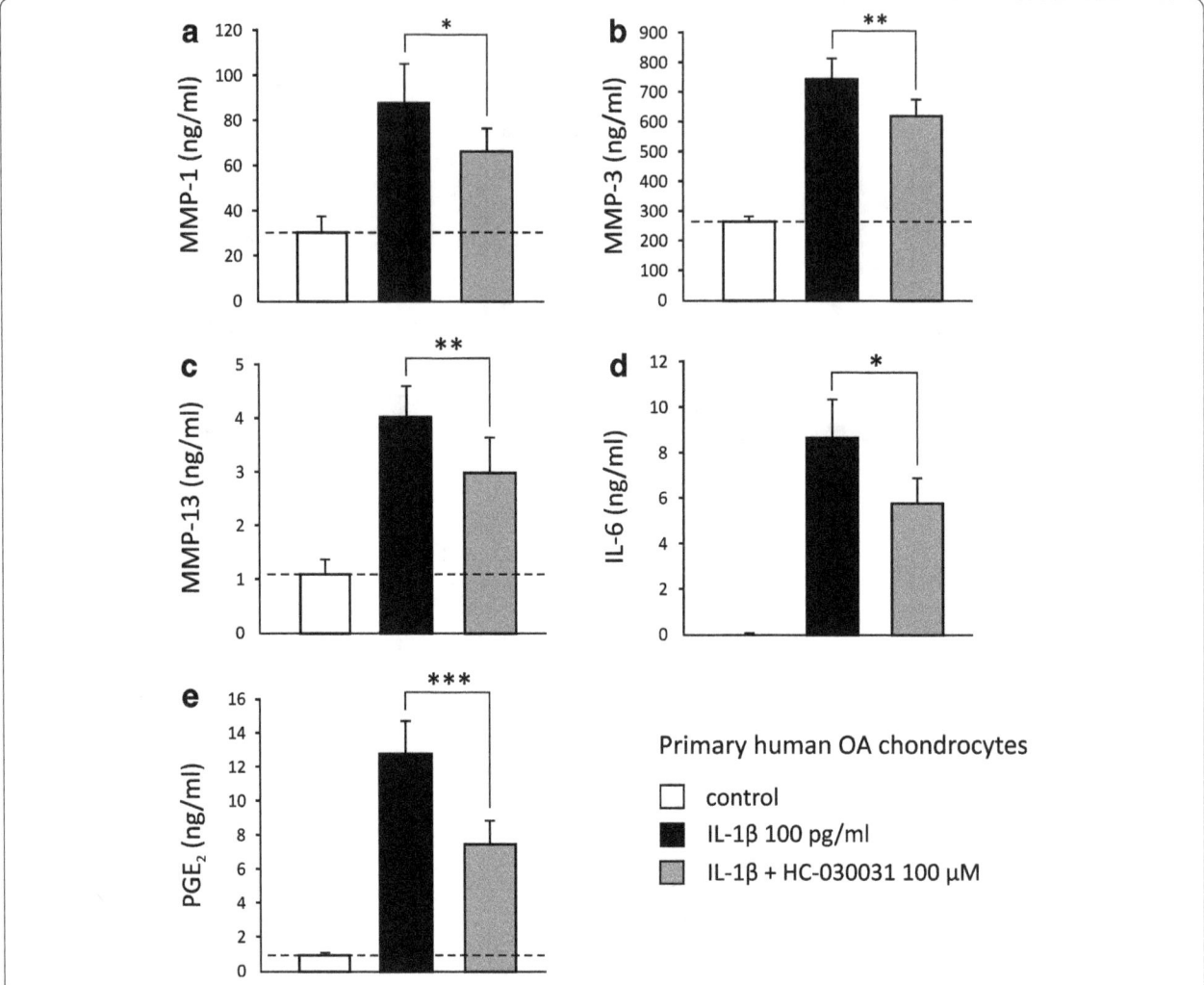

Fig. 6 IL-1β-enhanced expression of MMP-1 (**a**), MMP-3 (**b**), MMP-13 (**c**), IL-6 (**d**), and PGE$_2$ (**e**) in primary human OA chondrocytes is attenuated by pharmacological inhibition of TRPA1. Primary human OA chondrocytes were stimulated with IL-1β (100 pg/ml) in the presence and absence of the selective TRPA1 antagonist HC-030031 (100 μM) for 24 h. MMP-1, MMP-3, MMP-13, IL-6, and PGE$_2$ concentrations in the culture media were measured by immunoassay and the results are expressed as mean + SEM. Samples were obtained from eight patients and the experiments were carried out in duplicate. Paired t test was used in the statistical analysis; $^*p < 0.05$, $^{**}p < 0.01$, and $^{***}p < 0.001$ compared to the IL-1β-treated samples. *IL* interleukin, *MMP* matrix metalloproteinase, *OA* osteoarthritis, *PGE$_2$* prostaglandin E$_2$, *TRPA1* transient receptor potential ankyrin 1

factors are present in OA joints, and that TRPA1 mediates, at least partly, OA-related pain, inflammation, and cartilage destruction in neuronal and nonneuronal cells in the joint.

Conclusions

In conclusion, we found the TRPA1 cation channel to be functionally expressed in primary human OA chondrocytes and in part to mediate inflammatory and catabolic effects, which are both original findings. The inflammatory and hypoxic environment in the OA joint is conducive to enhance the expression and activation of TRPA1. The presence and effects of TRPA1 in human OA cartilage as found in the present study, together with the previous findings on TRPA1 in experimentally induced OA [27, 51] propose an intriguing role for TRPA1 as a mediator and drug target in OA.

Abbreviations

AITC, allyl isothiocyanate; ANOVA, analysis of variance; COX-2, cyclooxygenase-2; ELISA, enzyme-linked immunosorbent assay; H$_2$O$_2$, hydrogen peroxide; HIF, hypoxia-inducible factor; HRE, hypoxia response element; IL, interleukin; KO, knockout; LPS, lipopolysaccharide; MCP-1, monocyte chemotactic protein-1; MIA, monosodium iodoacetate; MIP, macrophage inflammatory protein; MMP, matrix metalloproteinase; MPO, myeloperoxidase; NF-kB, nuclear factor-kappa B; NO, nitric oxide; OA, osteoarthritis; PGE$_2$, prostaglandin E$_2$; qRT-PCR, quantitative reverse transcription polymerase chain reaction; SEM, standard error of the mean; TLR, toll-like receptor; TNF, tumor necrosis factor; TRPA1, transient receptor potential ankyrin 1; WT, wild-type

Acknowledgements

We wish to thank Ms Salla Hietakangas, Terhi Salonen, and Ella Lehto for excellent technical assistance and Ms Heli Määttä for skillful secretarial help.

Funding

The study was supported by grants from the Competitive Research Funding of the Pirkanmaa Hospital District, Finland; Tampere Tuberculosis Foundation, Finland; Finnish Cultural Foundation, Finland; Research Foundation of Rheumatic Diseases, Finland; and Patient Organization for Rheumatoid Arthritis (Tampereen Reumayhdistys), Finland. The funding bodies had no role in the design of the study, or collection, analysis, and interpretation of data, nor in writing the manuscript.

Authors' contributions

EN, MH, LJM, E-LP, RMN, TM, KV, and EM contributed to the design of the study and to the acquisition, analysis and interpretation of the data. EM conceived and supervised the study. EN drafted the manuscript and all authors revised the manuscript critically for important intellectual content and have approved the final version of the manuscript for submission.

Authors' information

Not applicable.

Competing interests

The authors declare that they have no competing interests.

Consent for publication

Not applicable.

Author details

[1]The Immunopharmacology Research Group, University of Tampere School of Medicine and Tampere University Hospital, Tampere, Finland. [2]Coxa Hospital for Joint Replacement, Tampere, Finland.

References

1. Chen J, Joshi SK, DiDomenico S, Perner RJ, Mikusa JP, Gauvin DM, et al. Selective blockade of TRPA1 channel attenuates pathological pain without altering noxious cold sensation or body temperature regulation. Pain. 2011; 152:1165–72.
2. McNamara CR, Mandel-Brehm J, Bautista DM, Siemens J, Deranian KL, Zhao M, et al. TRPA1 mediates formalin-induced pain. Proc Natl Acad Sci U S A. 2007;104:13525–30.
3. Bautista DM, Movahed P, Hinman A, Axelsson HE, Sterner O, Hogestatt ED, et al. Pungent products from garlic activate the sensory ion channel TRPA1. Proc Natl Acad Sci U S A. 2005;102:12248–52.
4. Bandell M, Story GM, Hwang SW, Viswanath V, Eid SR, Petrus MJ, et al. Noxious cold ion channel TRPA1 is activated by pungent compounds and bradykinin. Neuron. 2004;41:849–57.
5. Jordt SE, Bautista DM, Chuang HH, McKemy DD, Zygmunt PM, Hogestatt ED, et al. Mustard oils and cannabinoids excite sensory nerve fibres through the TRP channel ANKTM1. Nature. 2004;427:260–5.
6. Jaquemar D, Schenker T, Trueb B. An ankyrin-like protein with transmembrane domains is specifically lost after oncogenic transformation of human fibroblasts. J Biol Chem. 1999;274:7325–33.
7. Story GM, Peier AM, Reeve AJ, Eid SR, Mosbacher J, Hricik TR, et al. ANKTM1, a TRP-like channel expressed in nociceptive neurons, is activated by cold temperatures. Cell. 2003;112:819–29.
8. Nilius B, Appendino G, Owsianik G. The transient receptor potential channel TRPA1: from gene to pathophysiology. Pflugers Arch. 2012;464:425–58.
9. Bautista DM, Jordt SE, Nikai T, Tsuruda PR, Read AJ, Poblete J, et al. TRPA1 mediates the inflammatory actions of environmental irritants and proalgesic agents. Cell. 2006;124:1269–82.
10. Koivisto A, Chapman H, Jalava N, Korjamo T, Saarnilehto M, Lindstedt K, et al. TRPA1: a transducer and amplifier of pain and inflammation. Basic Clin Pharmacol Toxicol. 2014;114:50–5.

11. Anand U, Otto WR, Facer P, Zebda N, Selmer I, Gunthorpe MJ, et al. TRPA1 receptor localisation in the human peripheral nervous system and functional studies in cultured human and rat sensory neurons. Neurosci Lett. 2008;438:221–7.
12. Hatano N, Itoh Y, Suzuki H, Muraki Y, Hayashi H, Onozaki K, et al. Hypoxia-inducible factor-1alpha (HIF1alpha) switches on transient receptor potential ankyrin repeat 1 (TRPA1) gene expression via a hypoxia response element-like motif to modulate cytokine release. J Biol Chem. 2012;287:31962–72.
13. Yoshida T, Inoue R, Morii T, Takahashi N, Yamamoto S, Hara Y, et al. Nitric oxide activates TRP channels by cysteine S-nitrosylation. Nat Chem Biol. 2006;2:596–607.
14. Andersson DA, Gentry C, Moss S, Bevan S. Transient receptor potential A1 is a sensory receptor for multiple products of oxidative stress. J Neurosci. 2008;28:2485–94.
15. Taylor-Clark TE, Ghatta S, Bettner W, Undem BJ. Nitrooleic acid, an endogenous product of nitrative stress, activates nociceptive sensory nerves via the direct activation of TRPA1. Mol Pharmacol. 2009;75:820–9.
16. Zygmunt PM, Högestätt ED. Trpa1. Handb Exp Pharmacol. 2014;222:583–630.
17. Wang YY, Chang RB, Waters HN, McKemy DD, Liman ER. The nociceptor ion channel TRPA1 is potentiated and inactivated by permeating calcium ions. J Biol Chem. 2008;283:32691–703.
18. Jakobsson PJ. Pain: how macrophages mediate inflammatory pain via ATP signaling. Nat Rev Rheumatol. 2010;6:679–81.
19. Korhonen R, Kankaanranta H, Lahti A, Lahde M, Knowles RG, Moilanen E. Bi-directional effects of the elevation of intracellular calcium on the expression of inducible nitric oxide synthase in J774 macrophages exposed to low and to high concentrations of endotoxin. Biochem J. 2001;354:351–8.
20. Berridge MJ, Lipp P, Bootman MD. The versatility and universality of calcium signalling. Nat Rev Mol Cell Biol. 2000;1:11–21.
21. Moilanen LJ, Laavola M, Kukkonen M, Korhonen R, Leppanen T, Hogestatt ED, et al. TRPA1 contributes to the acute inflammatory response and mediates carrageenan-induced paw edema in the mouse. Sci Rep. 2012;2:380.
22. Fernandes ES, Russell FA, Spina D, McDougall JJ, Graepel R, Gentry C, et al. A distinct role for transient receptor potential ankyrin 1, in addition to transient receptor potential vanilloid 1, in tumor necrosis factor alpha-induced inflammatory hyperalgesia and Freund's complete adjuvant-induced monarthritis. Arthritis Rheum. 2011;63:819–29.
23. Caceres AI, Brackmann M, Elia MD, Bessac BF, del Camino D, D'Amours M, et al. A sensory neuronal ion channel essential for airway inflammation and hyperreactivity in asthma. Proc Natl Acad Sci U S A. 2009;106:9099–104.
24. Hox V, Vanoirbeek JA, Alpizar YA, Voedisch S, Callebaut I, Bobic S, et al. Crucial role of transient receptor potential ankyrin 1 and mast cells in induction of nonallergic airway hyperreactivity in mice. Am J Respir Crit Care Med. 2013;187:486–93.
25. Trevisan G, Hoffmeister C, Rossato MF, Oliveira SM, Silva MA, Ineu RP, et al. Transient receptor potential ankyrin 1 receptor stimulation by hydrogen peroxide is critical to trigger pain during monosodium urate-induced inflammation in rodents. Arthritis Rheum. 2013;65:2984–95.
26. Moilanen LJ, Hämäläinen M, Lehtimäki L, Nieminen RM, Moilanen E. Urate crystal induced inflammation and joint pain are reduced in transient receptor potential ankyrin 1 deficient mice–potential role for transient receptor potential ankyrin 1 in gout. PLoS One. 2015;10, e0117770.
27. Moilanen LJ, Hämäläinen M, Nummenmaa E, Ilmarinen P, Vuolteenaho K, Nieminen RM, et al. Monosodium iodoacetate-induced inflammation and joint pain are reduced in TRPA1 deficient mice – potential role of TRPA1 in osteoarthritis. Osteoarth Cartilage. 2015;23:2017–26.
28. Kapoor M, Martel-Pelletier J, Lajeunesse D, Pelletier JP, Fahmi H. Role of proinflammatory cytokines in the pathophysiology of osteoarthritis. Nat Rev Rheumatol. 2011;7:33–42.
29. Glyn-Jones S, Palmer AJ, Agricola R, Price AJ, Vincent TL, Weinans H, et al. Osteoarthritis. Lancet. 2015;386:376–87.
30. Nassini R, Pedretti P, Moretto N, Fusi C, Carnini C, Facchinetti F, et al. Transient receptor potential ankyrin 1 channel localized to non-neuronal airway cells promotes non-neurogenic inflammation. PLoS One. 2012;7, e42454.
31. Pfander D, Gelse K. Hypoxia and osteoarthritis: how chondrocytes survive hypoxic environments. Curr Opin Rheumatol. 2007;19:457–62.
32. Nummenmaa E, Hämäläinen M, Moilanen T, Vuolteenaho K, Moilanen E. Effects of FGF-2 and FGF receptor antagonists on MMP enzymes, aggrecan, and type II collagen in primary human OA chondrocytes. Scand J Rheumatol. 2015;44:321–30.

33. Altman R, Asch E, Bloch D, Bole G, Borenstein D, Brandt K, et al. Development of criteria for the classification and reporting of osteoarthritis. Classification of osteoarthritis of the knee. Diagnostic and Therapeutic Criteria Committee of the American Rheumatism Association. Arthritis Rheum. 1986;29:1039–49.

34. Goldring MB, Birkhead JR, Suen LF, Yamin R, Mizuno S, Glowacki J, et al. Interleukin-1 beta-modulated gene expression in immortalized human chondrocytes. J Clin Invest. 1994;94:2307–16.

35. Graham FL, Smiley J, Russell WC, Nairn R. Characteristics of a human cell line transformed by DNA from human adenovirus type 5. J Gen Virol. 1977;36:59–74.

36. Moilanen LJ, Hämäläinen M, Lehtimäki L, Nieminen RM, Muraki K, Moilanen E. Pinosylvin inhibits TRPA1-induced calcium influx in vitro and TRPA1-mediated acute paw inflammation in vivo. Basic Clin Pharmacol Toxicol. 2016;118(3):238–42.

37. Tsutsumi M, Denda S, Ikeyama K, Goto M, Denda M. Exposure to low temperature induces elevation of intracellular calcium in cultured human keratinocytes. J Invest Dermatol. 2010;130:1945–8.

38. Atoyan R, Shander D, Botchkareva NV. Non-neuronal expression of transient receptor potential type A1 (TRPA1) in human skin. J Invest Dermatol. 2009; 129:2312–5.

39. Kochukov MY, McNearney TA, Fu Y, Westlund KN. Thermosensitive TRP ion channels mediate cytosolic calcium response in human synoviocytes. Am J Physiol Cell Physiol. 2006;291:C424–32.

40. Fernandes ES, Fernandes MA, Keeble JE. The functions of TRPA1 and TRPV1: moving away from sensory nerves. Br J Pharmacol. 2012;166:510–21.

41. Ellman MB, Yan D, Ahmadinia K, Chen D, An HS, Im HJ. Fibroblast growth factor control of cartilage homeostasis. J Cell Biochem. 2013;114:735–42.

42. Hellwig-Burgel T, Rutkowski K, Metzen E, Fandrey J, Jelkmann W. Interleukin-1beta and tumor necrosis factor-alpha stimulate DNA binding of hypoxia-inducible factor-1. Blood. 1999;94:1561–7.

43. Rius J, Guma M, Schachtrup C, Akassoglou K, Zinkernagel AS, Nizet V, et al. NF-kappaB links innate immunity to the hypoxic response through transcriptional regulation of HIF-1alpha. Nature. 2008;453:807–11.

44. Koskinen A, Vuolteenaho K, Moilanen T, Moilanen E. Resistin as a factor in osteoarthritis: synovial fluid resistin concentrations correlate positively with interleukin 6 and matrix metalloproteinases MMP-1 and MMP-3. Scand J Rheumatol. 2014;43:249–53.

45. Tarkowski A, Bjersing J, Shestakov A, Bokarewa MI. Resistin competes with lipopolysaccharide for binding to toll-like receptor 4. J Cell Mol Med. 2010;14: 1419–31.

46. Nilius B. Transient receptor potential (TRP) cation channels: rewarding unique proteins. Bull Mem Acad R Med Belg. 2007;162:244–53.

47. Rech JC, Eckert WA, Maher MP, Banke T, Bhattacharya A, Wickenden AD. Recent advances in the biology and medicinal chemistry of TRPA1. Future Med Chem. 2010;2:843–58.

48. Jain A, Bronneke S, Kolbe L, Stab F, Wenck H, Neufang G. TRP-channel-specific cutaneous eicosanoid release patterns. Pain. 2011;152:2765–72.

49. Baraldi PG, Preti D, Materazzi S, Geppetti P. Transient receptor potential ankyrin 1 (TRPA1) channel as emerging target for novel analgesics and anti-inflammatory agents. J Med Chem. 2010;53:5085–107.

50. Wei H, Koivisto A, Pertovaara A. Spinal TRPA1 ion channels contribute to cutaneous neurogenic inflammation in the rat. Neurosci Lett. 2010; 479:253–6.

51. McGaraughty S, Chu KL, Perner RJ, Didomenico S, Kort ME, Kym PR. TRPA1 modulation of spontaneous and mechanically evoked firing of spinal neurons in uninjured, osteoarthritic, and inflamed rats. Mol Pain. 2010;6:14.

52. Okun A, Liu P, Davis P, Ren J, Remeniuk B, Brion T, et al. Afferent drive elicits ongoing pain in a model of advanced osteoarthritis. Pain. 2012;153:924–33.

53. Eid SR, Crown ED, Moore EL, Liang HA, Choong KC, Dima S, et al. HC-030031, a TRPA1 selective antagonist, attenuates inflammatory- and neuropathy-induced mechanical hypersensitivity. Mol Pain. 2008;4:48-8069-4-48.

54. Taylor-Clark TE, Undem BJ, Macglashan Jr DW, Ghatta S, Carr MJ, McAlexander MA. Prostaglandin-induced activation of nociceptive neurons via direct interaction with transient receptor potential A1 (TRPA1). Mol Pharmacol. 2008;73:274–81.

15

Association between biomarkers of tissue inflammation and progression of osteoarthritis

Fatemeh Saberi Hosnijeh[1], Anne Sofie Siebuhr[2], Andre G. Uitterlinden[1,3], Edwin H. G. Oei[4], Albert Hofman[3], Morten A. Karsdal[2], Sita M. Bierma-Zeinstra[5,6], Anne C. Bay-Jensen[2] and Joyce B. J. van Meurs[1*]

Abstract

Background: We aimed to investigate the prognostic value of two biomarkers of tissue inflammation, matrix metalloproteinase-dependent degradation of C-reactive protein (CRPM) and connective tissue type I collagen turnover (C1M), on the incidence and progression of radiographic osteoarthritis (OA) in the Rotterdam Study, a prospective cohort. Moreover, the independent effect of these biomarkers with respect to the established biomarkers of OA progression, like urinary type II collagen degradation (uCTX-II) and serum cartilage oligomeric protein (COMP), was evaluated.

Methods: Serum levels of C1M, CRPM, COMP and CRP of 1335 participants aged >55 years were measured in fasting serum using ELISA. The commercial ELISA detecting CTX-II was used in urine. Radiographs at baseline and 5-year follow-up were scored for OA stage by Kellgren-Lawrence grade. The associations between progression and incidence of OA and the baseline biomarkers were examined using logistic regression and generalized estimating equations adjusted for age, sex, BMI, and possible other confounders.

Results: The uCTX-II, COMP, and CRP concentrations were associated with the incidence and progression of OA. Moreover, OA progression was positively associated with CRPM (OR = 1.3, $p = 0.01$) and CRP (OR = 1.3, $p = 0.01$) levels with similar effect size as uCTX-II (OR = 1.3, $p = 0.01$) and COMP (OR = 1.2, $p = 0.02$). CRPM had prognostic value for progression of OA independent from the uCTX-II and COMP.

Conclusions: Our study confirmed the associations between uCTX-II and COMP concentrations and OA progression. Importantly, we showed for the first time that CRPM predicts the risk of OA progression independent of the established biomarkers uCTX-II and COMP.

Keywords: Osteoarthritis, Inflammation, Biomarker, CRP, Prospective cohort

Background

Osteoarthritis (OA), the most common form of arthropathy, is characterized by alteration of joint structure including progressive cartilage destruction, synovial inflammation, and changes to the subchondral bone [1]. The etiology of OA is not well understood although the knowledge in this respect has accumulated during the past decades. Beside genetic variation and biomechanical mechanisms [1], altered lipid metabolism [2] and inflammation [3] might also be important drivers of the molecular mechanism underlying OA.

It is clear that OA is heterogeneous in its etiology and disease course. Recent efforts are now focused on identifying subgroups of patients with distinct disease pathology, which will allow the development of new targeted therapies [1]. Circulating biochemical markers (biomarkers) have the potential to serve as a measure of the different pathological processes linked to OA.

* Correspondence: j.vanmeurs@erasmusmc.nl
[1]Department of Internal Medicine, Erasmus University Medical Center, P.O. Box 2040, Rotterdam 3000 CA, Netherlands
Full list of author information is available at the end of the article

However, very few biomarkers have been identified that can predict the course of OA. Up to now, only urinary C-terminal telopeptide of collagen type II (uCTX-II) and serum cartilage oligomeric protein (COMP) (both markers of cartilage and bone metabolism) have shown discriminative ability for diagnosis and prognosis of OA [4–10].

Compared to rheumatoid arthritis (RA) or seronegative spondyloarthritis, inflammation is less prominent in OA. There is no marked infiltration of inflammatory cells into joint tissues, and the synovial fluid usually contains few neutrophils [11]. C-reactive protein (CRP), a systemic biomarker for inflammation, has been shown to be elevated in some OA patients yet the evidence is conflicting [12]. Recent studies have suggested that local inflammation plays a prominent role in the pathogenesis, symptoms, and progression of OA [3, 13, 14]. Recently, a newly developed CRP measure was described. Matrix metalloproteinase (MMP)-dependent degradation of CRP (CRPM) can be measured in serum to quantify CRP fragments released from the inflamed tissue, after CRP has been synthesized in the liver and deposited in the joint and degraded by the proteolytic burden [15]. It has been shown that MMP-degraded CRP provides a more discriminative diagnostic potential compared to that of full-length CRP in ankylosing spondylitis (AS) patients [16].

Synovial inflammation (synovitis) is a common characteristic of inflammatory OA and is believed to stimulate the connective tissue turnover. Type I collagen, the most abundant structural collagen of the human body, is a collagen of the connective tissue, including the synovial membrane. The collagen biomarker C1M is a measure of MMP-driven soft tissue destruction [17]. In a recent study among RA patients, C1M levels were associated with progression of RA and were also shown to correlate with RA activity [18]. Moreover, elevated levels of C1M were found in OA patients with higher CRP [15] and CRPM levels [16]. It seems that inflammation is important in disease pathology in a subset of the OA population; however, the pathology of this subset is not well described and few longitudinal analyses of these patients have been presented [19, 20].

Due to a general lack of consistent evidence, differences between the populations studied (clinical trials vs. population-based cohorts), and differences in sample collection, future research is needed to validate the existing OA markers and to identify new candidates. The aims of the present study were to explore the prognostic value of two biomarkers of tissue-inflammation: C1M and CPRM. In addition, we examined the extent to which these two biomarkers could be considered to be independent of well-known markers of uCTX-II and COMP and demographic characteristics such as age, sex, and body mass index (BMI) for incidence and progression of radiographic OA in a large population of men and women. Moreover, we investigated whether CRPM has prognostic value for OA progression compared to the full-length CRP.

Methods
Study population
The Rotterdam Study (RS) is a population-based prospective cohort study ongoing since 1990 to investigate the occurrence and determinants of diseases in an aging population [21]. The Rotterdam Study consists of three subpopulations. The Rotterdam Study-I (RS-I) is the first cohort of 7983 persons aged 55 years and older living in the Ommoord district of Rotterdam in the Netherlands [21]. The RS-II started in 2000 when 3011 participants were recruited into the study when they became 55 years of age or moved into the study district. In 2006, a further extension of the cohort was initiated, the RS-III, in which 3932 subjects, aged 45–54 years, were included. The study has been approved by the institutional review board (Medical Ethics Committee) of the Erasmus Medical Center and by the review board of The Netherlands Ministry of Health, Welfare and Sports and all participants gave written informed consent.

Baseline measurements were obtained through a home interview and visits to the research center for physical examinations and laboratory assessments. Blood samples were drawn by venous puncture and stored at -20 °C at baseline. Weight-bearing anteroposterior radiographs of the knee and hip were obtained at baseline and after 5 years of follow-up. Radiographs were acquired with the knee extended and the patella in a central position. Radiographs of the pelvis were obtained with both feet in 10° internal rotation and the X-ray beam centered on the umbilicus. The present study includes RS-II cohort's participants for whom knee and hip radiographs at baseline and 5-year follow-up were available and scored. Subjects without baseline (n = 114) and follow-up radiographs (n = 1358), without informed consent (n = 1), without all biomarker data (n = 187), and subjects with AS (n = 2), with RA (n = 11), and with total joint replacement (TJR) due to fracture (n = 3) were excluded from the study. Therefore, out of 3011 participants, 1335 subjects were included in the current study.

Outcome assessment
Radiographs were scored for the presence of a TJR and OA of the hip and knee according to the Kellgren and Lawrence (KL) score. Radiographic OA (which we refer to here as OA) was defined as a KL score ≥ 2 of one or both joints or a TJR [22–25]. In addition, we defined TJR as grade 5. The incidence of knee and/or hip OA was defined as a combination of KL <2 at baseline and KL ≥ 2 at follow-up. As there is no consensus on the

definition of progression, we combined incidence and progression in one definition for the overall progression of osteoarthritis. This was defined as an increase in the KL score between baseline and follow-up of ≥1. In the case of a baseline score of zero, overall progression was defined as an increase of ≥2. Patients with scores of 4 and 5 at baseline were left out of the progression analysis. Controls were free of OA at the joint site studied but were allowed to have OA at other joint sites. For example, if knee OA was studied, controls had to be free of knee OA but were allowed to have hip OA. In total OA analyses, controls were free of both hip and knee OA.

Joint pain was determined to be present based on the answer (yes/no) to the questions if participants had had persistent joint pain and stiffness in the last 6 weeks.

Quantification of biomarkers

In order to ensure the reproducibility and performance of the assays, three genuine urine or serum samples, in addition to the kit controls, were added as quality controls on each microtiter plate, and the entire plate was rerun if any of the genuine controls were determined to have a concentration >20 % of the predetermined value.

uCTX-II measurement

Subsequent to overnight fasting, urine samples were obtained from all subjects at baseline and kept frozen at − 20 °C. Monoclonal antibody mAbF46, specific for CTX-II fragments, was used in a competitive enzyme-linked immunosorbent assay (ELISA) (Immunodiagnostic Systems Nordic, Copenhagen S, Denmark) following the instructions of the manufacturer. The concentration of uCTX-II (in ng/l) was standardized to the total urine creatinine (mmol/l), and the units for the corrected uCTX-II concentration are ng/mmol [7].

COMP measurement

Serum COMP (COMP®, AnaMar, Göteborg, Sweden) were measured using enzyme-linked immunosorbent assays based on a monoclonal antibody.

CRPM, C1M measurements

Biomarkers were analyzed from fasting serum by Nordic Bioscience, Herlev, Denmark. The markers were measured by validated ELISAs applying neoepitope-specific monoclonal antibodies (Nordic Bioscience, Herlev, Denmark). The technical data (reproducibility and stability) for the assays are described in the published technical articles on the assays. The technical data are available in the following articles: C1M [17], and CRPM [16].

CRP measurement

High-sensitivity (hs)-CRP was measured using Rate Near Infrared Particle Immunoassay (Immage Immunochemistry System; Beckman Coulter, Brea, CA, USA). This method can accurately measure protein concentrations from 0.2– 1440 mg/l with a within-run precision <5.0 %, a total precision <7.5 %, and a reliability coefficient of 0.995 [26].

Statistical analyses

Missing values of biomarkers [C1M: n = 39 (2.9 %); CRPM: n = 38 (2.8 %); CTX-II: n = 116 (8.7 %); COMP: n = 12 (0.9 %); CRP: n = 35 (2.6 %)], BMI (n = 6, 0.4 %), alcohol intake (n = 6, 0.4 %), smoking status (n = 1, 0.08 %), education (n = 20, 1.5 %), and diabetes (n = 5, 0.4 %) were imputed based on a maximum likelihood estimation method accounting for the correlation structure within the data [27]. In all analyses, levels of markers were $\log_{10}$-transformed to normalize their distributions. Standardized scores (Z score) were made for continuous variables; therefore the odds ratio (OR) is expressed as percentage of change per one standard deviation.

Pearson correlation coefficients were calculated to evaluate the correlation between biomarkers. A logistic regression model adjusted for confounding variables was used to calculate OR and 95 % confidence interval (CI) for incidence and overall progression of OA in relation to each biomarker. Age, gender, BMI [weight (kg)/height (m^2)], and presence of radiographic OA were included as confounding variables. The effect of diabetes, current smoking (self-reported), educational level, and alcohol intake (current, former, never) as potential confounding variables were examined, but did not appreciably change the risk estimates (less than 10 % change in the estimates) and, therefore, were not included in the final models. Moreover, through simultaneous modeling, we investigated whether the biomarker findings are independent of one another. Generalized estimating equation (GEE) models were further used for a joint-based analysis of knees and hips to fit the models for correlations between the right and left extremity in each individual. Evidence of statistical interaction of biomarkers with sex and age was evaluated by including cross-product interaction terms in the corresponding multivariable models. We further evaluated the association between the biomarkers and baseline joint pain among individuals with OA at baseline. In order to assess the discriminating power of the biochemical markers studied we generated receiver operating characteristic (ROC) curves for each model. Area under the curve (AUC) of the models including age, sex, and BMI after adding joint pain, baseline KL score, and the biomarkers were evaluated. Statistical analyses were performed using SPSS (IBM SPSS Statistics 21; IBM Corp., Armonk, NY, USA).

Results

The descriptive characteristics of study participants are presented in Table 1. Our study population was slightly

Table 1 General characteristics of the study participants

Baseline variables	Total cohort, n = 3011	Study subjects, n = 1335			
		All subjects at baseline	OA at baseline, n = 238	OA at follow-up, n = 326	No OA at follow-up, n = 955
Female, n (%)	1694 (56)	743 (55.7)	144 (60.5)	195 (59.8)	519 (54.4)
Age*	65.2 (8.43)	63.1 (6.48)	66.4 (7.90)	66.02 (7.72)	62.13 (5.71)
Body mass index, kg/m^{2*}	27.3 (4.23)	27.04 (3.85)	27.96 (4.11)	28.01 (4.29)	26.69 (3.65)
Current alcohol drinker, n (%)	2455 (81.5)	1146 (85.8)	205 (86.1)	277 (85)	822 (86.2)
Current smoking, n (%)	692 (23)	298 (22.3)	37 (15.5)	59 (18.1)	226 (23.7)
Low level of education, n (%)	424 (31.8)	999 (33.9)	74 (31.1)	103 (31.6)	298 (31.2)
Diabetes, n (%)	182 (6.0)	68 (5.1)	12 (5.0)	21 (6.4)	42 (4.4)
Knee pain, n (%)	725 (24.1)	328 (24.6)	96 (40.3)	128 (39.3)	185 (19.4)
Hip pain, n (%)	458 (15.2)	207 (15.5)	48 (20.2)	62 (19)	132 (13.8)
Knee OA, n (%)	339 (11.3)	185 (13.9)	185 (78.1)	185 (56.7)	-
Hip OA, n (%)	141 (4.7)	68 (5.1)	68 (28.7)	68 (20.9)	-
uCTX-II*, ng/mmol	-	2.3 (0.23)	2.42 (0.27)	2.40 (0.26)	2.27 (0.22)
COMP*, U/L	-	1.03 (0.10)	1.06 (0.10)	1.06 (0.10)	1.02 (0.10)
CRP*, mg/l	-	0.02 (0.49)	0.07 (0.48)	0.12 (0.49)	-0.02 (0.48)
CRPM*, ng/ml	-	1.01 (0.18)	1.01 (0.18)	1.02 (0.18)	1.01 (0.17)
C1M*, ng/ml	-	1.59 (0.17)	1.60 (0.18)	1.61 (0.18)	1.58 (0.17)

OA osteoarthritis, uCTX-II (urinary) type II collagen degradation, COMP cartilage oligomeric protein, CPR C-reactive protein, CRPM matrix metalloproteinase-dependent degradation of CRP, C1M connective tissue type I collagen turnover
*Mean (SD); levels of biomarkers are $\log_{10}$-trasformed

younger, less obese, less diabetic, and drank more alcohol than total population. OA cases at baseline and follow-up were older, more obese and diabetic, and smoked less than subjects who remained healthy at follow-up time.

Baseline levels of most of the biomarkers were higher in OA cases compared with subjects who remained free of OA during follow-up. At baseline, there were 68 and 185 hip OA and knee OA cases, respectively. At 5-year follow-up, 41 hips (32 new cases) and 111 knees (68 new cases) with incident OA were identified. Overall progression of OA was found in 170 out of 1295 participants who were eligible for OA progression analyses [knee OA cases (n = 122) and/or hip OA cases (n = 53)].

Biomarkers levels were significantly correlated to BMI and age except for uCTX-II with BMI ($p = 0.37$) and CRPM with age ($p = 0.54$) (data not shown). Moreover, there were significant differences in C1M ($p = 0.003$) and uCTX-II levels ($p < 0.0001$) between men and women. For age, gender, and BMI-corrected data, it was found that most of the biomarkers at baseline were significantly associated with each other, with the highest correlation between CRP, CRPM, and C1M (Table 2). Urinary CTX-II was not correlated to any of the inflammatory markers.

Incidence and progression analyses
We observed a significant increased risk for incident OA with higher levels of uCTX-II, COMP, and CRP, which

all remained significant in the full model including all markers and covariates (Table 3). Incident OA cases showed a trend toward higher levels of CRPM at baseline, but this did not reach significance level. Overall progression of OA was associated with uCTX-II, COMP, CRP, and CRPM levels. We found that the reported associations were independent of other biomarkers and remained significant in the full models.

We stratified the analysis for incidence and progression according to the affected joint (knee and hip OA). However, statistical power was limited per stratum leading to wider confidence limits and nonsignificant results

Table 2 Pearson correlations between biomarkers

		CRPM	CRP	COMP	uCTX-II
C1M	Correlation coefficient	0.330	0.580	-0.111	0.033
	p value	<0.0001	<0.0001	0.001	0.223
CRPM	Correlation coefficient		0.248	-0.015	-0.004
	p value		<0.0001	0.598	0.896
CRP	Correlation coefficient			-0.104	-0.041
	p value			0.0001	0.135
COMP	Correlation coefficient				0.159
	p value				<0.0001

The correlations were adjusted for sex, age, and body mass index
CRPM matrix metalloproteinase-dependent degradation of CRP, CRP C-reactive protein, COMP cartilage oligomeric protein, uCTX-II (urinary) type II collagen degradation, C1M connective tissue type I collagen turnover

Table 3 Adjusted odds ratios (OR) and 95 % confidence intervals (CI) from logistic regression models for incident and progression of osteoarthritis (OA) in relation to biomarkers levels

	Incidence of OA, n = 88/955[†]		Progression of OA*, n = 170/1125[‡]	
	OR (95 % CI)	p value	OR (95 % CI)	p value
uCTX-II	1.3 (1.0–1.7)	0.05	1.3 (1.1–1.5)	0.01
COMP	1.3 (1.1–1.6)	0.02	1.2 (1.04–1.5)	0.02
CRPM	1.2 (1.0–1.5)	0.07	1.3 (1.1–1.5)	0.01
C1M	1.1 (0.9–1.4)	0.23	1.1 (1.0–1.4)	0.10
CRP	1.5 (1.2–1.9)	0.0003	1.3 (1.1–1.5)	0.01
Full model				
uCTX-II	1.3 (1.0–1.7)	0.05	1.3 (1.1–1.5)	0.01
COMP	1.3 (1.0–1.6)	0.03	1.2 (1.02–1.5)	0.03
CRPM	1.2 (0.9–1.5)	0.17	1.2 (1.01–1.5)	0.04
C1M	0.8 (0.6–1.1)	0.11	1.0 (0.8–1.2)	0.67
CRP	1.8 (1.3–2.4)	0.0003	1.3 (1.02–1.6)	0.03

OA incident defined as Kellgren and Lawrence (KL) ≥2 at knee and/or hip; models were adjusted for age, sex, and body mass index; full models include all biomarkers adjusted for age, sex, and body mass index
uCTX-II (urinary) type II collagen degradation, *COMP* cartilage oligomeric protein, *CRPM* matrix metalloproteinase-dependent degradation of CRP, *C1M* tissue type I collagen turnover, *CRP* C-reactive protein
[†]Case number/control number; [‡]progressed/no-progressed; *additionally adjusted for prevalent OA

(Additional file 1). Additional joint-based generalized estimating equation analyses between incidence and progression of OA and individual or combined markers showed similar results (data not shown).

Cross-sectional logistic regression analyses adjusted for age, sex, and BMI between baseline OA status and CRPM (OR = 1.0, 95 % CI = 0.8–1.1, $p = 0.58$), CRP (OR = 1.0, 95 % CI = 0.8–1.1, $p = 0.70$), and C1M (OR = 1.0, 95 % CI = 0.9–1.2, $p = 0.92$) levels showed no significant associations. Moreover, we found a positive association, albeit non-significant, between hip pain and CRPM levels (OR = 1.6, $p = 0.14$), and between knee pain and CRP (OR = 1.3, $p = 0.10$), and C1M levels (OR = 1.3, $p = 0.09$) adjusted for age, sex, and BMI among OA baseline cases.

ROC curves of individual markers did not show higher discriminative ability for C1M, CRPM, or CRP models compared with uCTX-II in all OA analyses except a slightly higher prediction ability of CRP for total OA and hip OA incidence. ROC curves of the models including demographic variables resulted in an AUC of 0.68 for OA incidence (Fig. 1 and Additional file 2) and progression (Fig. 2 and Additional file 2). Adding the joint pain variable to the models did not improve it, while subsequent addition of all biomarkers added considerable predictive value for OA. Doubtful baseline KL score of one is the best predictor of future OA, even better than age, gender and BMI alone.

Discussion

We here evaluated two novel biomarkers for tissue inflammation (C1M and CRPM) for their ability to predict incidence and progression of OA after 5 years of follow-up in a population-based setting. We show that CRPM is associated with incidence and progression of OA. Moreover, CRPM had prognostic value for progression of OA independent from uCTX-II and COMP. In the full statistical model, CRPM and CRP proved to have similar prognostic value as uCTX-II and COMP. Together the biomarkers added significant prognostic power to the known risk factors of age, gender and BMI.

To date, several studies have reported that levels of uCTX-II and COMP are associated with OA and progression of OA, suggesting them as the most promising OA biomarkers [5, 7–10, 28–31]. Consistently, we found that uCTX-II and COMP levels were correlated with increased risk and progression of OA, confirming our previous finding among participants of RS-I [7, 10]. However, despite substantial clinical investigations, none of these markers have yet been proven to be of definite clinical value [32]. Different outcome measures and study designs as well as limited sample size of these studies have resulted in inadequate discriminating ability to differentiate between individual patients and controls (diagnosis) or between patients with different disease severities (burden of disease), and to predict prognosis in individuals with or without osteoarthritis (prognosis) [33].

Our study showed that CRP levels were related to the risk and progression of OA. In our previous study with RS-I participants, an association between CRP levels and incidence of hip OA was seen as well [12]. Data on hip OA progression was limited in that review. A recent review and meta-analysis of 32 studies showed no significant associations between CRP levels and progression of OA [defined as either exacerbation of joint space narrowing (JSN) or TJR], while CRP levels were significantly associated with pain and decreased physical function. Therefore, it was suggested that CRP may be elevated in OA patients, but probably plays a greater role in symptoms rather than radiographic changes in OA [14]. In our study, we observed no significant associations between knee and hip pain and CRP levels among prevalent cases at baseline when controlled for BMI. It should be noted that there was significant heterogeneity due to the quality and methodology of the studies included in the meta-analyses and the result should be regarded with caution.

It has been shown that the CRPM level is elevated in OA patients compared to the healthy adult reference range, and that the inflammatory burden is independent of disease severity (KL score) [15]. In our study, we observed progression of OA to be associated with higher levels of CRPM. Moreover, the association seemed to be

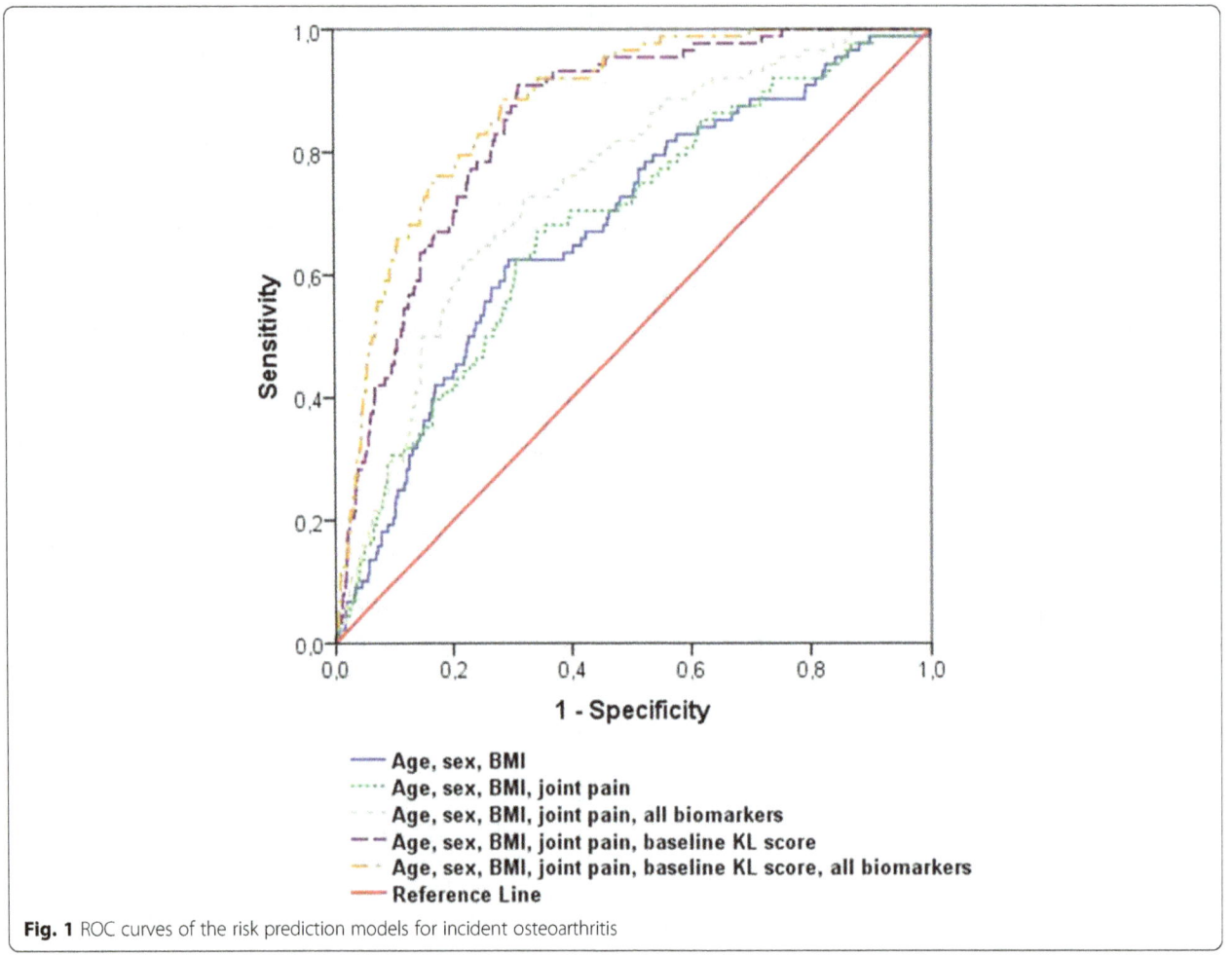

Fig. 1 ROC curves of the risk prediction models for incident osteoarthritis

independent of CRP. Previous studies did not support the role of systemic inflammation in OA etiology and progression [14], however, CRPM, a degradation product of CRP, and a possible biomarker of chronic tissue inflammation, might point toward a local low-grade inflammation to play a role in a subset of individuals with OA. Our results suggest that this subset is more prone to radiographic OA progression.

We observed no association between levels of C1M and incidence and progression of OA in both biomarker-specific and full models. The collagen biomarker C1M was found to be higher in OA patients with an elevated inflammatory burden as measured by high-sensitivity CRP [15] and CRPM [16]. Previous analysis of C1M in RA has shown that the biomarkers were associated with structural progression measured by JSN [15]. Moreover, a recent ex vivo experiment showed that under pro-inflammatory conditions serological biomarkers C1M, MMP-mediated degradation of collagen type III (C3M), and active MMP-3 may originate from the inflamed synovial membrane (Kjelgaard-Petersen CF, Bay-Jansen AC, Christiansen T,

Ladel C, Karsdal MA, Siebuhr AS. Novel synovitis biomarkers: TNF-α and IL-1β include MMP-mediated degradation of collagen type I and III and active MMP-3 and -9 in synovial membrane explants. 2014, Submitted). Our study showed significant positive linear association between C1M levels and CRPM, and CRP levels adjusted for age, sex, and BMI among baseline OA cases (data not shown). These findings illustrates that connective tissue turnover in OA (i.e., C1M levels) is increased with inflammation and, together with our findings of CRP and CRPM, provide more support to the importance of local inflammation in OA pathogenesis in a subgroup of patients.

Identification of subjects at a high risk of OA is necessary for preventive strategies. Biochemical markers might help in identification of subgroups of OA patients with higher risk of progression. Age, gender, and BMI are already rather strong predictors of OA risk and progression at older age in the population studied and in other investigations [10]. In a previous study among participants of RS-I, a prognostic model for incident knee OA was developed based on clinical, genetic and biochemical

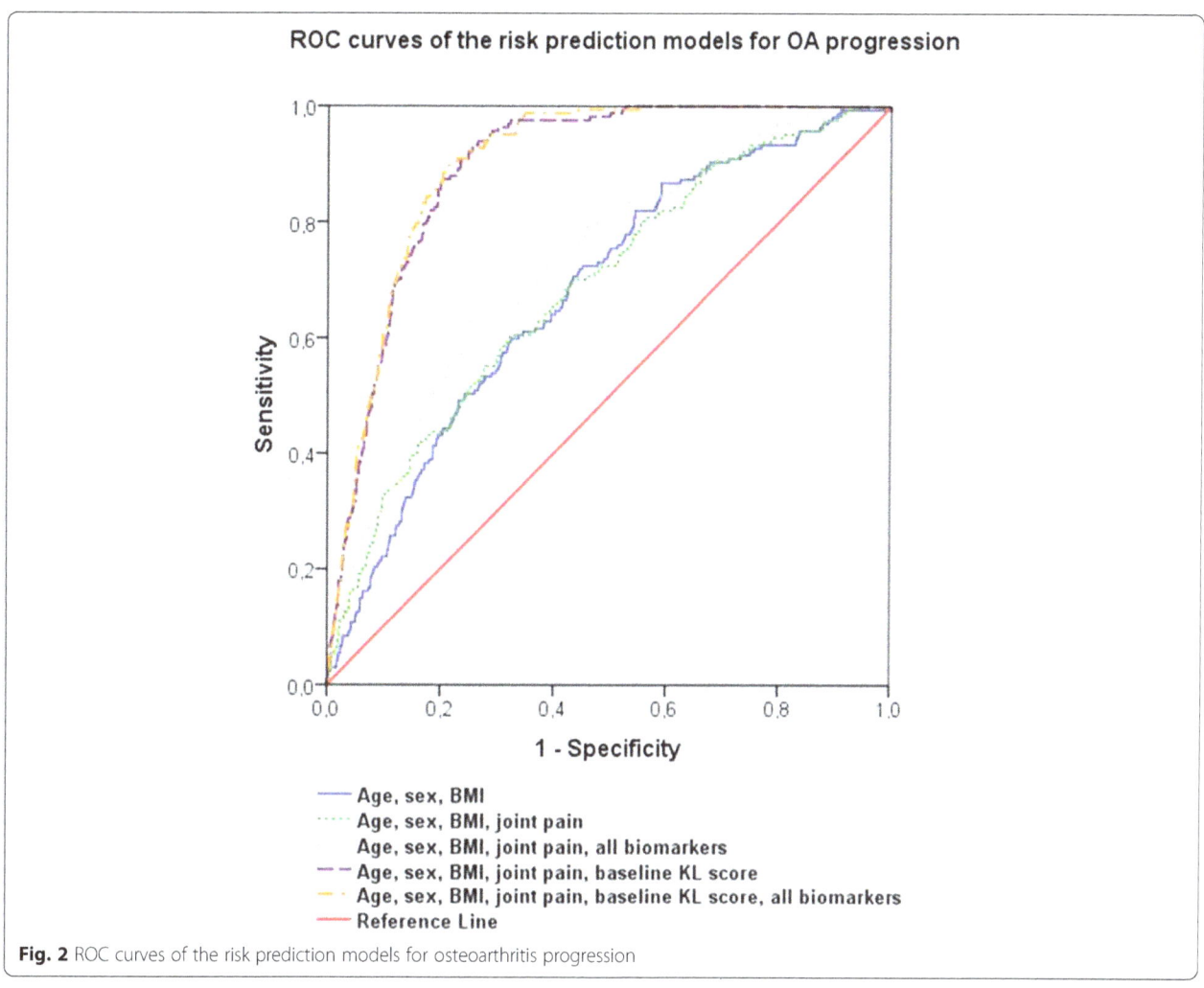

Fig. 2 ROC curves of the risk prediction models for osteoarthritis progression

(uCTX-II) risk factors [34]. The study showed that these risk factors combined had a relatively low predictive value for knee OA. In contrast, a model including doubtful minor radiographic degenerative features (KL score = 1) reached a good predictive value. Consistently, in our study, baseline KL score of one was the best predictor of future OA, and even better than age, gender and BMI alone. Addition of well-established biochemical markers together with tissue inflammation biomarkers added moderate predictive value to most of our models. Moreover, for the first time, we showed that a marker of MMP-dependent inflammation is able to predict progression of OA independent of established biomarkers uCTX-II and COMP. Future investigations are needed to identify the potential usefulness of the tissue inflammatory biomarkers in OA prediction in a clinical setting.

Radiographic OA bears little relationship to the illness characterized by joint pain and functional impairment [35, 36]. Different factors (i.e., bone marrow lesions, joint effusion, psychological factors, comorbidities) and mechanisms of joint pain (i.e., nociceptive pain, neuropathic pain, and central pain sensitization) have been described in OA patients [37, 38]. A recent study among OA patients showed the correlations between central pain mechanisms (temporal summation and pain modulation) and CRPM, independently of age, gender, BMI, and hsCRP [37]. Consistently, we found a positive association, albeit nonsignificant, between hip pain and CRPM levels, and between knee pain and CRP and C1M levels. These trends support the role of inflammation as a possible underlying mechanism of joint pain in OA, but more power is needed to definitely prove this suggestion.

There were considerable correlations between different markers reflecting turnover of cartilage (CTX-II, COMP, and C1M) and inflammatory markers (CRP and CRPM). Therefore, simultaneous modeling of several markers could provide more insight into the role of individual markers in OA progression. Moreover, due to the longitudinal design of the study, we were able to assess the potential predictive value of the markers to predict disease risk and progression. Controlling for confounder factors including age, sex, BMI, smoking status, education, and diabetes is another strength of our study. Our study, however, had some limitations that must be taken into account. First of all, biomarkers were only assessed in baseline samples. Serial biomarker assessments could also be very informative on the natural dynamics of each biochemical marker and on disease status. Moreover, the biomarker contributions from OA need to be distinguished from the contributions of normal and age-related bone and cartilage turnover, and other conditions affecting the biomarkers levels; this is currently a primary limitation for all systemic (serum and urine) biomarker measures [33]. However, individuals with rheumatoid arthritis or other inflammatory arthropathies were excluded from our analyses. Additionally, we adjusted the analyses for BMI and age, two major factors which affect the biomarkers levels. Second, OA definition was based on KL grades, which conflate osteophytes, and JSN and some studies have shown that biomarker associations can be different with respect to these related but different features [39]. Third, knee OA was defined using anteroposterior radiographs of the knee. Therefore, patellofemoral joint OA was not taken into account in the study. Moreover, uncontrolled occurrence of misalignment of the medial tibial plateau and central X-ray beam in standing anteroposterior radiographs of the knee might result in an underestimation of the rate and homogeneity of JSN in knee OA [40]. Fourth, pain was assessed by questionnaire and not by more precise methods such as Western Ontario and McMaster Universities Arthritis Index pain score or visual analog scale. Fifth, controls were free of OA at the joint site studied but were allowed to have OA at other joint sites. For example, if knee OA was studied, controls had to be free of knee OA but were allowed to have hip OA. In addition, the inference of the relevant relationships between serum or urine biomarker concentrations and disease of specific joints is complicated by the fact that our OA patients might have disease in other joints such as hands or spine joints. Sixth, several studies have suggested that risk factors for incidence of OA may be different from risk factors for progression [41]. This could be due to heterogeneity in OA structural pathology (e.g., bony proliferation versus cartilage loss), limitations of imaging, which may result in different sensitivities to the structural features, limited sample size of the studies that examined the risk factors, and that the risk factors may affect disease differently at different disease stages [41]. Although we had a reasonable sample size for total OA incidence and progression analyses, the statistical power was limited to identify which factors operate at different disease stages and for analyses of OA phenotypes leading to wider confidence limits. Finally, although we covered several confounding variables, we could not exclude bias due to unmeasured confounding factors as well as health-based selection bias as we used a subset of RS-II participants who had follow-up data. These subjects were probably more mobile to visit the center and survived in the follow-up period.

Conclusions

Our study confirmed that the uCTX-II and COMP concentrations are associated with incidence and progression of radiographic OA. Moreover, we showed for the first time that a MMP-dependent tissue-inflammation marker predicts the risk of OA progression independent of established biomarkers uCTX-II and COMP at the 5-year follow-up. This indicates that inflammation is associated with disease progression in OA and that inflammation has pathological relevance in OA. Further prospective studies are needed to confirm this association for OA.

Abbreviations

AS: ankylosing spondylitis; AUC: area under the curve; BMI: body mass index; C1M: connective tissue type I collagen turnover; CI: confidence intervals; COMP: cartilage oligomeric protein; CRP: C-reactive protein; CRPM: matrix metalloproteinase-dependent degradation of CRP; GEE: generalized estimating equation; hs: high-sensitivity; JSN: joint space narrowing; KL: Kellgren and Lawrence; MMP: matrix metalloproteinase; OA: osteoarthritis; OR: odds ratios; RA: rheumatoid arthritis; RS: Rotterdam Study; ROC: receiver operating characteristic; TJR: total joint replacement; uCTX-II: (urinary) type II collagen degradation.

Competing interests

ACBJ and MAK are full-time employees of Nordic Bioscience, a privately owned biotechnology company involved in biomarker development. ACBJ and MAK hold shares in Nordic Bioscience. ASS is a full-time employee of Nordic Bioscience. The remaining authors declare no competing financial interests. All authors declare no nonfinancial conflicts of interest.

Authors' contributions

FSH performed the statistical analysis, data interpretation, and drafted and revised the manuscript. JBJvM participated in the study design and coordination, data interpretation, and was involved in critically revising the manuscript for important intellectual content. SMBZ participated in the study design and coordination, data interpretation and helped to revise the manuscript. ASS designed and performed the experiments and helped to revise the manuscript. ACBJ designed and performed the experiments and helped to revise the manuscript. MAK designed and performed the experiments and helped to revise the manuscript. AGU participated in the study design and coordination and helped to revise the manuscript. EHGO participated in reading the X-rays and helped to revise the manuscript. AH participated in the study design and coordination. All authors read and approved the final manuscript.

Acknowledgments

The authors are grateful to the study participants, the staff from the Rotterdam Study and the participating general practitioners and pharmacists.

Funding source

The Rotterdam Study is supported by the Netherlands Organization of Scientific Research NWO Investments (number 175.010.2005.011, 911-03-012), the Research Institute for Diseases in the Elderly (014-93-015; RIDE2), the Netherlands Genomics Initiative (NGI)/Netherlands Organization for Scientific

Research (NWO) (project number 050-060-810) and the Erasmus Medical Center and Erasmus University, Rotterdam. This study is funded by the Dutch Arthritis Foundation (project number 13-1-201) and the Netherlands Society for Scientific Research (NWO) VIDI grant 917103521. The biomarker measurements were partly supported by the TreatOA consortium (FP7-HEALTH-2007-2.4.5-1), as well as the Danish Research Foundation (DFF under act 2013).

Author details

[1]Department of Internal Medicine, Erasmus University Medical Center, P.O. Box 2040, Rotterdam 3000 CA, Netherlands. [2]Biomarkers and Research, Nordic Bioscience, Herlev, Denmark. [3]Department of Epidemiology, Erasmus University Medical Center, Rotterdam, The Netherlands. [4]Department of Radiology, Erasmus University Medical Center, Rotterdam, The Netherlands. [5]Department of General Practice, Erasmus University Medical Center, Rotterdam, Netherlands. [6]Department of Orthopedics, Erasmus University Medical Center, Rotterdam, Netherlands.

References

1. Issa S, Sharma L. Epidemiology of osteoarthritis: An update. Curr Rheumatol Rep. 2006;8:7–15.
2. Masuko K, Murata M, Suematsu N, Okamoto K, Yudoh K, Nakamura H, et al. A metabolic aspect of osteoarthritis: lipid as a possible contributor to the pathogenesis of cartilage degradation. Clin Exp Rheumatol. 2009;27:347–53.
3. Hedbom E, Häuselmann HJ. Molecular aspects of pathogenesis in osteoarthritis: the role of inflammation. Cell Mol Life Sci. 2002;59:45–53.
4. Garnero P, Piperno M, Gineyts E, Christgau S, Delmas PD, Vignon E. Cross sectional evaluation of biochemical markers of bone, cartilage, and synovial tissue metabolism in patients with knee osteoarthritis: relations with disease activity and joint damage. Ann Rheum Dis. 2001;60:619–26.
5. Garnero P, Conrozier T, Christgau S, Mathieu P, Delmas PD, Vignon E. Urinary type II collagen C-telopeptide levels are increased in patients with rapidly destructive hip osteoarthritis. Ann Rheum Dis. 2003;62:939–43.
6. Garnero P, Ayral X, Rousseau JC, Christgau S, Sandell LJ, Dougados M, et al. Uncoupling of type II collagen synthesis and degradation predicts progression of joint damage in patients with knee osteoarthritis. Arthritis Rheum. 2002;46:2613–24.
7. Reijman M, Hazes JMW, Bierma-Zeinstra SMA, Koes BW, Christgau S, Christiansen C, et al. A new marker for osteoarthritis: cross-sectional and longitudinal approach. Arthritis Rheum. 2004;50:2471–8.
8. Hunter DJ, Li J, LaValley M, Bauer DC, Nevitt M, DeGroot J, et al. Cartilage markers and their association with cartilage loss on magnetic resonance imaging in knee osteoarthritis: the Boston Osteoarthritis Knee Study. Arthritis Res Ther. 2007;9:R108.
9. Dam EB, Loog M, Christiansen C, Byrjalsen I, Folkesson J, Nielsen M, et al. Identification of progressors in osteoarthritis by combining biochemical and MRI-based markers. Arthritis Res Ther. 2009;11:R115.
10. Valdes AM, Meulenbelt I, Chassaing E, Arden NK, Bierma-Zeinstra S, Hart D, et al. Large scale meta-analysis of urinary C-terminal telopeptide, serum cartilage oligomeric protein and matrix metalloprotease degraded type II collagen and their role in prevalence, incidence and progression of osteoarthritis. Osteoarthritis Cartilage. 2014;22:683–9.
11. Goldring MB, Otero M. Inflammation in osteoarthritis. Curr Opin Rheumatol. 2011;23:471–8.
12. Kerkhof HJM, Bierma-Zeinstra SMA, Castano-Betancourt MC, de Maat MP, Hofman A, Pols HAP, et al. Serum C reactive protein levels and genetic variation in the CRP gene are not associated with the prevalence, incidence or progression of osteoarthritis independent of body mass index. Ann Rheum Dis. 2010;69:1976–82.
13. Bonnet CS, Walsh DA. Osteoarthritis, angiogenesis and inflammation. Rheumatology (Oxford). 2005;44:7–16.
14. Jin X, Beguerie JR, Zhang W, Blizzard L, Otahal P, Jones G, et al. Circulating C reactive protein in osteoarthritis: a systematic review and meta-analysis. Ann Rheum Dis. 2015;74:703–10.
15. Siebuhr AS, Petersen KK, Arendt-Nielsen L, Egsgaard LL, Eskehave T, Christiansen C, et al. Identification and characterisation of osteoarthritis patients with inflammation derived tissue turnover. Osteoarthritis Cartilage. 2014;22:44–50.
16. Skjøt-Arkil H, Schett G, Zhang C, Larsen DV, Wang Y, Zheng Q, et al. Investigation of two novel biochemical markers of inflammation, matrix metalloproteinase and cathepsin generated fragments of C-reactive protein, in patients with ankylosing spondylitis. Clin Exp Rheumatol. 2011;30:371–9.
17. Leeming DJ, He Y, Veidal SS, Nguyen QHT, Larsen DV, Koizumi M, et al. A novel marker for assessment of liver matrix remodeling: An enzyme-linked immunosorbent assay (ELISA) detecting a MMP generated type I collagen neo-epitope (C1M). Biomarkers. 2011;16:616–28.
18. Siebuhr AS, Bay-Jensen AC, Leeming DJ, Plat A, Byrjalsen I, Christiansen C, et al. Serological identification of fast progressors of structural damage with rheumatoid arthritis. Arthritis Res Ther. 2013;15:R86.
19. Attur M, Belitskaya-Lévy I, Oh C, Krasnokutsky S, Greenberg J, Samuels J, et al. Increased interleukin-1β gene expression in peripheral blood leukocytes is associated with increased pain and predicts risk for progression of symptomatic knee osteoarthritis. Arthritis Rheum. 2011;63:1908–17.
20. Attur M, Statnikov A, Samuels J, Krasnokutsky S, Greenberg JD, Li Z, et al. Interleukin-1 receptor antagonist (IL-1Ra) plasma levels predict radiographic progression of symptomatic knee osteoarthritis over 24 months [abstract]. Arthritis Rheum. 2013;65 Suppl 10:804.
21. Hofman A, Brusselle GO, Murad S, van Duijn C, Franco O, Goedegebure A, et al. The Rotterdam Study: 2016 objectives and design update. Eur J Epidemiol. 2015;30:661–708.
22. Kellgren JH, Lawrence JS. Radiological assessment of osteo-arthrosis. Ann Rheum Dis. 1957;16:494–502.
23. Kellgren JH, Jeffrey MR, Ball J. The epidemiology of chronic rheumatism. Atlas of standard radiographs of arthritis. Oxford: Blackwell Scientific Publications; 1963.
24. Reijman M, Hazes JMW, Koes BW, Verhagen AP, Bierma-Zeinstra SMA. Validity, reliability, and applicability of seven definitions of hip osteoarthritis used in epidemiological studies: a systematic appraisal. Ann Rheum Dis. 2004;63:226–32.
25. Schiphof D, Boers M, Bierma-Zeinstra SM. Differences in descriptions of Kellgren and Lawrence grades of knee osteoarthritis. Ann Rheum Dis. 2008;67:1034–6.
26. Kardys I, de Maat MP, Uitterlinden AG, Hofman A, Witteman JCM. C-reactive protein gene haplotypes and risk of coronary heart disease: the Rotterdam Study. Eur Heart J. 2006;27:1331–7.
27. Lubin JH, Colt JS, Camann D, Davis S, Cerhan JR, Severson RK, et al. Epidemiologic evaluation of measurement data in the presence of detection limits. Environ Health Perspect. 2004;112:1691–6.
28. King KB, Lindsey CT, Dunn TC, Ries MD, Steinbach LS, Majumdar S. A study of the relationship between molecular biomarkers of joint degeneration and the magnetic resonance-measured characteristics of cartilage in 16 symptomatic knees. Magn Reson Imaging. 2004;22:1117–23.
29. Wisłowska M, Jabłońska B. Serum cartilage oligomeric matrix protein (COMP) in rheumatoid arthritis and knee osteoarthritis. Clin Rheumatol. 2005;24:278–84.
30. Sowers M, Karvonen-Gutierrez CA, Yosef M, Jannausch M, Jiang Y, Garnero P, et al. Longitudinal changes of serum COMP and urinary CTX-II predict X-ray defined knee osteoarthritis severity and stiffness in women. Osteoarthritis Cartilage. 2009;17:1609–14.
31. Van Spil WE, DeGroot J, Lems WF, Oostveen JCM, Lafeber F. Serum and urinary biochemical markers for knee and hip-osteoarthritis: a systematic review applying the consensus BIPED criteria. Osteoarthritis Cartilage. 2010;18:605–12.
32. Felson DT. The current and future status of biomarkers in osteoarthritis. J Rheumatol. 2014;41:834–6.
33. Lotz M, Martel-Pelletier J, Christiansen C, et al. Value of biomarkers in osteoarthritis: current status and perspectives. Ann Rheum Dis. 2013;72:1756–63.
34. Kerkhof HJM, Bierma-Zeinstra SMA, Arden NK, Metrustry S, Castano-Betancourt M, Hart DJ, et al. Prediction model for knee osteoarthritis incidence, including clinical, genetic and biochemical risk factors. Ann Rheum Dis. 2014;73:2116–21.
35. Dieppe PA, Lohmander LS. Pathogenesis and management of pain in osteoarthritis. Lancet. 2005;365:965–73.
36. Felson DT. The sources of pain in knee osteoarthritis. Curr Opin Rheumatol. 2005;17:624–8.
37. Schiphof D, Kerkhof HJM, Damen J, de Klerk BM, Hofman A, Koes BW, et al. Factors for pain in patients with different grades of knee osteoarthritis. Arthritis Care Res. 2013;65:695–702.
38. Arendt-Nielsen L, Eskehave TN, Egsgaard LL, Petersen KK, Graven-Nielsen T, Hoeck HC, et al. Association between experimental pain biomarkers and serological markers in patients with different degree of painful knee osteoarthritis. Arthritis Rheumatol. 2014;66:3317–26.

Permissions

List of Contributors

Ane Larrañaga-Vera, Ana Lamuedra, Sandra Pérez-Baos, Ivan Prieto-Potin, Gabriel Herrero-Beaumont and Raquel Largo
Bone and Joint Research Unit, IIS-Fundación Jiménez Díaz UAM, Avda. Reyes Católicos

Leticia Peña
Madrid 28040, Spain Clinical Analysis Department, HU-Fundación Jiménez Díaz, Madrid, Spain

Shinnosuke Hada, Haruka Kaneko, Mayuko Kinoshita, Hitoshi Arita, Jun Shiozawa, Yuji Takazawa, Hiroshi Ikeda, Ryo Sadatsuki and Ippei Futami
Department of Medicine for Orthopaedics and Motor Organ, Juntendo University Graduate School of Medicine, 2-1-1, Hongo, Bunkyo-ku, Tokyo 113-8421, Japan

Muneaki Ishijima and Kazuo Kaneko
Department of Medicine for Orthopaedics and Motor Organ, Juntendo University Graduate School of Medicine, 2-1-1, Hongo, Bunkyo-ku, Tokyo 113-8421, Japan
Department of Pathophysiology for Locomotive and Neoplastic Diseases, Juntendo University Graduate School of Medicine, 2-1-1 Hongo, Bunkyo-ku, Tokyo 113-8421, Japan
Sportology Center, Juntendo University Graduate School of Medicine, Tokyo, Japan

Lizu Liu
Department of Medicine for Orthopaedics and Motor Organ, Juntendo University Graduate School of Medicine, 2-1-1, Hongo, Bunkyo-ku, Tokyo 113-8421, Japan
Sportology Center, Juntendo University Graduate School of Medicine, Tokyo, Japan

Anwajan Yusup
Department of Medicine for Orthopaedics and Motor Organ, Juntendo University Graduate School of Medicine, 2-1-1, Hongo, Bunkyo-ku, Tokyo 113-8421, Japan
Research Institute for Diseases of Old Age, Juntendo University Graduate School of Medicine, Tokyo, Japan

Yasunori Okada
Department of Pathophysiology for Locomotive and Neoplastic Diseases, Juntendo University Graduate School of Medicine, 2-1-1 Hongo, Bunkyo-ku, Tokyo 113-8421, Japan

Takako Aoki
Sportology Center, Juntendo University Graduate School of Medicine, Tokyo, Japan

Tomohiro Takamura and Shigeki Aoki
Department of Radiology, Juntendo University Graduate School of Medicine, Tokyo, Japan

Hisashi Kurosawa
Department of Orthopaedics, Juntendo Tokyo Koto Geriatric Medical Center, Tokyo, Japan

Hui Li, Chao Zeng, Tuo Yang, Yi-lun Wang, Dong-xing Xie and Guang-hua Lei
Department of Orthopaedics, Xiangya Hospital, Central South University, #87 Xiangya Road, Changsha, Hunan Province 410008, China

Liang-jun Li
Department of Orthopaedics, Xiangya Hospital, Central South University, #87 Xiangya Road, Changsha, Hunan Province 410008, China
Department of Orthopaedics, Changsha Central Hospital, Changsha, Hunan 410000, China

Jie Wei
Health Management Center, Xiangya Hospital, Central South University, Changsha, Hunan Province 410008, China
Department of Epidemiology and Health Statistics, Xiangya School of Public Health, Central South University, Changsha, Hunan Province 410008, China

Robert Terkeltaub
VA San Diego Medical Center, San Diego, CA 92161, USA
Department of Medicine, UCSD, San Diego, CA 92161, USA

Hyon K. Choi and Yuqing Zhang
Division of Rheumatology, Allergy, and Immunology, Department of Medicine, Massachusetts General Hospital, Boston, MA 02114, USA

David J. Hunter
Rheumatology Department, Royal North Shore Hospital and Institute of Bone and Joint Research, Kolling Institute, University of Sydney, Sydney, NSW 2065, Australia

Yang Cui
International Medical Center, Xiangya Hospital, Central South University, Changsha, Hunan Province 410008, China

Jean-Pierre Pelletier, Jean-Pierre Raynauld and Johanne Martel-Pelletier
Osteoarthritis Research Unit, University of Montreal Hospital Research Centre (CRCHUM), 900 Saint-Denis, Suite R11.412, Montreal, QC H2X 0A9, Canada

François Abram
Medical Imaging Research & Development, ArthroLab Inc, Montreal, QC, Canada

Marc Dorais
StatSciences Inc, Notre-Dame-de-l'Île-Perrot, QC, Canada

Philippe Delorme
ArthroLab Inc, Montreal, QC, Canada

Thelonius Hawellek, Jan Hubert, Wolfgang Rüther and Andreas Niemeier
Department of Orthopaedics, University Medical Center Hamburg-Eppendorf, Martinistraße 52, 20246 Hamburg, Germany

Sandra Hischke
Department of Medical Biometry and Epidemiology, University Medical Center Hamburg-Eppendorf, Hamburg, Germany

Matthias Krause
Department of Osteology and Biomechanics, University Medical Center Hamburg-Eppendorf, Hamburg, Germany

Jessica Bertrand
Department of Orthopaedic Surgery, Otto-von-Guerricke-University Magdeburg, Magdeburg, Germany

Burkhard C. Schmidt and Andreas Kronz
Centrum of Geoscience, Georg-August-University Göttingen, Göttingen, Germany

Klaus Püschel
Department of Legal Medicine, University Medical Center Hamburg-Eppendorf, Hamburg, Germany

Ivan Shirinsky and Valery Shirinsky
Laboratory of Clinical Immunopharmacology, Federal State Budgetary Scientific Institution, Research Institute of Fundamental and Clinical Immunology, 6 Zalesskogo Street, 630047 Novosibirsk, Russia

Catherine Legrand and Cécile Lambert
Bone and Cartilage Research Unit, Arthropôle Liège, Institute of Pathology, Level 5, CHU Sart-Tilman, 4000 Liège, Belgium

Yves Henrotin
Bone and Cartilage Research Unit, Arthropôle Liège, Institute of Pathology, Level 5, CHU Sart-Tilman, 4000 Liège, Belgium
Department of Physical Therapy and Rehabilitation, Princess Paola Hospital, Vivalia, Marche-en-Famenne, Belgium

Attia Anwarand and Sabah Pasha
Warwick Systems Biology, University of Warwick, Clinical Sciences Research Laboratories, University Hospital, Coventry CV2 2DX, UK

Paul J. Thornalley, Usman Ahmed and Naila Rabbani
Warwick Medical School, Clinical Sciences Research Laboratories, University of Warwick, University Hospital, Coventry CV2 2DX, UK

Kashif Rajpoot
School of Computer Science, University of Birmingham, Birmingham, UK

Rose K. Davidson and Ian M. Clark
School of Biological Sciences, University of East Anglia, Norwich, UK

Élie Abed, Aline Delalandre and Daniel Lajeunesse
Unité de recherche en Arthrose, Centre de recherche du Centre hospitalier de l'Université de Montréal (CRCHUM), 900, rue Saint-Denis, Montréal, Québec H2X 0A9, Canada

Jason J. McDougall, Milind M. Muley, Holly T. Philpott, Allison Reid and Eugene Krustev
Department of Pharmacology, Dalhousie University, 5850 College Street, Halifax, NS B3H 4R2, Canada
Department of Anaesthesia, Pain Management & Perioperative Medicine, Dalhousie University, 5850 College Street, Halifax, NS B3H 4R2, Canada

Jean-Pierre Pelletier and Johanne Martel-Pelletier
Osteoarthritis Research Unit, University of Montreal Hospital Research Centre (CRCHUM), 900 Saint-Denis, Suite R11.412, Montreal, Quebec H2X 0A9, Canada

Jean-Pierre Raynauld
Osteoarthritis Research Unit, University of Montreal Hospital Research Centre (CRCHUM), 900 Saint-Denis, Suite R11.412, Montreal, Quebec H2X 0A9, Canada
Institut de rhumatologie de Montréal, Montreal, Quebec, Canada

André D. Beaulieu
Centre de rhumatologie St-Louis, Sainte-Foy, Quebec, Canada

Louis Bessette
Groupe de recherche en Rhumatologie et Maladies Osseuses Inc., Sainte-Foy, Quebec, Canada

Frédéric Morin
Centre de recherche musculo-squelettique, Trois-Rivières, Quebec, Canada

Artur J. de Brum-Fernandes
Service de rhumatologie, Centre hospitalier universitaire de Sherbrooke (CHUS), Sherbrooke, Quebec, Canada

Philippe Delorme, Patrice Paiement and François Abram
ArthroLab Inc., Montreal, Quebec, Canada

Marc Dorais
StatSciences Inc., Notre-Dame de l'Île-Perrot, Quebec, Canada

Charles B. Eaton
Alpert Medical School of Brown University, Providence, USA
School of Public Health of Brown University, Providence, USA

Center of Primary Care and Prevention, Memorial Hospital of Rhode Island, 111 Brewster Street, Pawtucket, RI 02860, USA

Syeda Ameernaz and Mary B. Roberts
Center of Primary Care and Prevention, Memorial Hospital of Rhode Island, 111 Brewster Street, Pawtucket, RI 02860, USA

Maria Sayeed
Department of Medicine, Memorial Hospital of Rhode Island, 111 Brewster Street, Pawtucket, RI, USA

John D. Maynard
Vera Light Inc., 800 Bradbury Dr SE # 217, Albuquerque, NM, USA

Jeffrey B. Driban and Timothy E. McAlindon
Division of Rheumatology, Tufts Medical Center, 800 Washington Street, Boston, MA, USA

Gladys Valverde-Franco, David Hum, Hassan Fahmi, Jean-Pierre Pelletier and Johanne Martel-Pelletier
Osteoarthritis Research Unit, University of Montreal Hospital Research Centre (CRCHUM), 900 Saint-Denis, R11.412B, Montreal, QC H2X 0A9, Canada

Bertrand Lussier
Osteoarthritis Research Unit, University of Montreal Hospital Research Centre (CRCHUM), 900 Saint-Denis, R11.412B, Montreal, QC H2X 0A9, Canada
Faculty of Veterinary Medicine, Clinical Science, University of Montreal, Saint-Hyacinthe, QC, Canada

Mohit Kapoor
Osteoarthritis Research Unit, University of Montreal Hospital Research Centre (CRCHUM), 900 Saint-Denis, R11.412B, Montreal, QC H2X 0A9, Canada. Division of Genetics and Development, Toronto Western Research Institute, University Health Network (UHN) and Department of Surgery, University of Toronto, Toronto, ON, Canada

Jiangping Wu
Laboratory of Immunology, University of Montreal Hospital Research Centre (CRCHUM), Montreal, QC, Canada

Adjia Hamadjida and Numa Dancause
Neurosciences Department, Faculty of Medicine, University of Montreal, Montreal, QC, Canada
Groupe de recherche sur le sytème nerveux central (GRSNC), Neurosciences Department, Faculty of Medicine, University of Montreal, Montreal, QC, Canada

Maha Jamal
Department of Pharmaceutical Sciences, MCPHS University, Boston, MA, USA

Ali Alquraini
Department of Pharmaceutical Sciences, MCPHS University, Boston, MA, USA
School of Pharmacy, Albaha University, Albaha, Saudi Arabia

Ling Zhang
Department of Emergency Medicine, Rhode Island Hospital, Providence, RI, USA

Gregory D. Jay
Department of Emergency Medicine, Rhode Island Hospital, Providence, RI, USA
Department of Biomedical Engineering, Brown University, Providence, RI, USA

Tannin Schmidt
Faculty of Kinesiology and Schulich School of Engineering, University of Calgary, Calgary, AB, Canada

Khaled A. Elsaid
Department of Biomedical and Pharmaceutical Sciences, Chapman University School of Pharmacy, Rinker Health Sciences Campus, 9401 Jeronimo Road, Irvine, CA 92618, USA

Elina Nummenmaa, Mari Hämäläinen, Lauri J. Moilanen, Erja-Leena Paukkeri, Riina M. Nieminen, Katriina Vuolteenaho and Eeva Moilanen
The Immunopharmacology Research Group, University of Tampere School of Medicine and Tampere University Hospital, Tampere, Finland

Teemu Moilanen
The Immunopharmacology Research Group, University of Tampere School of Medicine and Tampere University Hospital, Tampere, Finland
Coxa Hospital for Joint Replacement, Tampere, Finland

Andre G. Uitterlinden
Department of Internal Medicine, Erasmus University Medical Center, Rotterdam 3000 CA, Netherlands
Department of Epidemiology, Erasmus University Medical Center, Rotterdam, The Netherlands

Anne Sofie Siebuhr, Morten A. Karsdal and Anne C. Bay-Jensen
Biomarkers and Research, Nordic Bioscience, Herlev, Denmark

Albert Hofman
Department of Epidemiology, Erasmus University Medical Center, Rotterdam, The Netherlands

Edwin H. G. Oei
Department of Radiology, Erasmus University Medical Center, Rotterdam, The Netherlands

Sita M. Bierma-Zeinstra
Department of General Practice, Erasmus University Medical Center, Rotterdam, Netherlands
Department of Orthopedics, Erasmus University Medical Center, Rotterdam, Netherlands

Erica M. TenBroek, Laurie Yunker and Mae Foster Nies
Medtronic Inc., 710 Medtronic Parkway, Minneapolis, MN 55432, USA

Alison M. Bendele
Bolder BioPATH, Inc., 5541 Central Avenue, Suite 160, Boulder, CO 80301, USA

Fatemeh Saberi Hosnijeh and Joyce B. J. van Meurs
Department of Internal Medicine, Erasmus University Medical Center, Rotterdam 3000 CA, Netherlands

Index